POLICY ISSUES IN PERSONAL HEALTH SERVICES

Current Perspectives

Contributors

Thomas J. Bacon
David W. Dunlop
Laurel A. Files
Deborah A. Freund
Paul S. Jellinek
William F. Jessee
Suzanne J. Kotkin
James W. Luckey

Nancy Milio
George M. Neely
Barnett R. Parker
Harry T. Phillips
Leonard S. Rosenfeld
R. Gary Rozier
Nancy L. Tigar
James A. Wiley

POLICY ISSUES IN PERSONAL HEALTH SERVICES

Current Perspectives

Editors

Sagar C. Jain, Ph.D.

and

John E. Paul, M.S.P.H.

School of Public Health
University of North Carolina
at Chapel Hill

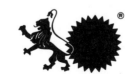

AN ASPEN PUBLICATION®
Aspen Systems Corporation
Rockville, Maryland
London
1983

Library of Congress Cataloging in Publication Data

Policy issues in personal health services.

Includes index.
1. Medical policy—United States. 2. Medical care—
United States. I. Jain, Sagar C.
RA395.A3P59   1983   362.1'0973   82-22702
ISBN: 0-89443-672-4

Publisher: John Marozsan
Editorial Director: Michael Brown
Managing Editor: Margot Raphael
Editorial Services: Jane Coyle
Printing and Manufacturing: Debbie Collins

Library of Congress Catalog Card Number: 82-22702
ISBN: 0-89443-672-4

Printed in the United States of America

1 2 3 4 5

Table of Contents

Preface

Personal health services are defined as all preventive, curative, supportive, and rehabilitative health services requiring direct interaction between recipient and provider. These services are intimately related to life and the well-being of people and generally are matters of great concern. They are a focus of continual discussion and debate regarding how they should be organized, financed, and delivered.

This book examines many aspects of current concerns and discussions pertaining to national policies on personal health services. It is not intended to be either a comprehensive report on these discussions or a textbook on the subject. It is simply a book of readings.

All chapters have been written specifically for this book, and the senior author of each chapter is a member of the faculty of the Department of Health Policy and Administration, University of North Carolina at Chapel Hill. Not all members of this faculty contributed chapters (only about one-third did). Each chapter reflects the contributing author's personal interest and expertise; all opinions, therefore, should be credited to the respective authors.

The book was written over a period of 18 months, starting in January 1981, with most of the chapters completed in the spring or summer of 1982. They thereby reflect information as well as mood current at that point.

The book is a labor of love. The participating authors spent hundreds of hours not only in writing their chapters in the midst of a major reorganization of the department but also in a series of meetings and seminars, especially organized to facilitate peer review. Each of them deserves a special note of thanks.

Two persons have earned medals: Jean Yates, director of the Reference Collection of the department, for doing a superb job of effectively and efficiently fielding innumerable requests for information of all sorts, and

Mary Johnson, my secretary, for readily and willingly taking on many chores that were beyond the call of duty. John Paul, my graduate assistant and doctoral student in our department, made so many contributions that he rightfully earned the title of assistant editor.

Sagar C. Jain, Ph.D.

July 1, 1982

Acknowledgments

The author of Chapter 7, Leonard S. Rosenfeld, wishes to acknowledge the help of Conrad Seipp for reviewing an early draft and for suggestions, Irene Rosenfeld for editing the text, and Pam McDonald for typing it.

The author of Chapter 10, Laurel A. Files, says that in addition to the several colleagues who constructively reviewed earlier drafts of that chapter, she owes special thanks to those who made possible her 1981–1982 stay at the University of Minnesota's Program in Hospital and Health Care Administration, Center for Health Services Research, and University Hospitals and Clinics. The hospitals' administrative staff, in particular, met all of her learning needs and she comments that she could not have written that chapter without their support.

Chapter 1

Policy Concerns and the Changing Role of Government in Personal Health: A Perspective

Sagar C. Jain, Ph.D.

Social policy issues arise when societal reality does not measure up to societal ideals, values, preferences, and aspirations. Policy issues reflect dissatisfaction with the state of things but, at the same time, denote societal determination to bring about desired corrections. Policy issues change with shifts in societal values; societal values and capability perceptions then are influenced by a variety of forces, including changes in size, distribution, and composition of population; socioeconomic development; resources; power balance; science and technology; communication; religion; state of well-being; political status and boundaries; and historical experience.

The greater the extent and the speed of these changes, the greater the likelihood of shifts in societal values and capability perception and, in turn, the greater the probability of new policy issues' gaining saliency. This chapter examines policy concerns pertaining to the role of government in personal health services in that conceptual framework.

THE BASIC VALUES AND CONCERNS OF THE U.S.

The United States is a large and complex society made up of people from a variety of nationalities, cultures, races, religions, and classes. It is a society characterized by multiple power centers, dynamism, and flux. In the face of so much variety, complexity, and change, it should be easy to say that Americans do not have a common value system and that various subgroups have different values. To a certain extent this is true but beneath

1

the surface Americans do have a strong, breathing, and living, common value system that makes them the unique people they are. The United States of America came into being as a nation asserting in the Declaration of Independence that ". . . all Men are created equal, that they are endowed by their Creator with certain inalienable Rights, that among these are Life, Liberty, and the pursuit of Happiness—That to secure these rights, Governments are instituted. . . ." Equality, life, liberty, and the pursuit of happiness continue to be the cornerstone of American values.

These values have not received equal attention throughout the nation's history, however. Initially, "equality at birth" was perceived as given, with no individual or group presumed to have a position of privilege as a birthright, but life, liberty, and the pursuit of happiness were rights to be secured by the government. Stated simply, every individual has a right to live and that life may not be taken away capriciously; furthermore, each individual has a right not only to live but to pursue happiness as that person deems fit, without direction, control, or interference from anybody.

For the people who came to this land of opportunity to escape religious, economic, social, or political oppression, to live without fear of persecution and death, and to be free to do their own things, to be in control of their own destinies, "life, liberty, and the pursuit of happiness" summarized all their hopes, dreams, and concerns. They came to be their own masters, and they would accept nothing less.

While all these rights have been important to individuals, until recently liberty has occupied the center stage of American history in all matters of social policy. Rightly, liberty was seen as a primary instrument of life and happiness, for without liberty to pursue happiness, life has little meaning. The greater the liberty, the greater the potential for fulfilling life. Protection and enhancement of liberty, therefore, became a central policy concern.

Led by this value orientation, the United States evolved into a classical laissez-faire society, with government essentially serving the role of night watchman, a society devoted to the institutions of private property, free enterprise, market, and competition. This social system, combined with the burning ambitions of the immigrants to find themselves a good life and the many bounties of the new land, produced a civilization of unprecedented prosperity. Unfortunately, these riches did not come equally to all. The system improved everybody's economic condition but favored those with enterprise, cunning, muscles, means of production, or sheer good luck.

With the passage of time, the rich got richer by exercising increasing control over the means of production and the gap between the haves and the have-nots became wider and wider. For these have-nots, liberty was an empty word. Without economic means they had no effective capability of exercising their right to life and pursuit of happiness. This situation was confounded further when the ranks of the have-nots were joined by penniless former slaves subjected to a plethora of laws and practices adapted to discriminate against people of the black race.

In the face of this situation, it no longer could be presumed that all men were born equal and that they enjoyed equal opportunities in life. In fact, the United States had become a society of institutionalized inequality supported by a set of interactive political, economic, and social arrangements. Unless these barriers to equality of opportunity were removed, the rights of life, liberty, and the pursuit of happiness could not be secured. Therefore, the government no longer could avoid focusing its attention on ensuring equality of opportunity to all, and the "Age of Reform" was launched (Hofstadter, 1955). It brought governmental action limiting laissez-faire and monopolistic practices in business, the individual income tax, and other legislation, all of which had the effect of strengthening government's role.

The realization of a new social reality and the resultant shift in value priorities toward equality, causing the "decline of laissez faire" (Faulkner, 1951), did not come suddenly and cannot be attributed to any single event or force; rather, several such factors cumulatively steered the shift from liberty to equality as the dominant guiding value of the nation. The Depression probably was the first major challenge to the soundness and efficacy of the free enterprise capitalistic system that was a product of the nation's liberty-dominated value precepts. In the same way, the New Deal was the first major move leading to a tilt toward equality. This trend gained noticeable momentum in the post-World War II years. Those were heady times for the United States. It had won the war and had established itself as the most powerful nation on the earth. In this process, it also had established the supremacy of its scientific, technological, and organizational know-how. It already was the richest nation. It could do anything and everything, and it set out to prove it.

Facing the cold war with the Soviet Union, it accepted the role of champion of the needy, poor, and oppressed all over the globe. It launched a massive program of assistance to rebuild Europe and Japan and to help the newly independent and underdeveloped countries in Asia, Africa, and Latin America to stand on their own feet.

For many of these initiatives to be effective, it was essential that American motives be perceived as legitimate and that the nation be accepted as a sincere advocate of democracy based on equality of opportunity. To gain such credence, the United States came under additional pressure to root out poverty, discrimination, and institutionalized inequality at home. A determined attack was mounted on these evils on many fronts. Much new legislation was enacted, old laws and practices were challenged, and a plethora of new social problems was introduced.

In its tilt toward equality, the country did not forsake its original commitment to liberty. In fact, liberty remained its supreme value but it was recognized that ensuring equality of opportunity was a necessary precondition for the effective exercise of the unalienable rights of life, liberty, and the pursuit of happiness. Consequently, it was not necessary to reject the social, economic, and political institutions based on liberty but to ensure that they provided for equality of opportunity.

To this end, a three-pronged strategy of regulation, expansion, and accommodation was evolved. This called for:

- regulations to ensure that there was no discrimination in the production of goods and services
- expansion of social services and benefits to remove historical disadvantages, and
- a systematic accommodation of the free enterprise system in the organization and delivery of new social programs.

This approach obviously produced visible and effective gains. As a result, today the United States is essentially a nation of well-to-do middle-class citizens, a nation in which the boundaries between the haves and the have-nots have become increasingly blurred, a nation in which equality of opportunity is a substantially realized value, and a nation that is ever vigilant in the protection of individual liberty.

While an emphasis on individual liberty produces minimum government, an emphasis on equality leads to a strong central government. To ensure equality of opportunity, all those factors that contribute to inequality must be identified and weeded out and all those that promote equality need to be cultivated, nurtured, and protected. Only a well-informed and powerful central government can carry out such a responsibility.

The proactive posture of the United States government to ensure equality of opportunity led to a rapid expansion in its role. One of the indicators of this change is seen in the fact that in 1927 governmental expenditures accounted for only 12.2 percent of the gross national product (GNP) (*Historical Statistics*, 1960); by 1960 this figure had risen to 28.3 percent and it has continued to rise—to 34.1 percent in 1970 and 36.9 percent in 1977 (*Statistical Abstract*, 1978). Similarly, while there were only 837,122 government employees at all levels—national, state, and local and including the military—in 1929 (*Historical Statistics*, 1960), their number increased to 6,402,000 in 1950 and 15,420,000 in 1977 (*Statistical Abstract*, 1978).

Yet another measure of this change is to be seen in the explosion in the number and types of regulatory activities of the government, as illustrated by expansion in the size of the *Code of Federal Regulations* from 23,000 pages in 1950 to nearly 84,000 pages in 1978, and of the *Federal Register* from 9,500 pages to more than 61,000 pages during the same period (Stenberg, 1981).

The progress toward equality has not been without costs. In fact, the financial expenditures have been significant and have been rising rather dramatically. The public expenditure on social welfare programs alone was nearly half a trillion dollars in 1982; in 1929, the total was $4.3 billion and in 1950, $24 billion. Looking at these expenditures in another way, in 1929 they accounted for 4.1 percent of the gross national product (GNP), in 1950 for 8.9 percent, and 1976 for 20.4 percent (*Historical Statistics,* 1960; Bixby, 1981).

Another example is found in the estimates of costs associated with complying with federal regulations. A study for the Joint Economic Committee by Murry L. Weidenbaum estimated these costs to be at least $100 billion during 1979; the Department of Commerce put the figure between $150 billion and $200 billion (Stenberg, 1981).

These large expenditures were perceived to be an essential price for the achievement of equality of opportunity, a necessary condition for an effective state of liberty. This thinking reflected the frame of mind of a people at a time when the country was flushed with a sense of omnipotence. It could do anything and everything and resources were not a real constraint.

Then came a series of major setbacks that shook the nation's confidence. First, the Russians gained a nuclear parity with the United States and became a world military power. They then launched Sputnik, challenging American leadership in science and technology. Nearer to home, the nation found itself unable to deal with Cuba and suffered the shame of the Bay of Pigs. These shocks were nothing in comparison to the humiliation in Vietnam; the Indochinese war not only placed a backbreaking strain on the American economy, it also damaged the spirit of the nation and produced a deep-seated self-doubt. Watergate and, more recently, Abscam produced concrete evidence that corruption had reached the highest levels of the government.

If these were not enough, the United States found itself helpless in the face of concerted action by the Organization of Petroleum Exporting Countries (OPEC) to increase the price of oil manyfold in the short period of five years, a step that had catastrophic effects on the economy, resulting in unprecedented trade and budget deficits, weakening of the dollar, damage to the international monetary system, and persistent "stagflation." While Vietnam and Watergate questioned the nation's morality, OPEC brought home its resource vulnerability. Add to these two other historical events, the rise of Japan as an economic superpower successfully challenging United States industrial power and the prolonged inability to free the embassy personnel taken hostage by Iran.

Things have not gone well at home, either. The rate of crime, especially violent crimes, continued to rise; unemployment hit 10.8 percent in 1982, an all-time high since the Depression; inflation seemed deeply rooted; double-digit interest rates continued to inhibit investment; the federal deficit seemed to be rising at an exponential rate (a projected deficit of $100+ billion during 1983 was being touted as a major achievement in fiscal responsibility); and the national debt already far exceeded the $1 trillion mark, requiring $125 billion a year in interest payments and forcing up the federal government's share of all borrowing in the United States to 52 percent (*U. S. News,* 1982).

These developments without doubt have had a strong impact on the American psyche and spirit and have created a siege mentality, an acute sense of vulnerability, resource consciousness, and caution. In turn, these have forced a reexamination of national values and priorities, with increasing attention given to financial and resource constraints.

HEALTH AND GOVERNMENT IN THE U.S.

Early Years: The Reign of Liberty

The role of government in the field of health, and the development and nature of health policies in the United States, mirrors the history of the evolution of the overall role of government in the country. The basic concerns of health policy have been the same as for overall social policy: life, liberty, and the pursuit of happiness; and the direction of these policies has been guided by the same values, events, and development. However, matters of health being closer to matters of life and happiness, issues pertaining to health at times seem to have been a potent force in the evolution of the overall role of government.

In the early years, when government's basic role was confined to that of securing life and liberty, such things as personal health, illness, and disability were considered to be largely matters of individual concern and responsibility (Tesh, 1982). The role of government in health matters was defined by the "harm-to-others" doctrine (Courtwright, 1980) and essentially was limited to sanitation and quarantine laws enacted by cities and states (Hanlon, 1974). Some states also provided for the care of indigent sick (Chapman & Talmadge, 1971).

Since the Constitution made no mention of health, Congress was considered to have little or no authority to act in this field. However, the widespread yellow fever epidemics of 1793 and 1794 led Congress to enact the quarantine law of 1796 by using the authority of the interstate commerce clause (Article I, Section 8) of the Constitution. This legislation, giving only a permissive role to the federal government, was passed by a narrow margin and after a long debate over state vs. federal authority.

In the first half of the 19th century, the United States experienced a great political and economic expansion but the role of government in the field of health saw little change. This was in spite of the fact that the lives and happiness of many were assaulted repeatedly by epidemics of smallpox, yellow fever, cholera, typhoid and typhus, tuberculosis, and malaria that took high tolls. However, it must be remembered that at that time medical knowledge regarding the etiology of these diseases still was rudimentary and that the golden age of bacteriology was yet to come.

The only initiative of significance at this time was the enactment of a federal law in 1813 requiring the president to appoint an agent who would ensure the high quality of cowpox vaccine and make it available free of charge to anyone requesting it. However, this law was repealed in 1822 after a federal vaccine agent by mistake sent a batch of smallpox vaccine, instead of cowpox vaccine, to North Carolina with dire results. A Congressional Select Committee investigating this matter concluded that the federal government would be unable to ". . . devise a system which will not be more liable to abuses in its operation and less subject to a prompt and salutary control, than such as may be adopted by local authorities" (Select Committee, 1822).

The next initiative was at the state level. In 1850, Massachusetts appointed a Sanitary Commission to inquire into conditions affecting the public's health in the Bay State. The Commission was chaired by Lemuel Shattuck, who helped produce a seminal document of far-ranging potentials. His recommendations called for the establishment of state and local boards of health; the development of systems for vital statistics; studies of the health of school children and of tuberculosis; control of smoke nuisance, food adulteration, and exposure of nostrums; and for health education. (It should be noted that several cities already had established local health departments: Baltimore, 1798; Charleston, S.C., 1815; Philadelphia, 1818; Providence, 1832; Cambridge, Mass., 1846 (*American Journal of Public Health,* 1945); however, no state level health department existed at that time.) Shattuck's additional recommendations included the establishment of nurses' training schools and the teaching of sanitary preventive medicine in medical schools. The Shattuck Report, however, received little attention and produced no direct action until 1869, when the Massachusetts Board of Health was established. After that there was rapid movement, with California establishing a state health department in 1870 and 36 other states following suit by the end of the 19th century (Hanlon, 1974).

Despite the establishment of local and state health departments, epidemics continued to break out and spread, generating a growing demand for effective federal quarantine measures. As a result, in December 1878 both houses of Congress appointed special committees to determine ways and means of controlling epidemics. The result was the passage of a law in 1879 creating a National Board of Health to be appointed by the president. The board was given extensive quarantine powers and also was charged with initiating a public health research program. Congress appropriated $500,000 to support the board's activities. However, the board fell victim to infighting and to battles over the balance between state and federal authority; it went out of business in 1884, when the authorizing legislation expired.

In 1886, the U.S. Supreme Court ruling on J. P. Morgan's *Louisiana and Texas Railroad & Steamship Co. v. Board of Health of Louisiana and State of Louisiana* clearly established the federal authority in the field of health. The Court noted:

> But it may be conceded that whenever Congress shall undertake to provide for the commercial cities of the United States a general system of quarantine, or shall confide the execution . . . of such a system to a national board of health . . . all state laws on the subject will be abrogated, at least so far as the two are inconsistent.

This ruling modified the Supreme Court's 1824 decision in *Gibbons v. Ogden* that had assigned the basic quarantine authority to the states. The new ruling provided the basis for an effective federal role in the health field. As a result, what started out as a battle over authority for quarantine ended up in a steady and effective expansion of federal authority, as evidenced by the following:

1887—A federal research body, the Hygiene Laboratory, was established in the Marine Hospital on Staten Island under the Marine Hospital Service. This was the beginning of the National Institutes of Health.

1893—The Marine Hospital Service, already having quarantine authority to investigate the origin and courses of epidemic diseases and to develop methods for their prevention and spread, was given additional authority for domestic quarantine and for inspection of all immigrants.

1901—The Hygiene Laboratory was upgraded to the National Hygiene Laboratory and funds were appropriated for a special building so its activities could be conducted properly.

1902—The Marine Hospital Service was reorganized as the Public Health and Marine Hospital Service under a surgeon general who was authorized to call an annual conference of state and territorial health offices to discuss and review health issues of common concern.

1906—The Pure Food and Drug Act was adopted.

1909—The first White House Conference on Children and Youth was held.

1912—The Public Health and Marine Hospital Service was renamed the Public Health Service in recognition of the fact that it was concerned with the health of all Americans.

1912—The National Hygiene Laboratory's role was broadened to the study of all human disease with a view to determining the causes of their origin and spread.

1912—The Children's Bureau was established under the Department of Labor to study all matters pertaining to the welfare of children, especially infant mortality, birth rate, diseases, employment, and similar issues.

1917—The National Leprosarium at Carville, La., was established, the Public Health Service given responsibility for the physical and mental examination of all aliens, and $25,000 was appropriated for studies and demonstrations in rural health to be undertaken by the Public Health Service in cooperation with the states.

1918—The Division of Venereal Disease in the Public Health Service was established to deal with health issues resulting from U.S. participation in World War I.

Despite this expansion, the federal role in health was rather small and was limited largely to serving the health needs of those groups for which it was directly responsible (e.g., the military and merchant seamen). As late as 1935, federal expenditures on health and medical programs for the civilian population were only $35 million while state and local expenditures that year were $625 million (*Historical Statistics,* 1960). However, the enactment of the Social Security Act in 1935 launched a new era of the federal government's role in health.

The Middle Years: Tilt toward Equality

The turn into the 20th century was noted for increasing public demands for economic reform and for better working conditions. Emerging trade unions gave special attention to issues pertaining to industrial safety and workers' compensation. As a result, between 1902 and 1914, 18 states passed worker compensation laws.

In 1906 a United States chapter of the International Association for Labor Legislation was organized as the American Association for Labor Legislation. This body rapidly became an important force behind a variety of social reform proposals. Building on the findings of the Russell Sage Foundation's 1910 study of European social and health insurance systems, the association in 1910 supported the idea of health insurance in the United States. This idea received a boost from the passage of the National Health Insurance Act in Britain in 1911.

In 1912 the Conference on Charities and Corrections joined the call for insurance against accident, sickness, old age, and unemployment (*Proceedings,* 1912). In the same year, Teddy Roosevelt's Progressive Party adopted a platform in support of a ". . . system of social insurance adapted to American use" (Progressive Party, 1912). Woodrow Wilson echoed similar sentiments in his Inaugural Address in 1913 when he said:

> There can be no equality of opportunity if men and women and children be not shielded in their lives, in their very vitality, from the consequence of great industrial and social processes which they cannot alter, control or simply cope with. (Wilson, 1926)

In 1916, health insurance bills based on the Model Health Insurance measures prepared by the American Association for Labor Legislation were introduced in the Massachusetts and New York Legislatures but failed to pass. These would have: (1) provided for cost sharing by employer, employee, and the state; (2) required compulsory participation; and (3) given administrative responsibility to mutual associations supervised by the state. No federal involvement was proposed.

In that year Meyer London, Socialist Representative from New York, introduced a resolution to appoint a commission to develop a plan for the establishment of a National Insurance Fund and for dealing with the problem of unemployment (House Joint Resolution, 1916). Opposed by organized labor and the insurance companies, the resolution was defeated, 189 yea, 138 nay, and 106 abstentions, with a two-thirds majority (288) needed for passage.

California, Illinois, New Jersey, Ohio, Pennsylvania, and Wisconsin appointed commissions to study and develop proposals for government-supported health insurance but none of these led to the enactment of such legislation.

These social reform initiatives calling for a major governmental role in health generated a backlash, most notably from the American Medical

Association (AMA). Formed in 1847, the AMA in its early years was a leader and supporter of governmental involvement in health. It recognized the need for a federal role in vital statistics, public health research, and quarantine, and pressured the states for the establishment of state boards of health. In 1872, it established a section of State Medicine and Hygiene and observed that:

> State Medicine consists in the application of medical knowledge and skill to the benefit of communities, which is obviously a very different thing from their application to the benefit of individuals in private or curative medicine. (Logan, 1872)

Reflected in this distinction between state medicine and private medicine, the AMA recognized the role of government at all levels in relation to the former but not to the latter.

The AMA attitude remained essentially unchanged until early 1900, when its leadership was captured by those who were impressed by the health insurance movement in Europe and Britain and who advocated similar programs for the United States. Under their influence, the AMA in 1916 appointed a Committee on Social Insurance to develop proposals for health insurance law; around that time, the *Journal of the American Medical Association* (JAMA) published editorials and papers favoring health insurance. The spokesman for the AMA even testified in favor of health insurance bills in Massachusetts and New York and of Meyer London's resolution in Congress (Chapman & Talmadge, 1971; Fishbein, 1947). However, by 1917 a determined voice of the AMA rank and file began to attack what it regarded as the organization's liberal posture and by 1920 succeeded in establishing AMA's opposition to compulsory health insurance as well as to any federal role in providing medical care services. This position was reiterated in 1922:

> The American Medical Association hereby declares its opposition to all forms of "state medicine" because of the ultimate harm that would come to the public weal through such form of medical practice.

> "State medicine" is . . . any form of medical treatment provided, conducted, controlled or subsidized by the federal or any state government, or municipality. . . . (JAMA, 1922)

Medical services provided by government to military personnel, indigents, and the mentally ill, as well as those needed to cope with communicable diseases and "such other services" were not considered "state medicine." Interestingly, this new definition of "state medicine" was very different from the one used by the AMA in 1872 (Logan, 1872). The old definition emphasized the control of communicable diseases, not government's medical treatment of nonindigents.

Opposition to government involvement in health insurance and medical care also came from sources other than the AMA. It was noted that the insurance industry was firmly opposed to proposals such as the Meyer London resolution. Organized labor saw such measures as undue governmental intervention in the collective bargaining process. Objections also were raised on the ground that compulsory contributions might be unconstitutional (Freund, 1917).

The growing opposition to a governmental role in health, combined with the spy scare and anti-Bolshevist hysteria in the postwar years, seemed to have effectively inhibited federal initiatives. The exception was the Sheppard-Towner Act of 1921, which provided for a federal grant-in-aid program to encourage and enable states to develop programs in maternal and infant care. Although by the time this act was passed 32 states already had developed the capability to provide such services, the measure provided valuable assistance to those states and helped 15 others to develop similar programs. However, the primary importance of the Sheppard-Towner Act was that it laid a foundation for a state-federal relationship in health. The grant-in-aid program allowed states full authority to initiate and administer their own plans, subject to federal approval.

The major breakthrough came in 1935 with the adoption of the Social Security Act (Public Law 74-271), legislation that has come to symbolize the beginning of both the tilt toward equality and the ascendancy of the federal government. The Social Security Act did not provide for any revolutionary measures in the field of health. Basically, it was legislation to provide economic protection to the retired, unemployed, and disabled, and to their dependents. It included only minor references to health.

Title V of the act strengthened the role of the Children's Bureau in maternal and child health, crippled children, and child welfare services. Title VI gave the Public Health Service additional authority and resources to help state and local governments improve their public health capabilities. However, by establishing a number of principles of governmental responsibilities for social welfare, this act set in motion many developments of far-reaching consequences.

The first of these principles pertained to the government's role and authority in compelling individual citizens to plan for their own long-term welfare. This was extremely important because it spoke directly to the questions of liberty as well as happiness. By instituting provisions for individuals' compulsory contributions toward unemployment insurance and retirement benefits, the act recognized that it was appropriate for government to constrain individual liberty in the short run to ensure individual happiness in the long run.

The second principle involved the relative authority of federal and state governments in matters concerning the general welfare. The act assigned the predominant role to the federal government, and when this was challenged in the courts, the Supreme Court held that under the general welfare clause of the Constitution (Article I, Section 8) "The Congress shall have the power to lay and collect taxes . . . , to pay the debts and provide for the common defense and general welfare of the United States . . . ," Congress had full authority to enact social welfare measures (*Steward Machine Co. v. Davis,* 1937). In another ruling it held that social welfare initiatives by Congress did not violate the Tenth Amendment ("The powers not delegated to the United States by the Constitution, nor prohibited by it to the States, are reserved to the States respectively, or to the people."). The Court said:

> Nor is the concept of the general welfare static. What is critical or urgent changes with time. . . . When money is spent to promote the general welfare, the concept of welfare or the opposite is shaped by Congress, not the States. (*Helvering v. Davis,* 1937)

The Helvering ruling also helped clarify a third principle implied in the Social Security Act, namely, the use of tax funds to support social welfare programs.

The fourth principle concerned federal authority to compel state and local governments to incur public expenditures for social welfare. This was dealt with by requiring those governments to share the cost of the public assistance programs provided for under the act.

Lastly, this act introduced a principle of entitlement that placed an obligation on the federal government to provide certain services and payments to all eligible citizens without a means test.

These principles of governmental responsibility for social welfare provided a strong basis for a proactive government posture in health. But opposition to governmental intervention was too powerful to allow any major initiative to bear fruit for several years.

The years immediately preceding and following the Social Security Act were marked by intense debate about government's role in personal health services. During this period several bills proposing compulsory health insurance and/or cost sharing by government were introduced with success. The primary arguments in favor of governmental intervention were threefold. First, many families could not afford the cost of medical care and therefore could not effectively pursue happiness. The comment by the United States Commission on Economic Security (1937) is typical of such observations:

> Tens of millions of families live in dread of sickness. Millions of families that are independent and self-sustaining in respect to the ordinary, routine needs of life sacrifice other essentials of decent living in order to pay for medical service. (p. 315)

The second line of argument was based on the observation that nonavailability of adequate and timely medical care was an important factor for disabled, blind, or dependent persons who were qualified for public assistance (Stevens & Stevens, 1974); therefore, it would be prudent for the government to provide necessary medical care to those who could not afford to pay for it.

The third argument pointed out that government already was active in the provision of personal health services but that the pattern of this involvement was fairly haphazard and patchy. For example, seamen and military personnel and their families were well covered by federal programs; federal health care services also were provided on Indian reservations. Further, many local governments were running public hospitals and dispensaries, largely for the benefit of the indigent. Public health departments at the state and local levels were increasingly active in providing a wide range of preventive care. However, these programs had many critical gaps; in addition, the categorical grants approach was resulting in two classes of personal health services, in which public programs were relegated to a low-quality, second-class status. It was argued that a single and comprehensive public financed health care system would remove inequities and would ensure the much-needed security and liberty to pursue happiness.

The opponents of governmental intervention had argued that very few persons were without adequate medical care (Delphey, 1917). When this argument could not be sustained, they asserted that the appropriate method for easing the financial plight was private, not public, insurance. The argument in favor of private insurance started to take hold. In the 1930s, Blue Cross and Blue Shield came into being and grew rapidly. The rapid expansion of private health insurance is seen in the fact that in 1940 only 9 percent of the civilian population had private coverage as compared to 51 percent by 1950 (Reed, 1967). In the light of this development, it was argued that private health insurance not only was desirable but was amply feasible.

In the 1940s, this debate seemed to have been boiled down to a rather simple formulation, namely, while the medical care needs of the well-to-do and the organized working population generally were well taken care of (through personal resources and private insurance), a large proportion of the population—the unorganized and the nonworking—did not enjoy such protection. Therefore, ways and means needed to be found to take care of these groups. The first step was the Social Security Amendments of 1950 (P.L. 81-734), which provided for limited medical services to those on public assistance under a federal-state cost-sharing arrangement based on grants-in-aid.

These amendments provided rather poorly for those on old age pensions. The medical plight of the aged became an increasingly important issue during the 1950s as this segment of the population gained increasing recognition as a growing voting block having special needs beyond its personal resources. There was general agreement that something needed to be done to provide relief but there were significant philosophical differences over approach and method.

At one extreme of the controversy were those who believed in the "entitlement approach," namely, the benefit should be provided to all eligible members of the population without any means test. They therefore favored a medical care program funded through increased employee and employer contributions to Social Security funds. At the other extreme were those who favored limited governmental action aimed at the indigent elderly; they therefore argued for expanded medical care through categorical public assistance. The Kerr-Mills Act of 1960 (P.L. 86-778) was a victory for the latter point of view insofar as its primary thrust was means-test-oriented public assistance. Under this act, the federal matching grants for medical care of old-age assistance beneficiaries were liberalized and a new federal grant-in-aid program was established to meet the medical needs of those elderly who were poor but not receiving cash assistance.

The passage of Kerr-Mills did not bring the controversy over government's role and responsibility for medical care to a rest. If anything, the debate became even more intense because the act turned out to be generally disappointing for a number of reasons, including uneven development of services in states, high emphasis on institutional care, and inability to provide assistance until medical indigency was achieved (Stevens & Stevens, 1974).

The Third Phase: Discovery of Limits

During the early years of United States history, the role of government in health was quite marginal; during the middle years (World War I to

1960) governmental intervention rose steadily but the primary initiative for developing and delivering services was at the state and local levels. However, the 1960s witnessed the emergence of federal government as the dominant actor in this policy arena. Starting with the Sheppard-Towner Act of 1921 and through Kerr-Mills in 1960, the federal role in personal health was limited largely to grants-in-aid to states; therefore, the primary initiative for development of programs and services was not at that level but at the state level.

During the 1960s, this approach continued but the federal sphere of influence kept growing with the steady introduction of new grants-in-aid programs for especially vulnerable groups. These included:

P.L. 87-510, Cuban refugees (1962)
P.L. 87-692, migrant farm workers (1962)
P.L. 88-164, those suffering from mental illness (1963)
P.L. 88-452, underserved central city and rural populations (1964)
P.L. 89-253, participants in Head Start programs (1965)
P.L. 89-4, residents of Appalachia (1965).

Simultaneously, the federal government also expanded its involvement in biomedical research, health manpower training, construction of health facilities, and development of capability for health planning and coordination through enactment of a series of new legislations and by amending those adopted previously.

But the real shift in the role of the federal government came with the passage of the Social Security Amendments Act of 1965 (P.L. 89-97), better known as the Medicare-Medicaid Act.

Part A of Title XVIII (Medicare) of the act provided for a specified amount of hospital and related institutional care for all participants in the Social Security program who were 65 years or older by raising the taxable wage base for Social Security contributions. Part B provided for a package of supplementary benefits including coverage of costs of physicians and related services; unlike Part A, participation in Part B was not compulsory. Title XIX (Medicaid) essentially extended Kerr-Mills to all recipients of public assistance, liberalized the scope of the covered medical care services, and made the federal grants-in-aid more generous.

This legislation, intended to be a giant step for social justice and equality of opportunity, resulted in strengthening the federal role in two ways. The first one was intended, insofar as the Medicare program was designed, as a national-level entitlement program with the federal government at the helm. The second, unintended, factor was the unforeseen rapid rise in the cost of Medicaid and Medicare programs. All initial assumptions as to demographic trends, participation rate, and medical care costs that had served as factual underpinnings of this act turned out to be grossly inaccurate. Both birth and death rates fell below projections and, as a result, the proportion of the elderly in the population rose faster than anticipated. On July 1, 1966, the Medicare program covered 19.1 million persons; the number had risen to 27.9 million by July 1, 1979 (Muse & Sawyer, 1982).

Participation in the Medicaid program is determined by how "eligible" is defined, and this was left to the states. Taking advantage of this situation several states adopted fairly liberal eligibility criteria. The extreme case was that of New York State, which qualified almost 45 percent of its population for Medicaid; if other states were to adopt similar definitions, close to 20 percent of the country's population could have been covered by the program (Stevens & Stevens, 1974).

Further, the states were given a relatively free hand in defining covered medical services. This discretion gave the states a license to go for broke and to seek as much of the easy federal money as possible. To top it all, utilization and the unit cost of hospital and physicians services rose much faster than anticipated. All of these factors resulted in a skyrocketing of total costs.

In 1965, it was estimated initially that Title XIX would increase the federal contribution by about $200 million in a full year of operation over that in the programs operating under then-existing law that were receiving a total of about $950 million a year (U.S. Congress, 1965). Within one year, this estimate had to be revised upward to $3 billion a year (U.S. Congress, 1966). By 1979, the federal expenditure for Medicare and Medicaid had soared to $29.2 billion and $12.1 billion, respectively (Bixby, 1981). This rapid growth in financial costs made the federal government the major fiscal agent in health services and, by exercising the inherent power of the purse strings, it gained the dominant role.

The 89th Congress (1965–1966), which enacted the Medicare-Medicaid legislation, was responsible for passing nearly a score of other laws, each of which added significantly to the federal role and authority in the health field. These included:

Appalachian Regional Development Act (P.L. 89-4)
Older Americans Act (P.L. 89-73)
Drug Abuse Control Act Amendments (P.L. 89-74)
Federal Cigarette Labeling and Advertising Act (P.L. 89-92)
Mental Retardation Facilities and Community Mental Health Centers Construction Act Amendments (P.L. 89-105)
Health Research Facilities Act Amendments (P.L. 89-115)
Housing and Urban Development Act (P.L. 89-117)

Public Works and Economic Development Act (P.L. 89-136)

Water Quality Act (P.L. 89-234)

Heart Disease, Cancer and Stroke Act (Regional Medical Programs) Amendments (P.L. 89-239)

Clean Air Amendments and Solid Waste Disposal Act (P.L. 89-272)

Health Professions Educational Assistance Act Amendments (P.L. 89-290)

Medical Library Assistance Act (P.L. 89-291)

Vocational Rehabilitation Act Amendments (P.L. 89-333)

Extended Comprehensive Health Planning and Public Health Service Act Amendments (P.L. 89-749)

Allied Health Professions Personnel Training Act (P.L. 89-751)

Demonstration Cities and Metropolitan Development Act (P.L. 89-754)

This increasing action posture of Congress in health matters continued to 1981, with each new piece of legislation directly or indirectly expanding and strengthening the federal presence. Initially, the primary policy concern was to make high-quality health services accessible to all, unhindered by any external factor such as ability to pay, location, race, gender, age, employment, or health condition. Another concern soon was added: cost containment.

The euphoria of the 1960s that produced a whole gamut of health programs also led to massive public expenditures for supporting these efforts. They rose from $11 billion in 1965 to $104 billion in 1980 (Gibson & Waldo, 1981); one estimate forecast that these expenditures would reach $207 billion in 1985 and $381 billion in 1990 (Freeland & Schendler, 1981). An equally important fact is that the shares of public and federal expenditures as proportions of total spending on health, after remaining stable for many years at around 26 percent and 13 percent, respectively, rose dramatically after 1965. By 1979, the share of public expenditures had risen by 65 percent and federal expenditures by nearly 120 percent (Table 1-1). These increases could be financed by new taxes, by shifting resources from other programs, or by deficit financing, described by Russell as "installment taxes" (see Russell, 1982).

Faced with the pulls and tugs of multiple power centers, Congress chose to use all three of these avenues. At the same time, it started to give increasing attention to keeping the costs of the programs within acceptable boundaries.

The Current Phase: Cost-Containment Pressure

By the mid-1970s, the cost containment alternative had become such a major concern in the discussion of health policy in the United States that

Table 1-1 Percent Distribution of Health Expenditures (by Sources of Funds for Selected Years, 1950 to 1979)

Source	1950	1955	1960	1965	1970	1975	1979
State and Local	14.4	14.4	13.5	12.7	13.7	14.6	14.4
Federal	12.8	11.3	11.2	13.4	23.5	28.1	28.7
Private	72.8	74.3	75.3	73.9	62.9	57.4	56.9

Source: Reprinted from "National Health Expenditures: Short-Term Outlook and Long-Term Projections" by Mark S. Freeland and Carol Ellen Schendler, *Health Care Financing Review,* Winter 1981, p. 114.

it seemed as if a new value, frugality, had taken hold of the country. However, frugality always has been considered an important virtue. (Remember: Cut your coat according to your cloth; a penny saved is a penny earned, etc.) As long as the country could afford new expenditures, the need for frugality remained dormant but concern started to surface as soon as resources became strained.

Some have argued that concern with cost is not recent but arose almost as soon as Medicare-Medicaid legislation was passed:

Title XIX was signed into law on July 30, 1965, with a blaze of publicity. Two-and-a-half years later, on January 2, 1968, its author and supporter, President Lyndon Johnson, was constrained to sign a bill which signalled the beginning of the demise of Medicaid. . . . In less than three years after its passage . . . the major cries were for cutbacks, both in programs and eligibility. By 1968 . . . [the] era of optimistic expansion was to be replaced by one of questioning retraction, and criticism. (Stevens & Stevens, 1974)

The reservations about Medicaid costs were not fully carried over to all public expenditures on health care until the second half of the 1970s. Up to that point the mood of the country still was very strongly for equality and, therefore, expansionist in the social welfare field. The early 1970s were marked by a flurry of national health insurance bills. In 1975 alone at least nine such measures were introduced (U.S. Congress, House, 1976). This is not to say that during this period there was no concern over the rising medical costs. In fact, some of the national health insurance proposals were put forward as ways of controlling these expenditures (Lewis & Keairnes, 1970). But by 1976, health containment of public expenditures on health became an official federal priority:

It is necessary, first, to be aware of the context. . . . The national economic scene has a major impact on the options and opportunities that are open. . . . A national public and private debt which now totals $2.7 trillion, aspirations far outdistancing resources as graphically portrayed by the recent services crises of New York City and New York State, and the emergence of the health industry as the number one industry of the country are but a few of the factors influencing possible actions related to health. . . . Overshadowing this scene as a major driving force is the rapidly growing cost of health care and the increasing public burden of paying that cost. . . . Until costs can be contained, Federal policymaking in health will be dominated by these basic economic considerations. Proposed solutions must address the total health care system. . . . Comprehensive national health insurance is such a total system approach, but health care cost escalation as well as externalities of economic and social policy make its timing and phasing uncertain.

It is within this context that priority must be set and set within the allocation of resources that will be actually available to us. Our priorities must reflect a broad concern for the health world [and] focus on keeping costs down. (PHS, 1976)

Despite this emphatic concern with containment of public health expenditures, two factors—"to help improve the health of the American people" and "to assure access to quality health care at reasonable cost"—were adopted as the goal and the primary objective of health planning for 1978–82 (PHS, 1976). It was noted that while great progress had been made toward improving access to services as well as in the public's overall health status, much still remained to be done. On the plus side, some of the major achievements were (PHS, 1981):

- Life expectancy at birth, as well as at 65 years, had continued to increase. In 1950, life expectancy at birth was 68.2 years and at age 65 it was 13.9; by 1968 these figures had risen to 73.3 and 16.3 years, respectively.
- Age-adjusted mortality rates continued to decline. Between 1950 and 1978, the mortality rate fell from 841.5 to 606.1 per 100,000 population.
- Between 1950 and 1978 the infant mortality rate dropped from 29.2 to 13.8 per 1,000 live births.
- Infants weighing 2,500 grams or less at birth per 100 total live births fell from 8.3 to 7.1 between 1966-68 and 1976-78.

- Between 1950 and 1979, rates of all major notifiable diseases with the exception of gonorrhea had fallen dramatically.
- Between 1974 and 1979, the percent of the population that self-assessed its health as fair or poor declined from 13.2 to 12.4.

However, a major concern remained: that these gains were not evenly distributed and that race, economic status, and location still were significant factors in access to services as well as in the determination of health status:

- Life expectancy at birth of nonwhites continued to be lower than that of whites (Table 1-2).
- Age-adjusted death rate from all causes continued to be significantly higher for the black population (Table 1-3).
- Infant mortality rate (24.1) in the black population was almost twice the 12.5 rate in the white population. A similar difference existed for infants weighing 2,500 grams or less at birth: black: 12.9, white: 6.0.
- Black and poor children 1 to 4 years of age had a poorer vaccination status than white and affluent children (Table 1-4).
- Race, income, and location continued to be significant factors in self-assessment of health status (Table 1-5).

Table 1-2 Life Expectancy at Birth by Sex and Race, 1978

Race	Male	Female
White	70.2	77.8
Nonwhite	65.0	73.6

Source: Adapted from *Health, United States,* U.S. Public Health Service, 1981, p. 111.

Table 1-3 Age-Adjusted Death Rate from All Causes by Sex and Race, 1978

Race	*(Per 100,000)* Male	Female
White	773.1	425.5
Black	1113.1	650.5

Source: Adapted from *Health, United States,* U.S. Public Health Service, 1981, p. 119.

Table 1-4 Vaccination Status of Children 1–4 Years of Age, by Race and Location, 1979

	Percentage of Population Vaccinated				
Characteristic	Measles	Rubella	DTP	Polio	Mumps
Race:					
White	66.2	64.7	69.0	63.6	57.5
Nonwhite	51.2	53.7	49.2	38.9	46.0
Location:					
SMSA Component					
Central City	57.8	58.0	58.0	52.1	49.5
Poverty Area	47.7	52.8	48.6	44.5	40.8
Nonpoverty Area	60.9	59.6	61.0	54.4	52.1
Remaining SMSA Areas	65.6	65.1	69.1	61.6	57.2
Non-SMSA Areas	66.1	64.1	67.7	62.6	58.5

Source: Adapted from *Health, United States,* U.S. Public Health Service, 1981, p. 146.

Table 1-5 Self-Assessment of Health Status as Fair or Poor, by Race, Income, and Location, 1979

Characteristics	Percentage of Population
Race:	
White	11.4
Black	13.0
Income:	
Less than $7,000	24.7
$7,000–$9,999	17.9
$10,000–$14,999	14.6
$15,000–$24,999	10.5
$25,000–or more	6.9
Location: Within SMSA	12.1
Outside SMSA	15.4

Source: Reprinted from *Health, United States,* U.S. Public Health Service, 1981, p. 148.

- An estimated 12 percent of persons under age 65 had no protection against the cost of hospital care, either through private insurance or a public program such as Medicare or Medicaid (Carroll & Arnett, 1981).

Further, despite the fact that the United States was spending at least as much money on health as did other industrialized countries, as measured by share of GNP, it did not enjoy a comparable health status; in fact, its status was one of the lowest (Table 1-6).

President Carter entered the White House in 1977 committed to work toward the removal of the remaining barriers to health services and to help Americans achieve a health status second to none. He had hoped to achieve these goals through remobilization and better management of available resources. At that time, many in Congress and at health meetings still talked about "impending national health insurance." But all this changed in the face of the economic and political realities that developed in the country. These included rapidly increasing oil prices, chronic trade deficits, the steep drop in the value of the dollar in international markets, persistent double-digit inflation and interest rates, the slowdown of the economy, growing federal budget deficits, unacceptable levels of unemployment, and graver doubt about the superiority of the U.S. industrial and defense capabilities (Cameron & Kirkland, 1980).

These developments forced final public recognition that the United States was not all-powerful and that it had finite capabilities. Under a system of competing claims on resources, the nation could afford the cost of any single goal at levels reflecting current aspirations but it could not

---

Table 1-6 Percentage of GNP Spent on Health, Infant Mortality Rates, and Life Expectancy at Birth

U.S. and Selected Industrialized Countries

Country	% GNP on Health	Infant Mortality Rates	Life Expectancy at Birth	
	1975	1978	1978 M.	F.
Canada	7.1	12.4	70.5	78.2
Denmark	—	8.9	71.7	77.7
England & Wales	5.6	13.1	70.2	76.3
France	8.1	10.6	69.9	77.9
Federal Republic of Germany	9.7	13.2	68.9	74.5
Japan	—	8.4	73.2	78.6
Netherlands	8.6	9.6	72.0	78.7
Sweden	8.7	7.8	72.5	79.0
Switzerland	—	8.6	72.0	78.9
U.S.A.	8.4	13.8	69.5	77.2

Sources: Data derived from "Health Care Expenditures in Nine Industrialized Countries, 1960–76" by Joseph G. Simanis and John R. Coleman, *Social Security Bulletin,* January 1980, pp. 3–8, and from *Health, United States,* U.S. Public Health Service, 1981, pp. 115–116.

accomplish all its aspirations at the same time. In coming to this realization, the public's long-standing faith in the ability of the federal government to surmount all problems—faith developed on the basis of the New Deal, WWII, the Korean War, the War on Poverty, Man-on-the-Moon—was seriously hurt. Opinion polls in 1977 and 1978 reported that a majority of the people had started to believe that government was incapable of solving the problems facing the country (Health Insurance Institute, 1978).

Health services suffered an additional black mark: costs consistently rose at a rate higher than the rate of inflation for the economy as a whole (Zubkoff, 1975; Raskin, Coffey, & Farley, 1978). Moreover, between 1960 and 1980 health care costs rose at an average annual rate of 11.7 percent when the GNP grew at an 8.6 percent rate. As a result, health expenditures took an increasing share of the GNP, reaching 9.4 percent in 1980 (Weichert, 1981).

In light of these facts, there was a growing question regarding the fair share for health in the national scheme of things. In other words, could the country afford to devote a larger share of its wealth to health services without jeopardizing other priorities? The answer to that question made cost containment the number one priority in health policy.

A PROPOSAL FOR RESTRUCTURING THE U.S. ROLE

Ever since financial constraint asserted itself as a high priority in health policy, explanations poured out for the rapid rise in cost of care as well as proposals for holding down those expenditures. The explanations ranged from (1) a fee-for-service/cost reimbursement profit-oriented free enterprise system, to (2) exponential growth of technology, to (3) the tyranny of regulations, to (4) separation of payment responsibility from the decision to seek care, to (5) undue emphasis on treatment and prolongation of life, to (6) the weak voice of consumers, to (7) a conspiracy of providers, to (8) the use of licensing and accreditation to establish monopolistic control, to (9) waste and fraud.

There were at least as many proposed solutions. These could be grouped into four broad categories: (1) design to control supply, (2) design to control demand, (3) design to provide incentive for efficiency, and (4) design to strengthen forces of competition and free market. Exhibit 1-1 lists, describes, and annotates the main proposals under each of these four categories.

Several of these proposals had been attempted, with varying results; others had not been made operational because of political opposition; a few still were under debate. Different as these proposals were in their

Exhibit 1-1 Summary of Major Health Cost-Containment Proposals

Nature of Proposal	Summary of Proposal	Selected References
1.0 **Supply Control**	The underlying argument is that demands expand to match supply, resulting in unnecessary utilization of health services. Demand being largely dictated by the providers, high supply does not result in lower cost. Therefore, it is argued that controlling the availability of health services should help in controlling cost.	Institute of Medicine, 1976a & b McClure, 1977 Klarman, 1978 Schweitzer, 1978
1.1 Certificate of need	This requires a formal justification and approval of all expansion of health facilities and all new investment in excess of specified amounts.	P.L. 93-641 P.L. 92-603. Sec. 1122 Klarman, 1978 Noll. 1975 Havighurst, 1975 Salkever & Bice, 1978, 1979
1.2 Ceiling on capital expenditures at state level	Each state, to correct the weakness of the certificate-of-need program, would be limited to a federally determined ceiling on capital expenditures.	Title II, H.R. 6575, 1977
1.3 Hospital conversion and closure	It is argued that elimination of excess bed capacity could offer large savings.	Institute of Medicine, 1976b McClure, 1977 Hanft, Raskin, & Zubkoff, 1978 Title III, H.R. 9717, 1977
1.4 Control over supply of physicians and other providers	An excess supply of physicians, dentists, and other providers leads to unnecessary utilization of health services. Therefore, it is necessary to control this supply.	Lyle, Citron, Snugg, & William, 1974 Congressional Budget Office, 1977 Morrow & Edwards, 1976 DHHS, 1980

Exhibit 1-1 continued

1.5 Improvement in clinician awareness of medical care cost	It is argued that providers often have little knowledge of the cost of the care they provide. Their training emphasizes know-how, not cost. Increased cost awareness on their part would result in conservative prescription of drugs and services.	National Commission on the Cost of Medical Care, 1978.
1.6 Systematic technology assessment	Cost-benefit and cost-effective data on technical advances would help in inhibiting indiscriminate purchase of new technology.	PHS, 1978
2.0 **Demand Control**	Less consumption equals less cost: hence reduce cost by reducing unneeded consumption.	
2.1 Cost sharing by consumer (deductibles, copayment, coinsurance, etc.)	The higher the direct cost to consumers, the greater their sense of responsibility in the utilization of health services.	Newhouse & Phelps, 1976 Beck, 1974
2.2 Utilization Review (PSRO)	This program calls for systematic monitoring and review of quality and cost-effectiveness of services. It is argued that this will discourage unnecessary utilization and unreasonable charges and will promote high quality.	Institute of Medicine, 1976a Congressional Budget Office, 1977 Health Services Administration, 1977 Schweitzer, 1979 Blumstein, 1978
2.3 Health promotion and disease prevention	Return on investments for health promotion and disease prevention activities is a lot higher than for treatment-related activities. The prevention/promotion investments also reduce the need for expenditures on treatment.	Quelch, 1980 Terris, 1977 Walker, 1977 PHS, 1976 Salmon & Berliner, 1980
2.4 Improvement in consumer ability to make better informed decisions on utilization (second opinion, systematic access to cost information, quality, and effectiveness)	Consumers freed from the dictates of the providers would use fewer and cheaper services.	Ingbar, 1978 National Commission on the Cost of Medical Care, 1978 McCarthy & Widmer, 1974 McCarthy, Finkel, & Kamons, 1977 Evans, 1974

3.0 Incentives for Efficiency	Instituting an adequate reward/punishment system can discourage waste and encourages efficiency.	Fein, 1981 Somer, 1978
3.1 Replace "customary, prevailing, and reasonable charges" (CPRC) with "maximum allowable charges" (MAC)	CPRC breeds inflation and forces an open-ended budget. MAC would encourage providers to be efficient and would provide a basis for prospective budgeting of expenditures.	Halahan, Scanlon, Hadley, & Lee, 1978 Glaser, 1976 Hadley & Lee, 1978 Redisch, 1978
3.2 Replace institutional cost reimbursement with prospective rate setting	This is an extension of the argument under 3.1 to hospitals and other institutions.	Hellinger, 1978 Bauer, 1978 Altman & Weiner, 1977
3.3 Hospital revenue ceilings	This is a more sophisticated version of 3.2. It would control the yearly revenues but leave the cost per unit of service unregulated.	Title I, H.R. 6575, 1977 Ginsburg, 1978
3.4 Prepaid Group Practices (PGPs) and HMOs	These should provide strong financial incentives to economize on the use of resources.	Davis, 1975 Schlenker & Ellwood, 1973 Gaus, Cooper, & Hirschman, 1976 Luft, 1978
4.0 Increase Competition a. among providers b. among insurers c. among services d. between service utilization and saving	It is argued the the free play of competitive forces will reduce waste, unnecessary utilization, and other inefficiencies.	Blue Cross, 1981 Greenberg, 1978 Enthoven, 1980 Enthoven, 1978a & b Ginzberg, 1980 Roemer & Roemer, 1982 Rushefskey, 1981

approaches to containing health costs, all suffered from one major common defect: they were focused so single-mindedly on frugality that they paid little or no attention to the other historically cherished values of equality and liberty. In fact, most of the cost-containment proposals tended to violate these historical values to some extent.

Almost all the proposals for control of supply and demand called for increased intervention by the federal government, which would subject the health system to an additional burden of regulation, expand the bureaucracy, and further contain liberty. Also, given the fact that most of these cost-containment approaches would not impact all sectors of the population equally and would affect the poor more acutely than the rich, they also did violence to equality. In their inability to satisfy the demands for liberty and equality lay the explanation for their political unacceptability and operational inadequacy.

What was true of the demand/supply proposals also was true very largely of the proposals that approached cost containment indirectly through carefully designed incentives. They also would strengthen the federal role, albeit to a lesser degree. An incidental advantage of these proposals might be that the nation would start to move toward a system of prospective budgeting of health services expenditures instead of simply paying the bills when they came due (Fein, 1981). This, in turn, could lead to a norm regarding the optimum level of health expenditures and produce a mind set of "living within a budget."

However, these proposals had a great deal of political difficulty in Congress and at other decision-making levels because they assigned a very powerful role to government. Out of all incentive-related proposals, those concerned with prepaid group practices and HMOs seemed to have greater harmony with the nation's overall value system. In actual practice, however, the high cost of recruiting and serving rural, nonworking, unorganized, elderly, and thinly scattered populations served as a powerful deterrent to bringing these groups under coverage of such programs. As a result, these plans seemed to fall short on the principle of equality.

Only after Ronald Reagan became President in 1981 did proposals to promote competition start to receive a serious hearing. These proposals reflected an idealized orientation toward the free enterprise system that gave primacy to liberty although they were being justified on the ground of cost containment.

However, little empirical evidence existed that these proposals would, in fact, achieve their avowed aim. The market for health services, not being the same as that for detergents or automobiles, did not behave in the classical model of Adam Smith. Based on the peculiarities of the health market, a plausible line of argument could be developed that the so-called

Policy Concerns and the Role of Government 29

procompetition proposals would generate more regulations and that instead of containing costs they actually would fuel the fires of inflation. Worst of all, these proposals might seriously limit access to services for those who already had difficulties with access. (Roemer & Roemer, 1982; Rushefsky, 1981; Fein, 1981).

It has been observed that cost-containment proposals are constructs of tinkerers and technocrats. Such an "expert" may be ". . . defined as one who knows every aspect of his job—except its ultimate purpose and social consequences " (Fein, 1981). The issues pertaining to organization, finance, and delivery of health services are not merely matters of technical concern; as noted earlier, they deal with some of the most basic social purposes: life, liberty, and pursuit of happiness. Equality is a fundamental prerequisite to liberty and, resources being finite, frugality is an inescapable responsibility; any arrangement of health services will be found wanting if it fails to meet this framework of values.

The history of the health system in the United States provides ample evidence that excessive emphasis on any one value tends to create a Hegelian antithesis; what is needed is a balanced approach, a Hegelian synthesis. Development and operationalization of such an approach should be the central focus of health policy debate during the next decade.

Since no model of health services that addresses all basic values is available, one would have to be developed from scratch. The first step in the development of such a model requires that essential parameters—do's and dont's—be specified. It might be argued that the critical parameters are as follows:

1. A healthy life is a fundamental right as well as the responsibility of each individual.
   Notes: a. Rights need protection of government.
   b. Responsibility places a moral and social burden that must be discharged through a good faith effort.
2. All individuals are free to pursue the goal of a healthy life on their own terms and in their own way.
   Notes: a. Freedom of choice is a very important value.
   b. Individuals are free to live as they choose but must accept the consequences of personal behavior and actions.
3. It is a responsibility of government to remove the conditions and barriers that cannot be surmounted by individuals and that stand in the way of a healthful life.
   Notes: a. The role of government is to help individuals achieve their goals.
   b. This helping process can be reactive or proactive.
   c. Conditions and barriers that come in the way of the indi-

vidual pursuit of a healthy life include ignorance, un-
healthy environment and food supply, lack of resources,
nonavailability of services on acceptable terms, and social
prejudices and discrimination.

d. Government cannot carry out this responsibility without
systematic, relevant, and timely information, effective
know-how, and adequate organizational and resource
capabilities.

4. Government, to meet its obligation to remove undesirable conditions
and barriers bearing oppressively on individuals pursuing health,
among other things should ensure universal, equitable, and effective
access to appropriate services.

Notes: a. Emphasis is on availability of and access to health services, not on mandatory utilization.

b. "Appropriate" is not necessarily equivalent highest quality. What is appropriate is contingent on context: situation, need, resources, historical experience, etc.

5. The health care system must be highly sensitive and responsive to
individuals' concerns, values, preferences, and priorities. This goal
is best achieved when the system is directly owned and managed by
citizens themselves.

Notes: a. The emphasis is on individuals and not on community.
The latter is seen as an instrument of individual well-
being—the servant and not the master.

b. It is recognized that individuals cannot function effectively without a communal life and that, next to family,
community tends to be the most important unit of organized activities.

c. The greater the distance between citizens and government, the greater the insularity, insensitivity, and callosity
of government. Remote government is distrusted and is
subject to indifference and hostility. To make and keep
government responsive to citizens is to develop and institute it at the grass-roots level and to elect it by democratic
process. Also, small is beautiful when it comes to government. Parkinson's Laws provide ample testimony that big
government tends to become bigger without becoming
effective and in this process tends to lead discourses on
social issues to degenerate into technical debates, resulting in burying the matter in a quagmire of regulations and
red tape.

d. The current socioeconomic climate indicates a high degree of concern with the rapidly rising cost of health care and with the extensive bureaucratic intervention based on voluminous regulations. There also is a general lack of confidence in the ability of professionals, bureaucrats, and remote politicians to resolve current and emerging health issues.

This list is not intended to be exhaustive; many other specifications could be added easily. There also is nothing sacrosanct about any of these items except that they seem to cover all of the basic values rather well and provide a nice balance in the relative importance of these values.

To continue the exercise, the next step in the development of the desired model is to prepare a trial sketch. Here a lot of energy could be saved if an existing model could be found that would more or less accommodate the just-cited specifications. Not only is the use of an existing model more cost-effective than de novo creation, it also offers an additional valuable benefit, namely, empirical data on efficacy. These data should go a long way in the development and review of the new model.

It is not necessary to look far and wide to find that the nation's public elementary and secondary education system meets most of the specifications to a remarkable degree. The similarities and differences between the characteristics of this system and the model specifications are as follows:

1. Both education and health are recognized as essential preconditions for the pursuit of happiness and, therefore, are considered basic rights and responsibilities of individuals.
2. Both systems recognize the importance of freedom of choice in the exercise of respective rights and responsibilities. However, in the public education model, this freedom is constrained insofar as a certain amount of formal schooling has been made compulsory for all children. This is done on the ground that education is too important in the achievement of happiness to be left to the personal circumstances, desires, and convenience of parents and their children.
3. Both systems require government to remove detrimental conditions and barriers to the exercise of these rights and responsibilities and to assure a universal, equitable, and accessible service system. Education has a long history of governmental effort toward achievement of this aim. It is worth noting that education not only is compulsory but also is available free of charge to all children (in public schools). However, pupils are not forced to attend public schools; they have an option to attend private schools if they are prepared to pay the required tuition and fees.

4. Both demand that the service system be highly responsive to citizens' needs, concerns, and priorities. To achieve this aim public education has developed an elaborate grass-roots system of organization and decision making. Its main features are:

   a. All elementary/secondary public education activities are organized by school district, usually a political unit smaller than or equal to local government.

   b. Each district elects a citizens' board, usually called the school board.

   c. The school board has direct and complete responsibility and authority for developing, organizing, and delivering all public education at the elementary/secondary level, within the constraints of federal, state, and local laws and regulations. It develops and approves educational programs and curricula, receives funds to finance educational activities under its jurisdiction, owns property, hires personnel, enters into contracts, and makes all policy decisions.

   d. Public education activities tend to be financed from the proceeds of a special purpose local tax supplemented by contributions by state government from general revenues and special project funds and by federal grants-in-aid. The school board does not have authority to levy taxes. Based on its budgetary needs, the school board requests suitable funds from the appropriate government, which considers this request in competition with all others within the constraint of available revenues and other financial requirements and the responsibility for balancing its own budget.

   e. Local, state, and federal governments have limited and relatively well-defined responsibilities in public education. These include:

Federal Government

1. to develop broad national goals and standards for education and to monitor progress
2. to help remove barriers to achievement of these goals and standards through grants-in-aid, research, and similar programs
3. to ensure that all federal laws, including those pertaining to civil rights and equality of opportunity, are fully implemented

State Government

1. to develop state-level goals, objectives, and standards for education
2. to develop an appropriate mechanism for organizing and delivering public education (school districts are to discharge this responsibility)

3. to ensure that needed financial, personnel, and other resources are available to achieve its goals, objectives, and standards for public education
4. to help all school districts in its jurisdiction achieve state educational goals, objectives, and standards through appropriate assistance
5. to monitor the progress of each school district
6. to enforce all relevant civil and criminal laws under its jurisdiction

Local Government
1. to develop local educational goals and standards
2. to be an active partner with state government to ensure that all reasonable requests for funds for public education are met
3. to levy and collect such special tax(es) as are legally permitted to finance public education
4. to enforce local codes and standards

It may be argued that the public education model is not a very sound one. It may be observed that the overall quality of public education in the United States actually is not very satisfactory and that schools, instead of preparing good citizens, have become fertile ground for crime and vandalism; that there is much inequality of opportunity in education; and that equity-oriented programs, including busing and affirmative action, can be very oppressive. None of these charges is without some merit.

However, in defense of this model it should be pointed out that despite its deficiencies the system has been remarkably successful in science and technology and in making public education an effective variable in social mobility. This system also has been very successful in containing costs and expenditures. Above all, as an effective model of grass-roots democracy and of balanced participation of local, state, and federal government, it addresses and resolves the issue of equity among multiple and at times competing values of society.

Unless a better model is presented, this one deserves serious consideration. Organization and delivery of health services on the model of public education would require a major shift in the focus of health policy debates but this alternative is not as radical as it may seem on first blush. The country already has the benefit of more than a century of experience in organizing and delivering services through state and local health boards. Their authorities and responsibilities could be restructured. Further, with the introduction of block grants, the federal-state relationship has been experiencing a major shift of program responsibilities to states. Some of the factors that led to the federal government's active role also have largely lost their original strength. These changes are:

1. Personal health services today, as was noted earlier, are more evenly distributed throughout the country than ever before, and this process is likely to continue with the steadily improving supply of health personnel and growing experience in the improvement of access.
2. Financial barriers to health services have been significantly lowered for the most vulnerable groups, viz., the poor and the aged.
3. The health information system already is quite sophisticated, comprehensive, and sensitive and is getting better. This has made it possible for federal and state, as well as local, governments to monitor the health system effectively and to correct its behavior through appropriate actions.
4. State and local governments have come to recognize and accept their roles and responsibilities for assuring high-quality personal health services to all their citizens and are increasingly active in this field.
5. The organizational and managerial capabilities of state and local governments have improved steadily with the growing professionalization of these functions. Many competent professionals now readily choose to work in state and local governments.
6. State and local governments have become increasingly sophisticated in dealing with pressures from power groups.
7. Mass media have gained a high degree of understanding and expertise in policy issues pertaining to personal health and are actively involved in reporting new developments as well as in exposing corruption, fraud, and unmet needs.
8. Citizens and health service consumers have an increasing understanding and awareness of their rights and obligations and increasingly are willing to assert themselves individually as well as in concert.

Despite these favorable developments, it would be naive to believe that a major restructuring of the federal-state-local role could be realized without a great deal of struggle. The pressure from a variety of vested interests, combined with the historical distrust of state and local governments in matters of social justice and social welfare, would form a powerful line of resistance. Issues regarding sources of new revenue for the financing of personal health services by these levels would have to be settled.

In view of the fact that the influence of the private sector in this field already is very significant and is growing rapidly, a serious discussion on public-private sector roles must be anticipated. Many other questions and problems would have to be resolved. Change and progress in a multipower-centered democracy comes neither rapidly nor easily but such societies survive, grow, and gain strength because of their ability to change.

REFERENCES

Acton, J.P. *Measuring the social impact of heart and circulatory disease program: Preliminary framework and estimates.* Santa Monica, Calif.: The Rand Corporation, 1975.

Altman, S., & Weiner, S. *Constraining the medical care system: Regulation as a second best strategy.* Paper presented at the Federal Trade Commission Conference on Computation in the Health Care Sector, Washington, D.C., June 1977.

American Journal of Public Health. Has Baltimore the oldest health department? Editorial, January 1945, *35*(1), 49.

American Medical Association. *Profile of Medical Practice, 1977.* Chicago: Author, 1977.

American Medical Association. Reference Committee on Legislation and Public Relations. Minutes of House of Delegates, May 25, 1922. *Journal of the American Medical Association,* 1922, *78,* 1715.

Atkinson, A.B., & Townsend, J.L. Economic aspects of reduced smoking. *Lancet,* 1977, *2,* 492–494.

Bardach, E., & Kagan, R.A. *Social regulations: Strategies for reform.* San Francisco: Institute for Contemporary Studies, 1982.

Bauer, K. Hospital rate setting—This way to salvation. In M. Zubkoff, I.E. Raskin, & R. Hanft (Eds.), *Hospital Cost Containment.* New York: Prodist, 1978, pp. 324–369.

Beck, R. The effects of copayment on the poor. *The Journal of Human Resources,* Winter 1974, *9*(1), 129–142.

Bixby, A.K. Social welfare expenditures, fiscal year 1979. *Social Security Bulletin,* November 1981, *44*(11), 3–12.

Blanpain, J., Delesie, L., Nys, H., Debie, J., & Luevens, J. *International approaches to health resources development for national health programs.* Hyattsville, Md: U.S. Public Health Service, National Center for Health Services Research, Contract No. HRA-230-75-0108, September 1976. (Executive Summary)

Blue Cross/Blue Shield Association. Bills in Congress present preview of new competitive health care system. *Urban Health,* July/August 1981, pp. 25–26, 44.

Blumstein, J. The role of PSROs in hospital cost containment. In M. Zubkoff, I.E. Raskin, & R. Hanft (Eds.), *Hospital Cost Containment.* New York: Prodist, 1978, pp. 461–485.

Burger, E.J., Health and health services in the United States: A perspective and a discussion of some issues. *Annals of Internal Medicine,* May 1974, *80,* 645–650.

Burney, I., & Gabel, J. *Reimbursement patterns under Medicare and Medicaid.* Prepared for the Conference on Research Results from Physician Reimbursement Studies, sponsored by the U.S. Department of Health, Education, and Welfare, Health Care Financing Administration, Office of Policy, Planning and Research, Washington, D.C., February 1978.

Cameron, J. & Kirkland, R.I., Jr., Five burdens that make a rich U.S. feel poor. *Fortune,* January 14, 1980, pp. 72–79.

Carroll, M.S., & Arnett, R.H., Private health insurance plans in 1978 and 1979: A review of coverage, enrollment, and financial experience. *Health Care Financing Review,* September 1981, *3,* 55–87.

Chapman, C.B., & Talmadge, J.M. The evolution of the right to health concept in the United States. *The Pharos of Alpha Omega Alpha,* January 1971, *34,* 30–51.

Cooper, B.S., & Rice, D.P. The economic cost of illness revisited. *Social Security Bulletin,* 1976, *39*(2), 21–36.

Courtwright, D.T. Public health and public wealth: Social costs as a basis for restrictive policies. *Milbank Memorial Fund Quarterly/Health and Society,* 1980, *58*(2), 268–282.

Davis, K. *National health insurance—Benefits, costs and consequences.* Washington, D.C.: The Brookings Institution, 1975.

Delphey, E.U. Arguments against the standard bill for compulsory health insurance. *Journal of the American Medical Association,* 1917, *68,* 1500–1501.

Dubnick, M.J. Government regulations: Advice and analysis. *Public Administration Review,* March/April 1981, *41,* 286–292.

Enthoven, A.C., Consumer-choice health plan (Part 1). *The New England Journal of Medicine,* March 23, 1978, *298*(12), 651–658. (a)

Enthoven, A.C., Consumer-choice health plan (Part 2). *The New England Journal of Medicine,* March 30, 1978, *298*(13), 709–720. (b)

Enthoven, A.C. *Health plan: The only practical solution to the soaring cost of medical care.* Reading, Mass.: Addison-Wesley Publishing Company, Inc., 1980.

Evans, G. Supplier-induced demand: Some empirical evidence and implications. In M. Perlman (Ed.), *The economics of health and medical care.* New York: John Wiley & Sons, Inc., 1974.

Faulkner, H.U. *The decline of laissez-faire, 1897–1917.* New York: Holt, Rinehart & Winston, Inc., 1951.

Fein, R. Social and economic attitudes shaping American health policy. In John B. McKinlay (Ed.), *Issues in Health Policy.* Cambridge, Mass.: The MIT Press, 1981, pp. 29–65.

Feldstein, M., & Taylor, A. *The rapid rise of hospital costs.* Washington, D.C.: Executive Office of the President, Staff Report for the Council on Wage and Price Stability, January 1977.

Fishbein, M. *History of the American Medical Association.* Philadelphia: W.B. Saunders Company, 1947.

Freeland, M.S., & Schendler, C.E. National health expenditures: Short-term outlook and long-term projections. *Health Care Financing Review,* Winter 1981, *3,* 97–138.

Freund, E. Constitutional and legal aspects of health insurance. *Proceedings of the National Conference of Social Work,* 1917, 553–558.

Gaus, C., Cooper B., & Hirschman, C. Contrasts in HMO and fee-for-service performance. *Social Security Bulletin,* May 1976, *39*(5), 3–14.

Gibson, R.M. National health expenditures, 1978. *Health Care Financing Review,* Summer 1980, *2,* 1–36.

Gibson, R.M., & Waldo, D.R. National health expenditures, 1980. *Health Care Financing Review,* September 1981, *3,* 1–54.

Ginsburg, P. Impact of economic stabilization program on hospitals: An analysis with aggregate data. In M. Zubkoff, I.E. Raskin, & R. Hanft (Eds.), *Hospital Cost Containment.* New York: Prodist, 1978, pp. 293–323.

Ginsburg, P., & Manheim, L. Insurance, copayment, and health services utilization: A critical review. *Journal of Economics and Business,* Spring/Summer, 1973, pp. 142–153.

Ginzberg, E. Competition and cost containment. *The New England Journal of Medicine,* November 6, 1980, *303*(19), 1112–1115.

Glaser, W. *Controlling costs through methods of paying doctors: Experience from abroad.* Paper presented at the Fogarty International Center Conference on Policies for the Containment of Health Care Costs and Expenditures, Bethesda, Md., June 1976.

Green, J. Responsibility for health. *Journal of Holistic Health,* 1977, pp. 76–79.

Greenberg, W. (Ed.) Competition in health care sector: Past, present and future. *Proceedings of a conference sponsored by the Federal Trade Commission, Bureau of Economics,* Washington, D.C., March 1978.

Gross, S. Professional disclosure—An alternative to licensing. *Personnel and Guidance Journal,* Spring 1977, pp. 568–588.

Hadley, J., & Lee, R. *Toward a physician reimbursement policy: Evidence from the economic stabilization period.* Washington, D.C.: The Urban Institute, July 1978. (Working papers)

Halahan, J., Scanlon, W., Hadley, J., & Lee, R. *The effect of Medicare/Medicaid reimbursement on physician behavior: A summary of findings.* Paper presented at the Conference on Research Results from Physician Reimbursement Studies, sponsored by the Department of Health, Education, and Welfare, Health Care Financing Administration, Office of Policy, Planning, and Research, Washington, D.C., February 1978.

Halper, T. The Double-edged sword: Paternalism as a policy in the problems of aging. In J.B. McKinlay (Ed.), *Issues in health care policy.* Cambridge, Mass.: The MIT Press, 1981, pp. 199–226.

Hanft, R., Raskin, I.E., & Zubkoff, M. Introduction. In M. Zubkoff, I.E. Raskin & R. Hanft (Eds.), *Hospital Cost Containment.* New York: Prodist, 1978.

Hanlon, J.J. *Public health: Administration and practice* (6th ed.). St. Louis: The C.V. Mosby Company, 1974, pp. 13–40.

Havighurst, C. Federal regulations of the health care delivery system. *University of Toledo Law Review,* Spring 1975, pp. 577–590.

Health Insurance Association of America. *Source book of health insurance data, 1981–82.* Washington, D.C.: HIAA, 1982.

Health Insurance Institute. *Current social issues: The public's view.* Washington, D.C.: HII, 1978.

Health Insurance Institute. *Health and health insurance: The public's view.* Washington, D.C.: HII, 1979.

Health Resources Administration. *Report on the graduate medical evaluation national advisory committee,* Vols. 1 and 3. (Department of Health and Human Services, U.S. Public Service, Publication Nos. (HRA) 81-651 and 81-653). Washington, D.C.: U.S. Government Printing Office, 1980.

Health Services Administration. *PSRO, An evaluation of the professional standards review organization* (Vol. 1). (Department of Health, Education, and Welfare, Office of Planning, Evaluation, and Legislation, Report No. OPEL 77-12.) Rockville, Md.: October 1977. (Executive summary)

Hellinger, F. An empirical analysis of several prospective reimbursement systems. In M. Zubkoff, I.E. Raskin, & R. Hanft (Eds.), *Hospital Cost Containment.* New York: Prodist, 1978, pp. 370–400.

Helvering v. Davis, 301 U.S. 619–646 (1937).

Hofstadter, R. *The age of reform: From Bryan to F.D.R.* New York: Alfred A. Knopf, Inc., 1955.

Ingbar, M. The Consumer's Perspective. In M. Zubkoff, I.E. Raskin, & R. Hanft (Eds.), *Hospital Cost Containment: Selected Notes for Future Policy.* New York: Prodist, 1978, pp. 103–165.

Institute of Medicine. *Assessing quality in health care, An evaluation.* Washington, D.C.: National Academy of Sciences, November 1976. (a)

Institute of Medicine. *Controlling the supply of hospital beds.* Washington, D.C.: National Academy of Sciences, October 1976. (b)

Jain, S.C. *Health services in North Carolina: An agenda for progress toward year 2000.* Paper prepared for the Commission on the Future of North Carolina. (Mimeographed), 1982, p. 10.

Jain, S.C. *Role of state and local governments in relation to personal health services.* Washington, D.C.: American Public Health Association, 1981.

Kavaler, F., Kelman, H.R., & Brownstein, A.P. Regulation of health care: prospects for the future. *Journal of Public Health Policy,* September 1980, *1,* 230–240.

Keeler, E., Morrow, D., & Newhouse, J. The demand for supplementary health insurance, or Do deductibles matter? *Journal of Political Economy,* August 1977, pp. 789–801.

Klarman, H. Health planning and progress: Prospects and issues. *Milbank Memorial Fund Quarterly/Health and Society,* Winter 1978, *56*(1), 78–112.

Koplin, A.N., Health departments in a National Health Service: An American perspective. *Journal of Public Health Policy,* September 1980, *1,* 241–257.

Lasch, C. *The culture of narcissism.* New York: W.W. Norton & Co., 1978.

Lecht, L.A. *The dollar cost of our national goals* (Research Report No. 1). Washington, D.C.: National Planning Association, Center for Priority Analysis, 1965.

Lewis C., & Keairnes, H. Controlling costs of medical care by expanding insurance coverage: A study of a paradox. *The New England Journal of Medicine,* June 18, 1970, *282*(25), 1405–1412.

Lilley, W., & Miller, J.C. The new social regulations. *The Public Interest,* Spring 1977, *47,* 49–61.

Logan, T.M. Report of the Committee on a National Health Council. *Transactions of the American Medical Association,* 1872, *23,* 46–51.

Luft, H.S. How do health maintenance organizations achieve their savings? *The New England Journal of Medicine,* June 15, 1978, *298*(24), 1336–1340.

Lyle, C., Citron, C., Snugg, W., & William, O. Cost of medical care in a practice of internal medicine: A study in a group of seven internists. *Annals of Internal Medicine,* July 1974, pp. 1–6.

Marmor, T. The politics of national health insurance: Analysis and perception. *Policy analysis,* Winter 1977, pp. 25–48.

McCarthy, E., Finkel, M., & Kamons, A. *Second opinion surgical programs: A vehicle for cost containment.* Paper presented to National Commission on the Cost of Medical Care. Chicago: American Medical Association, March 1977.

McCarthy, E., & Widmer, G. Effects of screening by consultants on recommended surgical procedures. *The New England Journal of Medicine,* December 19, 1974, *291*(25), 1331–1335.

McClure, W. *Reducing excess hospital capacity.* NTIS No. HRP-0015199/3, October 1977.

Morrow, J., & Edwards, A. U.S. health manpower policy: Will the benefits justify the costs? *Journal of Medical Education,* October 1976, pp. 791–805.

Muse, D.N., & Sawyer, D. *The Medicare and Medicaid Data Book, 1981.* (Department of Health and Human Services, Health Care Financing Administration, Publication No. (HCFA) 03128). Washington, D.C.: U.S. Government Printing Office, April 1980, p. 13.

National Commission on the Cost of Medical Care. *The national commission on the cost of medical care, 1976–77.* Chicago: American Medical Association, 1978.

Newhouse, J., & Phelps, C. New estimates of price and income elasticities of medical care services. In R. Rossett (Ed.), *The role of health insurance in the health services sector.* New York: National Bureau of Economic Research, 1976, pp. 261–313.

Noll, R. The consequences of public utility regulation of hospitals. In *Controls on Health Care,* Conference on Regulation in the Health Industry. Washington, D.C.: National Academy of Sciences, January 7–9, 1975.

Proceedings of Conference of Charities and Collections, 39th Annual Session, Chicago, 1912.

Progressive Party. A contract with the people. *Platform of The Progressive Party Adopted at Its First National Convention, Chicago, August 7, 1912.* New York: Progressive National Committee, 1912.

Quelch, J.A., Marketing principles and the future of preventive health care. *Milbank Memorial Fund Quarterly/Health and Society,* Spring 1980, *58*(2), 310–347.

Raskin, I.E., Coffey, R.M., & Farley, P.J. Cost containment. In *Health, United States, 1978.* (Department of Health, Education, and Welfare, U.S. Public Health Service, Publication No. (PHS) 78-1232.) Washington, D.C.: U.S. Government Printing Office, 1978, pp. 1–20.

Redisch, M. Physician involvement in hospital decision-making. In M. Zubkoff, I.E. Raskin, & R. Hanft (Eds.), *Hospital Cost Containment.* New York: Prodist, 1978, pp. 217–243.

Reed, L.S. Private health insurance: Coverage and financial experience, 1940–66. *Social Security Bulletin,* November, 1967, *30*(11), 3–22.

Relman, A.S. The new medical-industrial complex. *The New England Journal of Medicine,* October 23, 1980, *303*(17), 963–970.

Rice, D., & Wilson, D. The American medical economy—Problems and perspectives. In T. Hu (Ed.), *International health costs and expenditures.* (Department of Health, Education, and Welfare, National Institutes of Health, Publication No. (NIH) 76-1067). Washington, D.C.: U.S. Government Printing Office, 1976.

Roemer, M.I., & Roemer, J.E. The social consequences of free trade in health care? A public health response to orthodox economics. *International Journal of Health Services,* 1982, *12*(1), 111–129.

Rushefsky, M.E. A critique of market reform in health care: 'The consumer-choice health plan.' *Journal of Health Politics, Policy and Law,* Winter 1981, *5*(4), 111–129.

Russell, J. Endless budget deficits. *The Atlantic,* July 1982, p. 6.

Salkever, D., & Bice, T. Certificate-of-need legislation and hospital costs. In M. Zubkoff, I.E. Raskin, & R. Hanft (Eds.), *Hospital Cost Containment.* New York: Prodist, 1978, pp. 429–460.

Salkever, D., & Bice, T. *Hospital certificate-of-need controls.* Washington, D.C.: American Enterprise Institute, 1979.

Salmon, J.W., & Berliner, H.S. Health policy implications of the holistic health movement. *Journal of Health Politics, Policy and Law,* Fall 1980, *5*(3), 535–553.

Schlenker, R., & Ellwood, P. Jr., *Medical inflation: Causes and policy options for control* (Interstudy working paper). Minneapolis: InterStudy, March 1973.

Schweitzer, S. Health care cost-containment programs: An international perspective. In M. Zubkoff, I.E. Raskin, & R. Hanft (Eds.), *Hospital Cost Containment, Selected Notes for Future Policy.* New York: Prodist, 1978. pp. 57–75.

Scitovsky, A., & McCall, N. *Changes in the costs of treatment of selected illness, 1951–*

1964–1971. (Department of Health, Education, and Welfare, Health Resources Administration, Research Digest Series, Publication No. (HRA) 77-3161). Washington, D.C.: U.S. Government Printing Office, July 1976.

Simanis, J.G., & Coleman, J.R. Health care expenditures in nine industrial countries, 1960–76. *Social Security Bulletin,* January 1980, *43*(1), 3–8.

Solares, A. Midwifery licensing: Pitfalls, problems, and alternatives to licensing. In D. Stewart & L. Stewart (Eds.), *Compulsory hospitalization: Freedom of choice in childbirth?* Marble Hill, Mo.: National Association of Parents and Professionals for Safe Alternatives in Childbirth, 1979.

Somers, A. Health care financing: The case for negotiated rates. *Hospitals,* February 1, 1978, *53*(3), 49–52.

Stenberg, C.W. Federalism in transition, 1959–79. *The Future Federalism in the 1980s.* Washington, D.C.: The Advisory Commission on Intergovernmental Relations, 1981, pp. 27–38.

Stevens, Robert, & Stevens, Rosemary. *Welfare medicine in America.* New York: Free Press, 1974.

Steward Machine Co. v. Davis, 301 U.S. 548–618 (1937).

Synergy, Incorporated. Costs and benefits of regulation: A survey of studies. In *Regulatory Reform Seminar: Proceedings and Background Papers.* Washington, D.C.: U.S. Department of Commerce (Office of the Secretary) October, 1978.

Terris, M. Strategy for prevention. *American Journal of Public Health,* 1977, *67*(11), 1026–1027.

Tesh, S. Political ideology and public health in the nineteenth century. *International Journal of Health Services,* 1982, *12*(2), 321–342.

Ullman, D. Regulated freedom of choice: An alternative to licensure. *Holistic Health Review.* (forthcoming).

U.S. Bureau of the Census. *Historical statistics of the United States, Colonial times to 1957.* Washington, D.C.: U.S. Government Printing Office, 1960. (Historical Statistics, 1960)

U.S. Bureau of the Census, *Statistical abstract of the United States, 1978.* Washington, D.C.: U.S. Government Printing Office, 1979. (Statistical Abstract, 1978)

U.S. Commission on Economic Security. *Social Security in America: Factual background of the Social Security Act.* 1937, p. 315.

U.S. Congressional Budget Office. *Expenditure for health care: Federal programs and their effects.* Washington, D.C.: U.S. Government Printing Office, August 1977.

U.S. Congress, House, Committee on Ways and Means. *Limitations on federal participation under Title XIX of the Social Security Act.* Report 2224 to Accompany H.R. 18225, 89th Cong., 2d sess., 1966, p. 8.

U.S. Congress, House, Committee on Ways and Means. *National health insurance resource book.* Washington, D.C.: U.S. Government Printing Office, 1976, pp. 457–505.

U.S. Congress, House. *Report of the select committee . . . to inquire into the propriety of repealing the Act of 1813,* 17th Cong., 1st. sess., 1822, H. Rept. 93. (Select Committee, 1822)

U.S. Congress, Joint Resolution 1959, *Congressional Record,* 64th Cong., 1st sess., 1916, 53:2856.

U.S. Congress, Senate, Committee on Finance, *Social Security amendments of 1965.* 89th Cong., 1st sess., 1965, S. Report 404, p. 11.

U.S. Department of Health and Human Services. Health Resources Administration. *Report of the graduate medical evaluation national advisory committee* (Vols. 1 and 3). U.S. Government Printing Office, Washington, D.C.: DHHS Pub. No. (HRA) 81-651 and 81-653, 1980.

U.S. Public Health Service. *Forward plan for health, FY 1978–82.* (Department of Health, Education and Welfare.) Washington, D.C.: U.S. Government Printing Office, August 1976, pp. 1, 2. (PHS, 1976)

U.S. Public Health Service. *Health, United States, 1981.* Washington, D.C.: U.S. Government Printing Office, Department of Health and Human Services, December 1981. (PHS, 1981)

Wagner, J., & Zubkoff, M. Medical technology and hospital costs. In M. Zubkoff, I.E. Raskin, & R. Hanft (Eds.), *Hospital cost containment, Selected notes for future policy,* New York: Prodist, 1978, pp. 263–289.

Walker, R. Current issues in the provision of health care services. *Journal of Consumer Affairs,* 1977, *11*(2), 52–62.

Weichert, B.G. Health care expenditures. In *Health, United States, 1981.* (Department of Health and Human Services, Publication No. (PHS) 82-1232). Washington, D.C.: U.S. Government Printing Office, December 1981, p. 81.

Weidenbaum, M.L., & DeFine, R. *The cost of federal government regulation of economic activity.* Washington, D.C.: American Enterprise Institute, 1978.

Wikler, D.I. Persuasion and coercion for health: Ethical issues in government efforts to change lifestyles. *Milbank Memorial Fund Quarterly/Health and Society,* Summer 1978, *56*(3), 303–338.

Wilson, W. First inaugural address as President of the United States, March 4, 1913, The Public Papers of Woodrow Wilson. *The New Democracy,* Vol. 1, New York: Harper, 1926.

Wolfe, S.M. Economic cost of smoking. Washington, D.C.: Public Citizens Health Research Group, 1977. (Mimeographed)

Zubkoff, M. (Ed.). *Health: A victim or cause of inflation,* New York: Prodist, 1975.

Chapter 2

Financing and Cost Containment for Personal Health Services in the 1980s

Deborah A. Freund and Paul S. Jellinek

HISTORY OF PERSONAL HEALTH SERVICES FINANCING

The financing of personal health services in the United States has under-gone dramatic change in the last several decades. Major changes have occurred in the sources and methods of payment as well as in the level and sophistication of services purchased. These changes have brought to the fore a new array of complex problems, which in turn have led to a growing demand for innovative solutions. These are discussed in this chapter.

American medical practice prior to World War II was characterized by relatively simple payment methods. Typically, medical care was pur-chased directly from one's neighborhood general practitioner who was based in solo practice and provided a broad spectrum of primary care services. The use of hospital services was limited and those that were available were rather rudimentary by today's standards.

Physician and hospital charges generally were paid directly out of pocket by the patient. For those unable to pay, some philanthropic and public support (for example, in the form of tax-supported municipal hospitals) was available; in addition, it has been suggested that price discriminatory practices were followed by some providers as a means of cross-subsidizing low income patients (Kessel, 1958).

Insurance: From a Little to a Lot

The most striking feature characterizing the prewar era from a financing standpoint, however, was the relative absence of health insurance cover-age for either hospital or physician services. Table 2-1 provides data on trends in health insurance coverage for hospital, surgical, and physician

Table 2-1 Percent of U.S. Population with Types of Health Insurance Coverage

	Hospital Expenses	Surgical Expenses	Physicians' Expenses
1940	10.0	4.0	2.5
1950	40.0	15.6	5.9
1960	67.7	61.0	46.0
1965	77.0	74.0	63.0
1970	77.5	73.9	67.6
1979	83.0	78.8	74.3

Sources: Data derived from *The Source Book of Health Insurance Data 1980–81,* The Health Insurance Institute, Washington, D.C., © 1981, p. 12, and *U.S.A. Statistics in Brief, 1980,* U.S. Department of Commerce, Bureau of the Census, Washington, D.C. p. 2.

services since 1940. In 1940, roughly 10 percent of the population was covered for hospital expenditures, 4 percent for surgical, and 2.5 percent for physician charges. By 1950, those figures had risen to 40.0 percent, 15.6 percent, and 5.9 percent, respectively—a very substantial increase in each case, although still far below today's levels.

It is noteworthy that the increases in the 1940s and 1950s did not occur at the same rates across demographic groups. Table 2-2, for example, indicates that high-income urban residents and those working full time were most likely to have some form of health insurance. Furthermore, the gap in the proportion of individuals covered between upper and lower income and urban and rural populations appears to have widened during the 1940s, although substantial convergence is apparent by 1960.

Beginning in the 1950s and on into the early 1960s, medical practice and the financing arrangements that supported it began to undergo fundamental changes. Practice became technologically more sophisticated, more specialized, less personal, and, in the process, considerably more expensive. Table 2-1 indicates the steady upward trend in the proportion of the population covered by health insurance. Concurrently, the share of the gross national product (GNP) allocated to medical care rose from 4.0 percent in 1940 to 4.4 percent in 1950, and to 6.1 percent in 1965 to 9.7 percent in 1979 (Gibson, 1980).

Medicare and Medicaid

Perhaps the single most important change in contemporary medical care financing occurred in 1965 with the enactment of Medicare and Medicaid,

Table 2-2 Percent of Families with Health Insurance Coverage (by Selected Family Characteristics)

	1953	1958	1963
Income Level			
Lower	41	42	51
Middle	71	79	78
Upper	80	86	89
Residence			
Urban	70	73	77
Rural, Nonfarm	57	73	74
Rural Farm	45	44	54
Main Activity of Main Earner			
Working Full Time	69	78	82
Not Working Full Time	25	39	56

Source: Reprinted from *A Decade of Health Services* by Ronald Anderson and Odin Anderson by permission of The University of Chicago Press, © 1967, p. 77.

Titles XVIII and XIX of the Social Security Act (P.L. 89-97). Designed to improve access to hospital and physician services for the elderly and the poor, these two programs provided publicly subsidized health insurance coverage, with benefits to be paid out along traditional fee-for-service lines. By 1979, Medicaid alone provided coverage to almost 28 million beneficiaries (Health Care Financing Administration, 1982).

However, as Table 2-1 indicates, while the proportion of the total population with some form of coverage did increase for physician expenses, from 63.0 percent in 1965 to 67.6 percent in 1970, this did not hold true for either hospital or surgical coverage, suggesting that to some extent Medicare and Medicaid might have merely substituted public revenues for private funds, at least in the years immediately following their inception. Coverage for physician services continued to grow faster than for hospital and surgical expenses.

Certainly, these programs did bring about a dramatic increase in public expenditures for medical care, a development that in turn increased the government's stake in attempting to bring medical cost inflation under control. Ironically, it may well be that the federal entry into the medical market through Medicare and Medicaid provided the single greatest stimulus to those very costs it has been seeking so insistently to control ever since.

Table 2-3 shows both the absolute increase in medical expenditures between 1965 and 1979 and the relative increase in the government's share

Table 2-3 Public Health Expenditures, by Selected Third Party Payers, Type of Expenditure, and Amount

(Percent Distributions in Parentheses, (Figures in Millions)

	1979	1975	1970	1965
TOTAL	188,551	116,522	65,372	36,000
Direct Payments	59,973(31.8)	37,725(32.4)	26,128(40.0)	18,584(51.6)
Third Party Payments	128,577(68.2)	78,798(67.6)	39,244(60.0)	17,416(48.4)
Private Health Insurance	50,286(26.7)	31,077(26.7)	15,744(24.1)	8,729(24.2)
Philanthropy and Industrial Inplant	2,407(1.3)	1,539(1.3)	1,040(1.6)	788(2.2)
Government	75,884(40.3)	46,182(39.6)	22,460(34.4)	7,899(21.9)
Federal	53,311(28.3)	31,531(27.1)	14,561(22.3)	3,985(10.5)
Medicare	29,328(15.6)	15,588(13.4)	7,098(10.9)	—
Medicaid	11,770(6.2)	7,431(6.4)	2,795(4.3)	—
Other	12,213(6.5)	8,512(7.3)	4,669(7.1)	3,785(10.5)
State and Local	22,573(12.0)	14,650(12.6)	7,899(12.1)	4,114(11.4)
Medicaid	9,913(5.3)	5,873(5.0)	2,310(3.5)	—
Other	12,660(6.7)	8,778(7.5)	5,589(8.5)	4,114(11.4)

Source: Reprinted from "National Health Expenditures 1979," by Robert M. Gibson, Health Care Financing Review, Summer 1980, pp. 29–32.

of the burden over that same period. Equally noteworthy in the table, from the standpoint of cost control, is the continued decline in the proportion of direct out-of-pocket payments, counterbalanced by a steady increase in the proportion of both public and private third party payments.

Medical Cost Inflation

As noted, the evolution of personal health service financing from the straightforward out-of-pocket approach of the 1940s and 1950s to the highly complex public and private third party arrangements predominant today has given rise to a whole new array of equally difficult problems. Foremost among these clearly is medical cost inflation. The share of GNP allocated to medical care rose from 6.1 percent in 1965 to a startling 9.4 percent in 1980 (Gibson, 1980) and, perhaps even more significant, the average annual rate of increase in this GNP share climbed from 2.5 percent for 1950–1965 to 3.6 percent for 1965–1980.

The absence of any signs of reversal in these trends increased concern in the policy establishment, particularly with the advent in the late 1970s and early 1980s of an "era of scarcity" (Romani, 1980) and economic retrenchment. This slowdown in aggregate economic growth intensified intersectoral competition for both public and private dollars, thus stepping up the pressure on the medical segments to limit their share of GNP consumption.

In their efforts to develop viable responses to these pressures, health policy makers became increasingly interested with the potential of alternative delivery and financing systems for reducing inefficiencies and costs in the provision of medical care. These systems are discussed next.

THE ALTERNATIVE DELIVERY SYSTEM (ADS)

Under traditional third party fee-for-service insurance, the financing and provision of care are handled separately. Consumers, employees, or the government purchase contracts from an insurer. These contracts entitle the purchasers to obtain certain stipulated services from providers who are not employed by the insurer. It is argued that fee-for-service insurance reduces the out-of-pocket price to consumers while at the same time offering no incentives to providers to practice efficiently. This stimulates excessive demand for medical care by consumers and suppliers, and thereby drives total expenditures considerably higher than they would be under a direct out-of-pocket arrangement (Pauly, 1968).

In comparison, an alternative delivery system (ADS) to a greater or lesser extent consolidates the financing and provision of care within the same organizational entity. The consumer pays the ADS a fixed premium in advance and in return may obtain as much care as is desired for the length of the contract period, either free of charge or after paying a nomimal deductible or copayment. While the incentives facing the consumer after enrollment are essentially the same in an ADS as under fee-for-service (since in both cases there is no significant out-of-pocket cost), in choosing initially among available ADSs, it is in the consumers' interest to select the most efficient plan—that is, the plan that provides the greatest number of services of a given level of quality for the lowest price.

The history of ADSs in the United States dates back to the 1920s with the establishment of the Los Angeles Ross-Loos Clinic, the Elk City, Oklahoma, clinic, and the initiation of the first Kaiser plans in California in the 1940s (Jonas, 1977). However, it was not until the late 1960s to mid-1970s, as cost increases were beginning to accelerate, that ADSs began to flourish and multiply in numbers, and, as Table 2-4 indicates, this trend has continued into the 1980s.

Originally, the most common type of ADS was the prepaid group practice or, as it later came to be called, the health maintenance organization (HMO) (Elwood, 1971). More recently, variations of HMOs have emerged, including the primary care network (PCN), individual practice association (IPA), and health care alliance (HCA). While data on the number of PCNs and HCAs in operation in 1982 were sparse and unreliable, Table 2-4 indicates that the number of IPAs has almost doubled between 1978 and

Table 2-4 Growth of Alternative Delivery Systems

	Number of Alternative Delivery Systems	Number That Were IPAs	Total Enrollment (in millions)
1974	142	NA**	5.3
1975	178	NA**	5.7
1976	175*	NA**	6.0
1977	165*	NA**	6.3
1978	167	58	7.4
1979	173	65	8.2
1980	236	97	9.1
1981	243	111	10.3

*Decline from 1975–76 and from 1976–77 due to delicensure of HMO plans in California.

**NA—Data not collected prior to 1978.

Source: Personal communication: Kenneth Linde, Director of Qualification, Office of HMOs, U.S. Dept. of Health and Human Services, October, 1982.

1981 and that enrollments in all forms of ADSs have doubled between 1974 and 1981.

The types of ADSs are described next.

Health Maintenance Organization

The HMO, which, as indicated, is the most common type of ADS in operation, fully integrates the provision and financing of services. Services generally are provided by a large multispecialty group of physicians and may be available either at a single location or at multiple sites. The HMO is its own insurer although it may choose to carry reinsurance. Expensive high-technology services with a low probability of use may be purchased by the plan from fee-for-service specialists as needed but at no additional cost to the patient.

While the specifics of the financing arrangements vary from one HMO to another, in general the physician group is at risk—the higher the expenditures out of the overall group revenue pool, the lower the physicians' incomes.

Individual Practice Association

An IPA blends prepayment with traditional fee-for-service payment. Enrollees prepay a fixed premium in exchange for "free" care from the IPA's physicians; the doctors, on the other hand, are reimbursed on a fee-for-service basis and most frequently also retain fee-for-service practices. In an IPA, the provision and financing company collects premiums, pays providers, and markets the plan, while the IPA, which generally is a regional grouping of physicians, produces the services and maintains responsibility for determining the membership.

In an IPA, the physician is rewarded for seeing more patients, at least in the short run. However, if costs do outrun revenues, the physician ultimately must take a reduction in reimbursement. In an IPA: (1) physicians retain responsibility for the organization and delivery of care, (2) members conduct peer review to ensure appropriate utilization, and (3) enrollees maintain freedom of choice of physician (Egdahl, Taff, Friedland, & Linde, 1977).

Primary Care Network

In a PCN, enrollees designate a participating primary care physician to serve as coordinator of all their services. The physician directly provides all needed primary care and refers the enrollee to specialists or to the hospital as necessary. The physician thus serves as the enrollees' primary provider and financial manager. In terms of financial coverage, each PCN physician is rated individually by an insurance company, with which the doctor then shares the risk for all physician and nonphysician (including hospital) services.

Typically, a PCN physician's account consists of two parts:

1. The direct services of the physician: payment out of this "pot" is made on a fee-for-service basis until the physician reaches some threshold number of enrollees (for example, under the SAFECO-United Health Care plan the threshold was 200), at which point the method of payment converts to negotiated capitation.
2. Referral and hospital care: bills for these services must be authorized by the primary care physician, with actual payment handled by the insurance company.

PCN physicians share in both the surpluses and deficits of the part II accounts so they have an incentive for cost-consciousness (Moore, 1979).

Health Care Alliance

An HCA is structurally simpler than the other ADSs. HCA enrollees agree to obtain all of their medical care from a given panel of physicians, who may be organized as a large multispecialty group or perhaps simply as an association of individual doctors in private practice. As in an IPA, participating physicians may continue to have fee-for-service patients along with the HCA enrollees. In addition, the physicians face no financial risk in an HCA.

HCA premiums simply reflect the cost of the benefits package offered. Responsibility for establishing premium levels, collecting payments, and marketing the plan is delegated to an insurance company (National Chamber Foundation, 1978).

Preferred Provider Organization

The newest type of ADS is the Preferred Provider Organization (PPO). PPOs are groups of hospitals and physicians that contract on a fee-for-service basis with employers, insurance companies, or third party administrators to provide comprehensive medical services to subscribers (Federation of American Hospitals Review, 1982, p. 12). In return for using a preferred provider, subscribers receive economic rewards such as reduced coinsurance and copayments.

General features of PPOs include the use of a closed provider panel, a negotiated fee that reflects a discount, utilization review, and more rapid payment by insurance carriers. Unlike HMOs, capitation payment is not used and subscribers are not "locked in" to the plan for any given period of time.

Because their development is so recent, there is thus far no published review of their success in reducing costs. To date, PPOs have been established in Detroit, Denver, and California.

COST-CONTAINMENT POLICY

While the development of ADSs constitutes an important approach to resolving medical cost inflation, it is in many regards a microlevel step. The object is to arrive at a new organizational and financial structure that will improve the operational efficiency of individual medical care "firms." However, it has become clear that many providers are reluctant to participate in such new structures unless they have some clear-cut incentives to do so. Why bother restructuring a practice, and in the process sacrifice a certain amount of professional autonomy and perhaps even income, unless, in effect, forced to? In other words, while the various ADSs provide a means for cutting costs, they do not provide a reason to do so. The reason for cutting costs, it appears, must be brought to bear on the system by a full-fledged macrolevel cost containment policy.

While many specific cost-containment strategies have been proposed, at both state and federal levels, each of these generally can be classified as being of one of two broad generic types: regulatory or competitive. Both seek to reduce costs by encouraging greater efficiency in the production and consumption of care but the means for accomplishing this objective are decidedly different. Under regulation, decision-making authority over resource allocation, which includes determination of the price, quantity, and quality of medical care available, is shifted from providers to government agencies and the market incentive structure may be left unchanged. Under competition, decision-making authority over resource allocation stays with the provider, and the incentive structure of the medical market is changed.

Advocates of regulation tend to argue that the medical market is inherently monopolistic because the physician inevitably acts as both supplier and demander (as the patient's "agent") of care; advocates of competition maintain that the critical monopoly features of the market are legal rather than inherent and thus are subject to reform.

A second, more pragmatic, set of assumptions that separates the two camps has to do with the political feasibility of inducing physicians to participate voluntarily in any serious cost-cutting program. Those favoring regulation assume that physicians will refuse voluntary participation, thus forcing the government to impose mandatory controls, while those favoring competition assume that doctors will adopt the competitive approach once they become convinced that the only other alternative left to them is mandatory control.

The question of political feasibility is extremely complex and interesting in its own right but beyond the scope of this chapter. While limited strides have been taken to implement both approaches at state and federal levels, all efforts to establish a full-scale national policy embodying either regulation or competition have failed. Unfortunately, the reasons for the apparent failure of the regulatory process do not yield themselves to traditional empirical research in any obvious ways and thus no obvious answers to the problem can be suggested.

On the other hand, the question of whether or not regulation or competition can succeed in economic terms—that is, whether regulation or competition, once implemented, can reduce costs and improve efficiency—is, at least in principle, subject to empirical investigation. A review of some of the existing empirical evidence on this crucial question of economic efficacy follows.

THE REGULATORY APPROACH

Evidence on three kinds of regulatory programs is analyzed: certificate of need (CON), professional standards review organizations (PSRO), and rate review. While all three programs are targeted at the hospital sector (which consumes the largest share of the medical care dollar), it is presumed that the results can be generalized to other sectors of the medical market as well.

Certificate of Need

CON legislation is designed to control hospital capital expansion. The assumption underlying this approach is that capital expansion pushes up costs, especially because of what is referred to as "Roemer's Law," which hypothesizes that "a built bed is a filled bed" (Roemer & Shain, 1959). CON legislation seeks to control the number and distribution of hospital beds, as well as major capital equipment purchases, in a community.

Federal support for CON was provided with the passage of the National Health Planning and Resources Development Act of 1974 (P.L. 93-641), which created a national network of health systems agencies (HSAs) to administer the program at the local level. By February 1980, all but three states had enacted CON laws.

Additional measures to regulate hospital capital expansion include Section 1122 of P.L. 92-603 (The Social Security Act Amendments of 1972), which gave regulators the authority to withhold federal reimbursement (such as Medicare and Medicaid funds) from hospitals violating established capital expansion limits. Various Blue Cross and Blue Shield programs also have sought to exercise the same kind of leverage with their powers of reimbursement.

Empirical research on the effectiveness of capital expansion regulation has generated surprisingly consistent results. Whether measured on a per capita, per case, or per diem basis, CON programs have not been successful in holding down hospital costs. In a seminal study done in 1974 and published in 1976, Salkever and Bice discovered that when constrained by a CON ruling from increasing the number of beds, hospitals tended instead to increase investment in other forms of capital so that the capital-to-bed ratio increased substantially and no net reduction in costs was observed (Salkever & Bice, 1976). Similar findings were reported by Steinwald and Sloan (1981) and by Coelen and Sullivan (1980).

It is worth noting that a number of studies of CON effectiveness detected an increase in hospital investment with the advent of this legislation. Various explanations have been offered for this rather unsettling finding, including

- the possibility of an ''anticipatory response'' by hospitals (Steinwald & Sloan, 1981),
- the relative ''immaturity'' of regulatory bodies in their initial phase of operation (Steinwald & Sloan, 1981), and, perhaps most interesting,
- the possibility that under certain circumstances hospitals may actively seek CON regulation as a means to create barriers to market entry by potential competitors, thus creating a pseudomonopoly environment for themselves (enabling them to raise prices above the competitive equilibrium level.)

Evidence supporting this third explanation is reported by Wendling and Werner (1980).

Utilization and Quality Review (PSROs)

Utilization and quality review, in contrast to other regulatory efforts, directly involve physicians. As a self-policing mechanism designed to ascertain the necessity of prescribed care, utilization review has been pursued by numerous hospitals for many years. In the mid-1960s, utilization review was made mandatory for hospitals seeking Medicare and Medicaid reimbursement, and in 1972 this policy was supplanted by the establishment, under P.L. 92-603, of PSROs. It was the responsibility of PSROs, which ranged in size from small local groups to large statewide organizations, to provide for local review of the quality and appropriateness of hospital care.

Much of the research on PSROs and traditional utilization review programs has taken the form of case studies, which tend to preclude straightforward generalization of the results. Nevertheless, some of the findings are instructive. For example, a study of New Mexico's Experimental Medical Care Review Organization (a precursor to PSRO) suggested the program had no impact on hospital days, admissions, or length of stay (Brook, Williams, & Rolfe, 1978). Similar findings were reported by Gertman, Monheit, Anderson, Engle, and Levenson (1979) and by Coelen and Sullivan (1980) in studies of the Medicare population.

The most comprehensive evaluation of PSROs has been carried out by the Health Care Financing Administration (HCFA, 1980). The HCFA study used multivariate analysis (a statistical procedure used to study hospital utilization as a fraction of multiple patient, hospital program factors) to compare hospital utilization by Medicare patients in 108 areas with PSROs to 81 areas without PSROs. No statistically significant differences in utilization were found. It also reported that when the results were disaggregated by region, statistically significant differences among regions were found. Negative effects were strongest in the East and West, positive effects in the South. Further research will be required to explain these rather intriguing regional differences.

Rate Review

While CON and PSRO are relatively well-defined programs, specifically mandated by federal law and more or less homogeneous from location to location, rate review is a generic designation embracing a highly diverse array of rate-setting and revenue negotiation programs imposed on hospitals by all levels of government.

A common feature that distinguishes most rate review programs from other regulatory measures is the use of prospective reimbursement. That is, instead of billing third party payers after the services have been provided—the method used under traditional retrospective reimbursement—the hospital receives a fixed payment in advance, or prospectively. Two other rate review programs that did not incorporate prospective reimbursement were President Nixon's Economic Stabilization Program (ESP), which ran from 1971 to 1974, and the hospital industry's own Voluntary Effort (VE), which began in 1977.

Prospective Reimbursement

The essence of the prospective reimbursement (PR) is that it shifts the responsibility for absorbing costs from the third party payer to the hospital. In principle, hospitals that overrun their prospective reimbursement must sustain the loss, while those underspending their reimbursement are permitted to keep some fraction of the cost saving. Actual reimbursement levels may be established by formula, by negotiation or, as is increasingly the case, by a combination of the two. PR is used most commonly by state governments, although a number of individual insurers such as Blue Cross have adopted it as well. Consequently, there is variation across programs regarding which reimbursements are involved.

The empirical literature evaluating the effectiveness of PR is more comprehensive and methodologically more sophisticated than that on CON and PSRO. Biles, Schramm, and Atkinson (1980) found from descriptive evidence that, for 1977 and 1978, expenses per admission and per patient day were several percentage points lower in states that used mandatory PR than in those that did not. More rigorous multivariate analyses by Sloan (1981), by Coelen and Sullivan (1980), by Steinwald and Sloan (1981), and by the Congressional Budget Office (1979) confirmed these findings. The Sloan (1981) study, which controlled for program age, is of special interest. The estimates indicated that older programs, those that had been in existence longer, reduced costs by 7 to 20 percent while younger ones had no impact at all. This may help to account for the absence of significant impact reported by some of the early studies of PR effectiveness.

Economic Stabilization Program

The ESP part of President Nixon's wage and price controls pertained to hospitals. Under the ESP, annual growth of hospital revenues was limited to 6 percent and all wage and price increases required special justification.

Research findings on the effects of ESP are similar to those described for PR programs (Ginsberg, 1978). Because the ESP was part of a unique program covering the entire economy and hence an unlikely candidate for medical care cost control per se, these findings are not reviewed here.

Voluntary Effort

The VE was the hospital industry's counterproposal to the mandatory cap on hospital cost inflation proposed by the Carter Administration. Administered by 50 state-level committees charged with monitoring each individual hospital's performance, VE's objective was to reduce costs by some specified amount each year.

Little evidence regarding its effectiveness is available. A multivariable analysis by the Congressional Budget Office indicated a statistically insignificant saving of approximately 1 percent (Steinwald & Sloan, 1981; Sloan, 1981). On the other hand, a significant negative impact per adjusted admission and a positive impact on hospital profits were reported, a somewhat surprising but perhaps encouraging result.

THE COMPETITIVE APPROACH

Advocates of competition point to what they consider the disappointing results of regulation as evidence that a new solution is needed. In their view, such a solution must meet certain criteria, two of which are:

1. Consumers must be induced to make cost-effective choices of health insurance plans and services.
2. Providers must be induced to deliver care more efficiently. Efficient providers should be able to attract patients to their practice from inefficient providers and thus increase their incomes.

Enthoven (1980) suggested that one way to meet the first criterion might be to provide consumers with fixed dollar employer or government contributions to their medical insurance and at the same time to offer options from which they could choose. To meet the second criterion, he proposed that reorganized systems of care be formed that would not be dependent on the traditional fee-for-service mode of payment—in other words, that ADSs be widely adopted as a central feature of the medical care markets.

It is perhaps worth repeating at this point that ADSs are not inconsistent with either the regulatory or competitive approaches. Advocates from both camps favor these alternative systems as a means of producing medical care more efficiently at the individual practice level.

Nevertheless, it is clear that while ADSs are not inconsistent with the regulatory scenario, they are absolutely critical to the competitive plan.

Thus, in attempting to evaluate the prospects for a national cost containment policy predicated on competition, evidence on ADSs' effectiveness in containing costs must be reviewed.

Cost Trends under Alternative Systems

On the face of it, the evidence on whether or not ADSs contain costs is unambiguous: they do, particularly those that follow the pure prepaid group model, such as HMOs. Based on an extensive analysis of the empirical literature on this question, Luft (1978) concluded that total per capita costs were some 10 percent to 40 percent lower for prepaid group enrollees than for patients of traditional fee-for-service practices.

Unfortunately, this answer alone satisfies almost nobody. If costs are indeed reduced by such a substantial amount, then the critical question becomes: how? Or, to put it perhaps even more bluntly: at whose expense do these savings occur? Are providers taking a loss by being forced to produce more efficiently, and if so, which providers? Or are consumers being short-changed with lower quality care? Answers to these and a number of related questions are considerably less clear-cut, yet ultimately they are equally important to the case for competition-based cost containment as the simple finding that ADSs do save money.

Economies of Scale

One way that an ADS might reduce total costs would be to reduce costs per unit, or, put differently, to improve its efficiency in production. To do this, the ADS could avail itself of potential "economies of scale," by either purchasing inputs more cheaply or combining them more efficiently than do competing fee-for-service practices (Luft, 1980).

In an attempt to ascertain whether ADSs actually did achieve their savings in this way, Luft analyzed data from the Federal Employees Health Benefits Plan and the California State Employees Health Insurance Plan, where beneficiaries were given the option of enrolling in a commercial fee-for-service plan, Blue Cross and Blue Shield, or in an HMO (Luft, 1978). Based on a comparison of the premium growth trends for each of the packages offered, Luft concluded that the cost savings to HMO enrollees were not attributable to lower per-unit costs.

Because total expenditures are the product of per-unit costs times the number of units produced, Luft's conclusion that ADSs did not reduce per-unit costs implied that they must produce fewer units of care than their fee-for-service counterparts. But did they reduce hospital or ambulatory care services, or some combination of the two?

Hospital Utilization

Hospital utilization can be reduced by limiting average length of stay, number of admissions, or both. Gaus, Cooper, and Hirschman, in comparing hospital utilization by 8,000 Medicaid beneficiaries enrolled in HMOs, IPAs, or the standard Medicaid plan, found that the HMO enrollees reported half as many patient days (where patient days = admissions × length of stay) as those enrolled in the standard Medicaid plan (Gaus et al., 1976). (While the Medicaid population is atypical of the United States as a whole, there is no obvious reason to suspect that the relative utilization differences between the HMO and standard plan enrollees cannot be generalized.)

The findings by Gaus et al. for IPA hospital utilization were not as unequivocal. One explanation suggested by Egdahl et al. (1977) and Broida, Lerner, Lohrenz, and Wentzel (1975) was that because IPA physicians often continued to see a large number of fee-for-service patients along with their IPA subscribers, their incentives to improve their operating efficiency—including the use of costly hospital care—were more muted than under pure prepaid group conditions. A second explanation might simply be that since IPA physicians were reimbursed on a fee-for-service basis, they perceived less of an incentive to reduce costs, especially in the short run.

Egdahl et al., in the most definitive work to date on IPA hospitalization rates, reported on three case studies: Employer's Insurance of Wausau (Wisconsin), the San Joaquin (California) Foundation for Medical Care, and the Physician's Association of Clackamas County (Oregon).

The Wausau study reported that the first enrollees permitted to join that plan were employees of Employer's Insurance of Wausau, a group that previously had been covered by an indemnity plan underwritten by the employer. Thus, the investigators had access to hospitalization data for these employees before and after they joined the Wausau plan. The enrollees thus served as their own control group, thereby eliminating the common problem of self selection bias. (Self-selection bias might arise if those who enrolled in the prepaid plan generally were in better health than those in the fee-for-service control plan.) The Wausau data indicated that after one year in the plan, hospital days dropped by 68 percent and that this drop resulted almost entirely from a decrease in average length of stay (from 7.4 to 4.5 days) rather than to reduced admission rates. This decrease persisted when membership in the plan was opened to the community at large.

Similar findings for the San Joaquin and Clackamas County Programs suggested that under certain circumstances IPAs could reduce hospital utilization to the same extent as could HMOs.

Data on hospital utilization by PCNs are extremely difficult to come by because they represent a relatively new form of organization. One study that is available, by Moore (1979), compared hospitalization rates for United Health Care (a PCN) in Seattle, Washington, with those for the

Group Health Cooperative of Puget Sound (an HMO) and for Blue Cross-Blue Shield of Washington State. It found that the PCN outperformed both the HMO (by 17 percent) and Blue Cross-Blue Shield (by 59 percent), again strictly by reducing average length of stay (in fact, the admissions rate was somewhat higher for United Health Care than for the other plans). [However, these results must be viewed with some caution; since this text was written, United Health Care has gone out of business. Final evaluation of these results should await further understanding of United Health Care's lack of success.]

In summary, the available evidence, as represented here, suggested that ADSs did reduce hospital utilization rather substantially, especially by shortening the average length of stay. HMOs in general appeared to be slightly more successful in this than IPAs but it was too early to generalize about the effectiveness of PCNs.

Ambulatory Care Utilization

Given that ADSs reduce hospital utilization, two opposing hypotheses regarding their use of ambulatory care suggest themselves. Either ambulatory care is a substitute for hospital service, in which case it should rise as hospital care is reduced, or it is a complement to hospital use (for example, if it is used for follow-up treatment after hospitalization), in which case it should fall as hospital care is reduced.

The evidence, unfortunately, is ambiguous. Luft (1978), in his comprehensive review, found that in 18 out of 26 cases, ambulatory care utilization was lower under an ADS than under fee-for-service plans, with eight cases (including the five IPAs in the sample) pointing the other way. Similar research for PCNs has, thus far, not been conducted.

Self-Selection

The problem of self-selection, already mentioned in connection with the Wausau IPA study, is central to almost all comparative research on the efficacy of ADSs and therefore merits further discussion. Simply stated, the question in dealing with self-selection is this: are individuals who enroll in an ADS systematically sicker or healthier than those who do not?

Either possibility appears plausible. On the one hand, an ADS might actively seek to enroll healthier populations in order to keep costs low and maintain a competitive edge. This sometimes is referred to as "cream-skimming." On the other hand, sicker individuals might be attracted to the ADS by the more comprehensive coverage offered.

The severe complexity of the problem of skewed enrollee populations has been noted by Rossiter and Freund (1982) and by Luft (1981). Data describing the actual health status of individuals as well as their attitudes toward their health at the time of enrollment are almost nonexistent (the Wausau data are a partial exception and are valued accordingly). Instead, a measure of actual utilization following enrollment in the plan is used as a proxy for health status at the time of entry under the assumption that actual health status and utilization are highly correlated. Using such proxy data, a test is made to determine the direction and strength of the relationship between ADS enrollment and high utilization. A statistically significant positive relationship would suggest adverse selection while negative relationships would suggest cream-skimming.

An obvious problem with this proxy variable approach is, of course, that providers may influence utilization in the plan—the very assumption on which the entire ADS approach is predicated. Thus, the use of utilization data as a proxy for initial health status ought to introduce substantial bias into the results.

Taking this bias directly into account, Rossiter and Freund compared federal employees who selected high option Group Health (an HMO) with those who chose high option Blue Cross-Blue Shield and found, in line with the work of others, no evidence of adverse selection into the HMO. By isolating the high option enrollees, the investigators presumably identified populations with roughly similar initial health status and attitudes toward health.

It should be noted, however, that the self-selection issue was by no means resolved. A study by Eggers (1980) on the enrollment of Medicare beneficiaries in the Group Health Cooperative of Puget Sound (an HMO) came to the conclusion that HMOs do cream-skim.

Future of Personal Health Financing

This review has looked briefly at some of the history of contemporary health care financing, some of the problems that have emerged, and some of the solutions that have been offered in response at both the micro- and macrolevels. The one overriding point that should be abundantly clear is that the future of health care financing remains essentially unresolved.

While the most recent data available indicate no reversal whatsoever in the growth of the medical share of GNP, it is inevitable that at some point the tide must turn, or at the very least be halted. Where that turning point will come and how the brakes will be applied remains, for the moment, the great mystery that bedevils health policy makers, providers, and consumers alike.

There is a growing body of experience and evidence on alternative methods of restraining costs but, by and large, the evidence raises as many questions as it answers. Not only are there many detailed questions about the specific costs and benefits of particular financing arrangements and to whom those costs and benefits accrue but also there are broader questions—perhaps more in keeping with political philosophy than with the economic approach that has been pursued here—regarding the failure of any of these strategies to gain a broad national constituency, questions that may lead ultimately to a reevaluation of the true role of medical care in the American economy and culture.

As to the more immediate question of how to contain costs as painlessly and expeditiously as possible, it appears that while regulatory approaches by no means have been uniformly impressive, some forward strides have been made under prospective reimbursement. Meanwhile, HMOs and other types of ADSs also appear to be successful in reducing per-unit costs. However, it is unlikely that either approach can succeed ultimately unless major additional policy steps are taken to restructure the health care delivery system.

If prospective reimbursement is truly to succeed, either each of the 50 states individually would have to adopt a rigorous program like that of New York or Maryland or the federal government must assume full regulatory responsibility. Each of these programs entails setting reimbursement rates by a predefined formula. Since the formula is objective, and the rates are actually set by a quasi governmental body rather than through negotiation with individual hospitals, the system is less likely to be manipulated. In addition, these states are traditionally very stringent on which costs are deemed allowable and hence will be reimbursed. A hotly debated proposal advanced by the Reagan Administration for a federal takeover of Medicaid shortly before this writing and recently passed Congressional legislation mandating prospective reimbursement for the Medicare program may make substantial inroads into the second approach. At the state level, it has been the unbridled increase in Medicaid expenses that has driven several states, constitutionally prohibited from having a deficit, to impose mandatory prospective reimbursement.

For competition to succeed on a large scale will require major reforms. The individual consumer must be given a fixed dollar subsidy and a multiple choice among health plans, yet multiple choice has been offered only rarely and certain Congressional proposals to cap tax write-offs for health insurance premiums (for example, the Gephardt and Durenberger proposals) have thus far met with fierce resistance from business and labor as well as from the medical lobby.

Thus, the system seems for the moment to have reached an impasse of sorts. It is doubtful whether simply gathering more information about how regulatory or competitive programs operate will, by itself, be sufficient to pull the system out of this impasse—there do not appear to be any "silver bullets" waiting to be discovered. Rather, the impasse is more likely to break under the cumulative impact of continued massive cost increases.

It is at that point, when the need to respond finally becomes unavoidable and the policy establishment is forced to take major steps, that all the research findings, painstakingly collected over many years, will become of vital importance in establishing viable new methods of personal health services financing.

REFERENCES

Biles, B., Schramm, C.J., Atkinson, J.G. Hospital cost inflation under state role-setting programs. *The New England Journal of Medicine,* September 1980, *303*(12), 664–668.

Broida, J., Lerner, M., Lohrenz, F., & Wenzel, F. The impact of HMO membership in an enrolled prepaid population on utilization of health services in a group practice. *The New England Journal of Medicine,* April 10, 1975, *295*(15), 780–783.

Brook, R.H., Williams, K., & Rolfe, J.E. Controlling the use and cost of medical services: The New Mexico experimental medical care review organization—A four-year case study. *Medical Care,* September 1978, *16*(9) (Supplement).

Coelen, C., & Sullivan, D. *An analysis of prospective reimbursement programs on hospital cost.* Abt Associates, 1980. (Mimeographed)

Congressional Budget Office. *Controlling rising hospital costs.* Washington, D.C.: Government Printing Office, 1979.

Egdahl, R.H., Taff, C.H., Friedland, J., & Linde, K. The potential of organization of fee-for-service physicians for achieving significant decreases in hospitalization, *Annals of Surgery,* September 1977, *186*(3), 388–399.

Eggers, P. Risk differential between Medicare beneficiaries enrolled and not enrolled in an HMO. *Health Care Financing Review,* Winter 1980, 4, 91–99.

Elwood, P. Health maintenance organizations: Concept and strategy. *Hospitals,* March 16, 1971, *45*(6), p. 53.

Enthoven, A.C. *Health plan: The only practical solution to the soaring cost of medical care.* Reading, Mass.: Addison-Wesley Publishing Company, Inc., 1980.

Federation of American hospitals review, July/August 1982, *15*(6), p. 12.

Gaus, C., Cooper, B., & Hirschman, F. Contrasts in HMO and fee-for-service performance. *Social Security Bulletin,* May 1976, *39*(5), 3–14.

Gertman, P.M., Monheit, A.C., Anderson, J.J., Engle, J.B., & Levenson, D.K. Utilization review in the United States: Results from a 1976–77 national survey of hospitals. *Medical Care,* August 1979, *17*(8) (Supplement).

Gibbons v. Ogden. Reports of cases argued and adjudged by the Supreme Court of the United States (Wheaton). 9:1-222 (February term, 1824), p. 203.

Gibson, R.M. National health expenditures, 1980. *Health Care Financing Review,* September 1981, 3, 18–19.

Health Care Financing Administration. *The medicare and medicaid data book.* Washington, D.C.: The Department of Health and Human Services, 1982, p. 4.

Health Care Financing Administration. *Professional standards review organization: Program evaluation.* Washington, D.C.: Department of Health and Human Services, 1980.

Helvering v. Davis, Commissioner of Internal Revenue. United States Reports. 301:619–646 (May 24, 1937).

Jonas, S. *Health care delivery in the United States.* New York: Springer Publishing Co., 1977.

Kessel, R. Price discrimination in medicine. *The Journal of Law and Economics,* October 1958.

Louisiana and Texas Railroad and Steamship Company v. Board of Health of the State of Louisiana and the State of Louisiana. U.S. Supreme Court Reports (Lawyers' Edition) 30: 237–243 (May, 1886).

Luft, H. How do health maintenance organizations achieve their savings? Rhetoric and evidence. *The New England Journal of Medicine,* June 15, 1978, *298*(24), 1336–1343.

Luft, H. Trends in medical care costs: Do HMOs lower the rate of growth? *Medical Care,* 1980, *18*(January 1), 1–16.

Luft, H. *Health maintenance organizations: Dimensions of performance.* New York: Wiley and Sons, 1981.

Moore, S. Cost containment through risk sharing by primary-care physicians. *The New England Journal of Medicine,* June 14, 1979, *300*(24), 1359–1362.

National Chamber Foundation. *A national health care strategy: How business can stimulate a competitive health care system.* Washington, D.C.: National Chamber Foundation, 1978.

National HMO Census. (Department of Health and Human Services, Washington, D.C.: Publication No. DHHS 80-50159, Office of Health Maintenance Organizations). U.S. Government Printing Office, June 30, 1980, p. 1.

Pauly, M. Economics of moral hazard. *The American Economic Review,* June 1968.

Roemer, M., & Shain, M. *Hospital utilization under insurance.* Chicago, American Hospital Association, 1959.

Romani, J. Public health: Notes on the state of our union. *American Journal of Public Health,* March 1980, pp. 260–263.

Rossiter, L., & Freund, D.A. *Adverse selection in the market for health insurance: A simultaneous logit approach.* Mimeographed.

Salkever, D.S., & Bice, T. The impact of certificate of need controls on hospital investment. *Milbank Memorial Fund Quarterly/Health and Society,* Spring, 1976, *54*(1), pp. 185–214.

Shattuck, Lemuel, et al. *Report of the sanitary commission of Massachusetts* (Boston: Dutton & Wentworth State Printers, 1850). (Reprinted in 1948 by Harvard University Press, Cambridge, Mass.)

Sloan, F.A. Regulation and the rising cost of hospital care. *Review of Economics and Statistics,* November 1981, *23*(4), 479–487.

Sloan, F.A., & Steinwald, B. *Insurance regulation and hospital costs.* Lexington, Mass.: D.C. Heath and Company, 1980.

Steinwald, B., & Sloan, F.A. Regulatory approaches to hospital cost containment: A synthesis of the empirical evidence. In M. Olson (Ed.), *A new approach to the economics of health care.* Washington, D.C.: American Enterprise Institute, 1981, 273–307.

Stewart Machine Co. v. Davis, Collector of Internal Revenue. United States Reports. 301:618 (May 24, 1937).

U.S. Congress. *American act for the promotion of the welfare and hygiene of maternity and infancy and for other purposes.* P.L. 67-97. Sixty-seventh Congress. 1st Sess. Pub. Stat. at Large. 42(1):224–226 (November 23, 1921).

U.S. Congress. American act to extend and improve coverage under the federal old-age, survivors and disability insurance system. . . to provide grants to the states for medical care for aged individuals of low income. . . . P.L. 86-778. Eighty-sixth Congress. 2nd Sess. Pub. Stat. at Large. 74:924-997 (September 13, 1960).

U.S. Congress. *American act to prevent the introduction of infectious or contagious diseases into the United States, and to establish a national board of health.* Forty-fifth Congress. 3rd Session. Pub. Stat. at Large. 20:484–485 (March 3, 1879).

U.S. Congress, House. *H.R. 6575, Transitional system of hospital cost containment.* 95th Congress. (April 25, 1977).

U.S. Congress, House. *H.R. 9717, Transitional system of hospital cost containment.* 95th Congress. (October 21, 1977).

Wendling, W., & Werner, J. Nonprofit firms and the economic theory of regulation. *Quarterly Review of Economics and Business,* Fall 1980, *20*(3), 6–18.

Chapter 3

Assuring the Quality of Health Care: Policy Perspectives

William F. Jessee

The decades of the 1960s and 1970s saw a major reawakening of public and professional interest in the quality of health care services. The increasing complexity of medical technology, growing pressures from the legal system, and increasing concerns for the costs of health care generated an unparalleled interest in approaches to evaluating and improving the quality of the services being provided. Despite this flurry of interest, quality assurance in health care has historical roots that may be traced back as far as 2000 B.C. and that provide an important basis for understanding the current public policy focus on this issue.

The *Code of Laws,* produced around 1700 B.C. by Hammurabai in Mesopotamia, contains what are perhaps the earliest references to sanctions for poor quality. The *Code* stipulates,

> If a physician performed a major operation on a nobleman with a bronzed lancet and has caused the nobleman's death, or he opened the eyesocket of a nobleman and has destroyed the nobleman's eye, they shall cut off his hand.

These rather severe penalties were substantially reduced, however, if the patient was of lower social rank. In such cases, the physician was required to make good, slave for slave, for a death, or to pay one-half the value of the slave in silver if an eye were destroyed.

Many centuries later, Florence Nightingale (1820–1910) developed a quality assessment mechanism that she used for evaluating the outcomes of care provided to British soldiers during the Crimean War. To demonstrate the poor quality of care and lack of sanitation in British Army field hospitals, she collected statistics of disease-specific case fatality ratios, demonstrating conclusively that more soldiers were dying of pneumonia,

65

dysentery, and other infectious diseases than as casualties of the war itself. This resulted in profound changes in British public policy toward health services for the military and stands as an early example of the relationship between evaluation of health care outcomes and public policy response.

In the United States, the roots of organized quality assurance activity may be traced to the early 1900s with the beginning of an effort by the Clinical Congress of Surgeons of North America to develop a system for nationwide evaluation of hospitals, along the lines of Abraham Flexner's famous study of medical education (Flexner, 1910). The surgeons proposed that hospitals be judged individually according to objective measurement of their performance, based on a systematic analysis of individual cases treated (Wetherill, 1915). A Boston surgeon, E.A. Codman, was instrumental in influencing the Clinical Congress of Surgeons to implement his method of "end results analysis" in its evaluation of hospitals (Committee on Standardization of Hospitals, 1914).

In a now-classic monograph, Codman described his approach to evaluating the outcomes of surgical care and published an abstract of every case treated in his hospital during the years 1912–1916 (Codman, 1916). For each case, he classified the results as favorable or unfavorable and assigned responsibility for the latter to errors in diagnostic or technical ability, poor surgical judgment, inadequate care or equipment, the natural history of the disease, or the patient's refusal of treatment. His system required at least one evaluation of the case a year or more following hospitalization, until a condition of stability permitting a final judgment had been reached. Prophetically, Codman pointed out that the analyses he made himself of cases cared for in his hospital

> cannot carry the weight they would if the Trustees of an Endowed Hospital had had them audited as they do financial accounts. . . . they . . . rely on what the staff is said to be able to do, not what it actually does do, to the patients.

The strength of Codman's argument that hospitals should be evaluated on the basis of the results they produced for patients gained a considerable degree of acceptance from leading surgeons at the time.

The entrance of the United States into World War I temporarily interrupted the process of hospital standardization and Codman appears to have given up his "end results" technique to return to the Massachusetts General Hospital following service in the war. The American College of Surgeons (ACS) in 1918 assumed responsibility for conducting a survey of hospitals to determine the adequacy of their performance in patient care

(Bowman, 1920). It is apparent from information that has survived that the College intended to use objective criteria to evaluate the outcomes of care provided in the institutions surveyed (Bowman).

However, neither the criteria employed nor the survey findings ever were published nor are they preserved in the files of the ACS. It is known that of 692 hospitals of 100 beds or more, only 89 apparently met the ACS standards (American College of Surgeons, 1946). It has been stated that the facts elicited by the first survey were so shocking that the ACS, at its annual meeting in 1919, ordered the reports on each individual institution destroyed (Lembke, 1967). This decision was based on the rationale that the public interest would be better served by not publishing the findings until the individual hospitals had had an opportunity to review the results and make efforts to improve their performance.

Subsequently, the ACS began to conduct hospital surveys that relied not on the outcomes of care provided but rather on structural measures of quality such as the adequacy of the physical plant, the qualifications of the medical staff and nursing personnel, the completeness of medical records, and the facilities for radiologic and laboratory diagnosis (American College of Surgeons, 1946). It was not until the 1970s that the profession began to move away from strict reliance on structural quality control measures and turned instead toward a reexamination of process and outcome assessment as a mechanism for assuring the public that the services provided in health care institutions were, indeed, of acceptable quality.

This chapter develops a definition of quality in health care services and examines alternative approaches to achieving that end. Subsequently, individual structure, process, and outcome-oriented public policies aimed at controlling the quality of health services are examined. Finally, suggestions are offered for the future direction of public policies designed to assure the quality of health services.

QUALITY OF CARE DEFINED

One of the great stumbling blocks that has faced programs designed to evaluate and improve the quality of services has been the difficulty in arriving at a generally acceptable definition of quality of health care. The concept that ''quality is in the eye of the beholder'' has been pervasive throughout the health care industry and often has been used by practitioners as a response to the question of why quality assurance programs have not been implemented.

Brook and Williams (1975) defined quality symbolically as follows:

$$Q = T + A + (T)(A) + \epsilon$$
where Q = quality of health care;
T = technical care;
A = art of care; and,
ϵ = a random error factor.

As expressed by this equation, the quality of care includes not only aspects of the technical practice but also the human psychosocial aspects (the art of care) as well as the interaction between the two. Finally, the error factor is important in the Brook and Williams definition as a means of noting that some outcomes of health care, to at least some degree, may be determined by random chance.

One of the most extensive attempts to evaluate and define the concept of quality of health care was a book by Donabedian (1980). He explored numerous findings from research on health care quality as well as discourses on the philosophy of health services in an attempt to arrive at a unifying model. It is interesting to note that Donabedian's extensive conceptual framework incorporated the concepts of benefits, risk, and volume of services provided as essential components of any prescription for quality. He also explored such factors as client and provider satisfaction.

An earlier work by the present author (Jessee, 1979) presented the thesis that quality of care in hospitals could be defined operationally by the objectives of an integrated quality assurance system. Three discrete but interrelated objectives can be postulated; when considered together, they constitute an operational definition of quality:

1. optimal achievable benefits of health care for each patient, within the biologic constraints imposed by the person's illness, age, or underlying chronic diseases and within the limitations imposed by the individual's own choices in complying with health care recommendations
2. the minimal expenditure of resources necessary to achieve these benefits
3. the avoidance of injury or additional disability resulting from the provision of health care services

This definition, like the more extensive work by Donabedian (1980), incorporates the elements of benefits, volume of services, and risks, and attempts to unify these three elements.

Much of the substantial literature of the 1960s and 1970s focused on the first element of this definition (optimal achievable benefits). Unfortunately, less attention has been paid to the relationship between benefits and costs or risks, with the assumption often being made that cost and quality of services are positively and linearly related. Increasing evidence, however, suggests that this may not be the case (McLamb & Huntley, 1967; Steel, Gertman, Crescenzi, & Anderson, 1981).

Figure 3-1 presents the hypothetical relationship between benefits of health care, cost of services, and patient risk. The contemporary literature suggests that, as a nation, the United States may well be approaching the flat portion of the curve in which further increases in the volume of services or costs of care will produce only marginal benefits and may, when increased risk is taken into account, actually reduce benefits to the patient.

For instance, three studies of the risk of iatrogenic illness in patients treated in hospitals have used very similar methodologies to identify the incidence of unexpected outcomes of hospitalization. The earliest of these (Schimmel, 1964) found a reported incidence of 20 percent in 1964. Three years later, a similar study in another hospital reported almost identical findings (McLamb & Huntley, 1967).

A 1981 study (Steel, Gertman, Crescenzi, & Anderson) reported that 36 percent of all patients on the general medical service of a university hospital suffered injury as a result of treatment; that this injury was life threatening in 9 percent of the patients; and that the injury contributed to death in 2 percent of those studied. This apparent increasing trend in the frequency of patient injury may well be a reflection of the progress in medical technology between 1964 and 1981. If so, a fourth factor might be added to the abscissa of the diagrams in Figure 3-1 showing technologic sophistication and the increasing risk attendant to that sophistication. As the capacity of modern medicine to provide increasingly advanced technologies to patients, with their attendant benefits, has increased, so has the risk associated with the application of those technologies. The magnitude of these risks, their relation to potential benefits, and the exact shape of these hypothetical curves remain central issues for future research to guide the formulation of appropriate public policy toward new technology.

Although an issue of considerable concern in formulating public policy to assure quality of services, the definition of quality has not received widespread attention in the professional literature other than in the works of Donabedian and Brook. The operational definition offered earlier (optimal benefits, minimal expenditure, at minimal risk) is appealing both professionally and intellectually but might provoke controversy in the health professions, particularly surrounding the inclusion of an emphasis on containing resource expenditures or costs. If this operational definition is accepted, however, it then becomes possible to construct a conceptual

Figure 3-1 Hypothetical Relationship between Benefits, Risks, and Volume (or Cost) of Health Services

(After Donabedian, 1980)

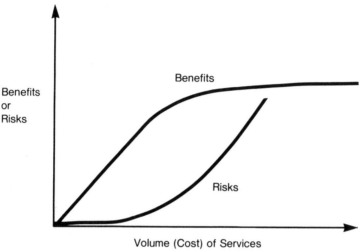

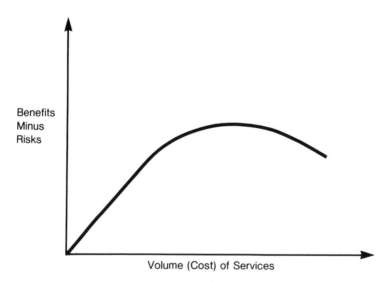

Source: Author. Adapted from *The Definition of Quality and Approaches to Its Assessment* in *Explorations In quality assessment and monitoring* (Vol. I) by A. Donabedian, by permission of Health Administration Press, © 1980.

framework within which public policy may be formulated for the development of systems designed to assure the quality of health services in a variety of settings.

TOWARD A QUALITY ASSURANCE SYSTEM

A substantial body of literature during the early 1970s described alternative procedures for assessment of the quality of health services. However, it is only since the middle of that decade that substantial attention has been devoted to the development of systems for quality assurance. It is important to emphasize that "assessment" and "assurance" are not synonymous; the latter term, when applied in medical care review programs, implies actions to eliminate substandard performance and to improve the efficacy or efficiency of the system for providing services (Jessee, 1977a).

FUNCTIONS SUBSYSTEMS

To be effective, any system for quality assurance must perform three interdependent functions: (1) monitoring of care, (2) assessment of problems, and (3) improvement of services. When all three components are in place they form a cybernetic system (Figure 3-2). Until about 1980, most quality assurance activities focused on the assessment component of the system, with substantially less attention to monitoring and improvement. Underdevelopment of these components markedly reduced the effectiveness of quality control activities, resulting in gradual evolution toward the current concept of a systems approach. Consideration of each of these assurance functions is an essential prerequisite to the development of effective quality control activities in health care programs.

Monitoring of Care

Monitoring is a continuing process for the evaluation of important measures of professional performance, effectiveness of resource utilization, and patient risk. Monitoring is intended to function as an early warning system that can immediately identify out-of-the-ordinary occurrences that represent potential failures in quality. Monitoring activities, however, do not define the causes of the adverse findings; that is the function of the second component of the system—in-depth assessment of potential problems.

Figure 3-2 Cybernetic Quality Assurance System

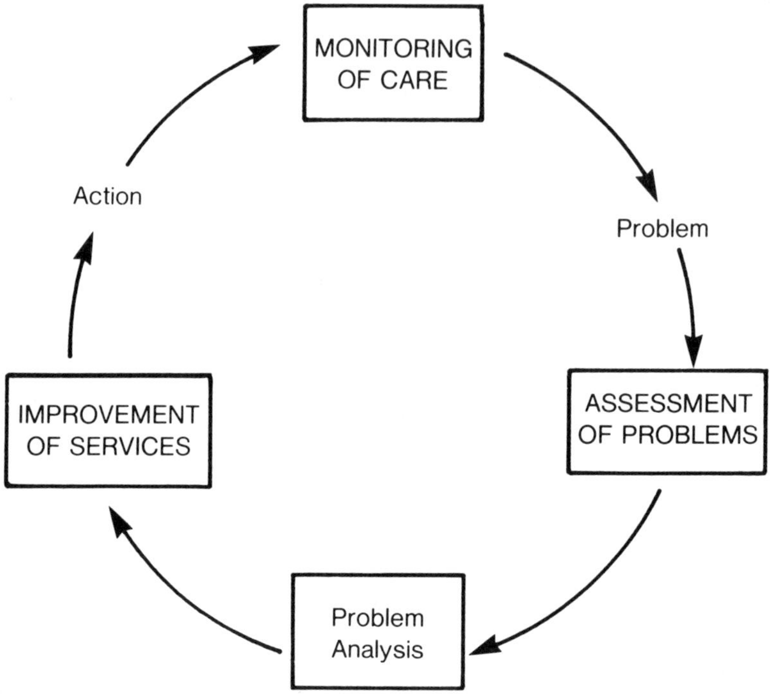

Monitoring in health care is analogous to the monitoring activities conducted in a modern aircraft. Just as the flight crew continuously evaluates
data coming from a variety of measuring systems to ensure that the
mechanical, hydraulic, and electrical functions of the aircraft are under
control, so, too, must the health care institution have a variety of measures
of aspects of quality that can be evaluated continuously to ensure that
diagnostic and therapeutic processes and outcomes are acceptable.

When the flight crew identifies an unusual value, it triggers an evaluation
of the situation to determine whether there is, indeed, a functional problem
or whether there is merely a false positive warning. Similarly, findings
from monitoring the quality of health services that indicate a potential
problem require that further in-depth evaluation (assessment) be conducted in order to validate the problem and determine its severity and
extent, or to ascertain whether the results merely represented a false
positive signal.

A variety of techniques may be used to identify potential problems in the quality of health services. These may be grouped into five generic categories (Jessee, 1982a):

1. *Variation from Norms:* This category requires that quantitative measures of the performance of health care delivery be available from which ''norms'' (i.e., usual or average performance) may be developed. Performance that varies markedly from a normative value then may be viewed as a potential problem in quality of care. A variety of health care data routinely collected by health care providers, fiscal intermediaries, and other health agencies can be used for the development of such norms. Typically, such data as length of stay, death rates, cost or charges, surgical rates, nosocomial infection rates, normal tissue rates, etc., are used to develop norms. Values that depart significantly from the mean, median, or mode then are defined as representative of potential problems requiring further assessment.

2. *Criteria-Based Screening:* A variety of other approaches are based on the concept that performance that varies from explicit written criteria requires careful peer review and analysis. Such criteria-referenced problem identification methods may utilize either process or outcome measures and usually employ data abstracted from patient records. These techniques focus on the establishment of criteria defining optimal levels of health care and then compare actual performance with those definitions. They differ from norm-referenced techniques primarily in that each individual case is considered by comparison with the criterion statement, rather than relying upon statistical descriptions of performance. However, the technique becomes very similar to the norm-referenced methods in that patterns of variation from criterion statements also should be considered in determining whether or not the variation represents a real problem or merely a false monitoring finding.

3. *Multifactorial Indexes:* Several investigators have developed ''indexes of the quality of care'' that combine elements of both criteria-based and normative approaches. These techniques require that a variety of aspects of provider performance be evaluated against explicit written criteria, that a quantitative compliance score be computed for each patient in the sample, and that statistical distributions of these scores then be developed for practitioners or institutional providers to determine which ones fall significantly above or below the mean. This combination of criteria-referenced and norm-referenced techniques into a multifactorial index holds substantial promise as a

more sophisticated technique for identifying true positive problems in the quality of care.

4. *Small Group Methods:* These techniques, in contrast to the others described, rely primarily on qualitative perceptions rather than on quantitative measures. They are intended to use providers' experience in identifying barriers to good quality patient services and in setting priorities for investigation and resolution of such potential problems.

5. *Survey Methods:* Surveys attempt to collect either a set of uniform information or critical incident data on individual problems from a large group of respondents. Surveys of patients, practitioners, and staff members have been used in a variety of settings to pinpoint potential quality problems. Again, like the small group methods just discussed, surveys depend on qualitative perceptions rather than quantitative measures of quality.

All of these methods are of value primarily in highlighting potential problems for further analysis. None provides an absolute measure for determining the quality of services. For that reason, none of them should be used independently of the judgment process required during the assessment phase, described next.

Assessment of Problems

Once a potential problem has been identified through any of these monitoring techniques, the next function in a systems approach is the in-depth evaluation, or assessment, of the potential problem. This step is designed to validate the existence of the problem; to identify its causes, extent, and severity; and to lead to recommendations for action to eliminate it. Before conducting such an assessment, it is important to define the objectives. They must be measurable, explicit, time limited, and related directly to the problem under study.

Once the objectives are stated, a method for collecting the data necessary to allow in-depth assessment of them must be selected. Many assessment methods are based on review of medical records. Four broad categories of assessment methodologies are:

1. *Document-Based Review:* This consists of in-depth assessment of either the processes or outcomes of care based upon information in written documents. Medical audit methods are the most familiar example of this category. Other forms of assessment using incident

reports, utilization review data, financial information, or other documents as the primary sources of information also are included.

2. *Direct Observation Studies:* No documentation is readily available to allow accurate assessment of the quality of services provided in many care processes. Under such circumstances, either direct human or electronic (videotape) observation of the care process may be necessary in order to assess the degree of compliance with established criteria. For instance, accurate evaluation of the quality of services during an event such as cardiopulmonary resuscitation is possible only through direct observation of that process.

3. *Interviews:* Interviews or direct discussion with practitioners or patients can provide information about the process or outcome of care and about the reasons for problems that may have been identified through other techniques. Such face-to-face discussion may provide information that cannot be obtained through any other approach.

4. *Experiments:* An experimental design may be the most appropriate approach to investigation for some selected problems. However, caution should be exercised since experimentation often involves ethical issues and may be substantially costlier than other simpler approaches to problem assessment.

Selection of the specific approach in assessing a particular problem must be individualized to that situation. For instance, document-based review may suffice to determine whether or not weights are being recorded on infants seen in the emergency room for a diagnosis of gastroenteritis. However, direct observation or interviews may be needed to determine why these weights are not being recorded, if that is the fact. As a general rule, the simplest, fastest, and least expensive method that can yield the needed information should be used. Ingenuity may well be required in the design of an assessment that is able to respond to the objectives that have been set from the review of the monitoring information.

Improvement of Services

The final function of a quality assurance system is the planning and implementation of changes in individual or organizational behavior so as to improve health care. Although quality assurance programs that do not lead to improvement are pointless, this component of a system is perhaps the least well developed in the health care industry. Coming to grips with concepts of individual or organizational change is critical to the success of any quality assurance program. Attention to identification and analysis of problems, without equal focus on their solution, is destined to produce frustration and to reduce the impact of the programs in any setting.

Approaches to improving both individual (Jessee, 1982b) and organizational (Jessee, 1981) behavior have been presented in detail elsewhere. In summary, success in improving care depends on knowledge of theories and methodologies for encouraging change in individual and organizational behavior. This is as critical to quality assurance as is an understanding of the technical concepts discussed earlier for monitoring and assessment of health care problems. By incorporating skills from the fields of organization development, planned change, adult learning, and the behavioral sciences into health care organizational management, quality assurance programs can strengthen their potential for success in improving services.

CONTENT SUBSYSTEMS

A systems approach to quality assurance also must include three content subsystems that conform to the operational definition of quality discussed earlier. Specifically, mechanisms for evaluation of professional performance, utilization of resources, and patient risk are essential.

Performance Evaluation

If, indeed, the results of patient encounters with the health care delivery system are influenced by the service processes provided, then evaluation of the performance of individual professionals is an essential component of an effective quality assurance program. Although the strength of the relationship between processes of care and their outcomes has been questioned (Brook & Appel, 1973), empirical evidence would dictate that evaluation of the performance of the various health services providers is an important tool for assuring that patients obtain optimal results in their encounters with the delivery system.

Although the physician's performance is of major concern, it must be kept in mind that health care delivery requires the coordinated efforts of a variety of professionals, all of whom play a role in achieving optimal results for each patient. For this reason, the performance evaluation component of a quality assurance system must include mechanisms for assessing the performance not only of physicians but also of nurses, therapists, and other practitioners.

Resource Utilization

As the proportion of the gross national product devoted to health services continued to approach 10 percent, public concern over the resources consumed in the provision of that care also increased (Havighurst, 1977). The public policy effort to promote competition as a means for containing health care costs (Enthoven, 1980) was a response to the recognition that in many instances resources were being used unnecessarily, producing both waste and potential adverse patient results because of the increased risk associated with unnecessary utilization of services.

Based on the definition presented earlier, it is essential that a quality assurance system include a component designed to monitor, assess, and improve utilization so as to achieve a better match between patient needs and resource consumption. Many might take the position that reduction in the utilization of services is equivalent to reduction in quality. However, if the definition of quality discussed above is accepted, this is not necessarily the case. Appropriate quality assurance systems must include mechanisms for identifying inappropriate usage—whether underutilization or overutilization—and taking corrective action to improve the match between patient needs and resources used.

Risk Management

The final content component of the quality assurance system must be a mechanism for monitoring patient risk, particularly the frequency of client injury, and taking actions to reduce risk where it is excessive. At some point on the curve relating patient benefit to resources used (Figure 3-1, supra), the risk of additional utilization begins to exceed the marginal benefit, requiring that action be taken to reduce the likelihood of injury as a result of care. The medical liability system, which is discussed in detail later, has acted as an important pressure to assure that the evaluation of patient risk is a component of quality control activities.

Figure 3-3 illustrates the nine-celled matrix which is created when these functions and content subsystems interact. Ideally, public policy should ensure that health care institutions engage in quality assurance programs involving each of the nine cells. This conceptual framework can also serve as a useful guide to individual facilities in ensuring that the quality assurance program addresses each of the nine essential activities defined by the cells of this matrix.

PUBLIC POLICIES FOR QUALITY CONTROL

Donabedian (1966) formulated the concept that quality in health services could be evaluated by three alternative approaches: structure, process, or outcome.

Figure 3-3 Quality Assurance Matrix

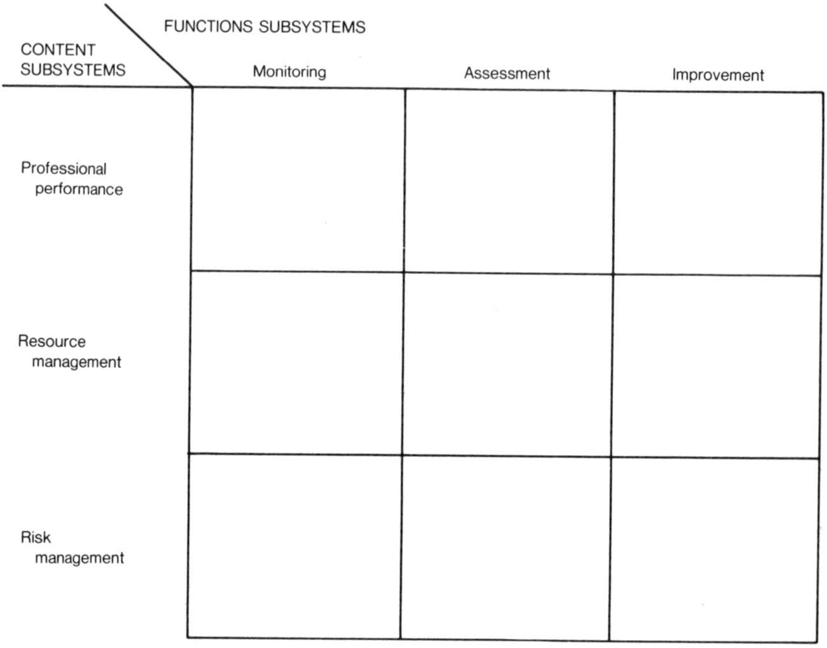

Matrix illustrating the interaction of content and functions of a comprehensive quality assurance system. Activities in each of the nine cells of the matrix are critical to an effective system.

Structure refers to the inputs into a health care delivery system, including the physical and organizational settings in which providers work. The concept includes the human, physical, and financial resources needed to provide medical care, as well as the number, distribution, and qualifications of professional personnel. The number, size, equipment, and geographic distribution of facilities also are included. As an additional input, the organization and financing of services may be included as a structural determinant of quality. Structural measures of quality, then, may be considered to be indirect measures that influence the final outcomes of health services.

The set of activities in which health care providers engage with patients may be referred to as the "process" of care. This includes the complex of diagnostic and therapeutic procedures undertaken (i.e., what is done to the patient). Evaluation of the quality of care using process measures attempts to formulate specific steps of indicated (and contraindicated) diagnostic and therapeutic procedures that should be provided (or not provided) to patients, given the presence of specific conditions or circumstances. Quality is then evaluated in terms of compliance with this set of process criteria. Traditional methods of medical audit focused heavily on process measures of care, although later trends included outcome measures as well as process in such studies.

Clearly, the outcomes of care are the most critical component of any patient's encounter with the delivery system. These are the results that are achieved for the patient and, consistent with the earlier definition of quality, are a key element in deciding whether the quality of care provided is acceptable. Unfortunately, however, outcomes often are temporally remote from the individual patient/practitioner encounter and therefore are more difficult to measure. For that reason, many quality control activities have focused more heavily on processes than on results.

Structure, process, and outcome measures of health care quality may be readily understood by analogy with cooking. In determining where to find a good meal, a diner might look for a restaurant that has been highly recommended by a local critic, where the chef is Cordon Bleu trained, and where the ingredients used are always fresh, carefully selected, and of uniformly high quality. These would be structural measures of the potential quality of the meal.

Process evaluation of the meal would consist of direct observation to assure that ingredients were prepared correctly and in the right amounts, that cooking was performed at the right temperature for the right period of time, and that the coordination of the various events leading to the preparation of the repast proceeded in an orderly and coherent fashion in accordance with the specifications contained in the recipes being followed. However, the most critical test of the quality of the restaurant would be the look, smell, and taste of the food ultimately presented. This, then, is the outcome measure of the quality of the restaurant.

Similarly, structural measures of health care include licensure and certification status of the facilities and practitioners. Process measures evaluate the degree to which the provision of services complies with generally accepted practices of good care. But the critical factor is whether or not the patients' original condition is relieved or improved, or their health status maintained, as a result of the encounter with the system.

Public policies have been developed to attempt to control quality through all three of these approaches. Structural measures for quality control include licensing of personnel, certification of professionals, continuing medical education, and licensure and accreditation of health facilities. These are considered next.

STRUCTURAL POLICIES

Licensing of Personnel

Attempts to regulate the quality of services provided through the licensure of professional personnel are based on the constitutional authority of the states to protect the health and welfare of the public. Traditionally, this has represented a unique partnership between defined professional groups and state government in which the latter has granted authority to license to groups of professionals of the discipline involved. Although the licensing body represents the public interest, the determination of whether particular educational programs are acceptable to the entity lies, to a great extent, in the hands of nonpublic groups. For instance, accreditation of medical schools is a function of the Liaison Committee on Medical Education, which consists of representatives from the American Medical Association, the Association of American Medical Colleges, and other medical professional groups.

This tendency toward performance of quasi-governmental functions by the group being regulated has led to charges that licensure leads to elements of guildism. It might be argued that the ability of members of a professional group to protect their economic position by restricting the entry of others into that field has resulted in increased medical care costs and virtually eliminated competition. It has even been proposed that state licensure of physicians be eliminated as a means to stimulate greater economic competition in the health care industry.

As of 1977, 35 health professions and occupations were licensed by one or more states (U.S. Health Resources Administration, 1977). Individual licensing is based strictly on attainment of educational requirements and/ or passing a state-required examination or equivalent. In addition, many states require that the applicant have no record of conviction for a felony and that supportive letters of recommendation from others licensed to practice the same profession be produced.

Persons unable to meet these requirements are not permitted to practice their profession legally within the state. In particular, the practice of medicine without the required state license constitutes felony assault and battery.

Historically, there has been virtually no direct public accountability for or public participation in the licensing activities of any state. However, in response to widespread public demands for increased accountability, by 1980, 24 states had added public members to their medical licensing boards (Derbyshire, 1980).

The concept of health professional licensure represents a minimal standard that must be met in order to permit an individual to offer services to the public. Unfortunately, the entire health professional licensure system is based on the unfounded assumption that persons who are qualified for licenses will continue to be able to meet minimum standards of competence throughout their professional careers. Generally, licensure, once achieved, is lifelong and subject to revocation only in the event of conviction for a felony or other evidence of incompetence or moral turpitude. In response to this problem, some states (i.e., Maryland) established separate state boards responsible for assuring the adequacy of the professional competence of licensed individuals. Such agencies may include substantial consumer representation. In California, the Board of Medical Quality Assurance is, in fact, administratively responsible to the state's Division of Consumer Affairs. These agencies investigate complaints of poor quality or inappropriate performance and provide for substantially increased accountability to the public for the performance of practitioners licensed by the state.

Certification

Certification is a structural quality control mechanism developed by professional groups both to separate and identify their profession and to provide some minimal standard of education and competence for membership in those bodies. The certification process is most closely associated with medical specialties. Various specialty boards require completion of at least three years of postgraduate training and the passage of a special examination in order to receive the imprimatur of board certification in the particular medical specialty.

Recognizing that procedures for testing cognitive and analytic skills may not be related to clinical competence, medical specialty boards increasingly are developing alternative methods for assuring that their certification represents some measure of actual competence in clinical practice. There also has been a growing trend throughout the medical specialties toward periodic recertification, usually based on reexamination. At least one board (the American Board of Family Practice) now requires that records of selected cases be submitted for review as part of the recertification process. This allows at least some evaluation of the process and outcome of care provided by the physician, as reflected in the medical record, as part of the recertification operation.

Like licensure, such board certification may be criticized on the ground that private voluntary certifying authorities, consisting of physicians practicing the specialty in question, are in charge of the approval process. The power of specialty boards is derived in large part from the fact that many hospitals do not permit a physician to practice in a particular field unless certified by the appropriate board.

Many allied health disciplines have developed certification programs for their members as a means of upgrading the professional image of the field, as well as for formulating some minimal standard of competence as a quality control mechanism. Here, as with medical specialty certification, the quality control mechanisms are completely structural in that certification is based on completion of educational requirements and ability to pass a written examination.

In many allied health fields, the educational requirements have been waived for individuals who were practicing the profession before enactment of the certification requirements by the specialty organization (grandfathering). For this reason, individuals who are certified by a variety of allied health disciplines represent a checkerboard of educational backgrounds. Professional societies' designations include "accredited" (i.e., accredited records technician [ART]); "registered" (registered respiratory therapist [RRT]), and "certified" (certified registered nurse anesthetist [CRNA]). All of these designations connote structural quality control by a professional self-regulatory organization.

Continuing Medical Education

Out of the concern that health practitioners keep up with the rapid changes in medical technology, a variety of professional organizations, including several medical specialty boards and some state licensing agencies, have moved toward requiring certain numbers of hours of continuing education in order to maintain either certification or licensure. For instance, the Maryland State Board of Medical Examiners requires that physicians complete 100 credit hours of continuing medical education (CME) every two years for renewal of their license. By 1976, 14 of the state boards of medical examiners either had implemented or were considering mandatory continuing medical education for licensure. Many state medical societies had begun to require continuing medical education for maintaining membership (Felch, Jessee, Mangun, Mason, Stern, & Wildgen, 1976).

The impact of these compulsory continuing education requirements on the competence of physicians and other health professionals is largely unknown. Without question, the number of accredited continuing education offerings has proliferated tremendously. In fact, continuing health education has become a multimillion-dollar industry. It also is likely that more physicians and allied health professionals are participating in more formal courses as a result. However, the continued growth of these requirements as a means of controlling the quality of services has been criticized by a variety of authors as a generally ineffective solution to the problem (Libby, Weinswig, & Kirk, 1975; Brown & Uhl, 1970; Jessee, 1977b; Miller, 1967; Stein, 1976).

Although there is substantial evidence that well-designed and well-conducted continuing education programs can improve practitioners' knowledge and skills, there is little to support the concept that such deficiencies are the major cause of problems in the quality of services. Rather, many more quality problems appear to relate to attitudes, habits, and environmental constraints in the organization. Nonetheless, mandatory continuing education continues to play an important role in both state licensure and professional certification programs as a structural method for attempting to assure the public of acceptable quality services.

Facility Licensure and Accreditation

Licensure also has been applied to a variety of health care facilities. In particular, hospitals and nursing homes must be inspected and licensed by agencies in all the states. Licensure surveys generally focus on the adequacy of the physical plant, particularly sanitation and safety. In addition, however, structural components of the organization of the facility's employees and medical staff are considerations in determining the institution's adequacy for licensure purposes.

As of 1977, 17 different types of medical or residential care health related facilities were subject to licensure in the United States (Bureau of Health Planning, 1977). Although the statutory boards involved in determination of adequacy for licensure usually include representatives from the type of facility being approved, they are much less likely to be dominated by providers than are the statutory boards that license individual health practitioners. Licensing generally represents compliance with minimal standards designed to assure a baseline of protection from health and environmental hazards.

Accreditation of health care facilities, like certification of individual practitioners, is a voluntary system for structural quality control. The major agency involved in accreditation of health care facilities is the Joint Commission on Accreditation of Hospitals (JCAH). The JCAH, organized in 1952, is the successor to the original hospital standardization program originated by the American College of Surgeons discussed earlier. JCAH members include the American Medical Association, the American Dental

Association, the American College of Physicians, the American College of Surgeons, and the American Hospital Association.

Although accreditation is not mandatory, there are strong incentives for achieving such status that lend a quasi-public role to the process. For instance, approved internships and residencies may be conducted only in hospitals that are accredited by the JCAH. In addition, the Medicare program accepts JCAH accreditation as evidence that the institution complies with the standards set for participation in that effort. In 1978, 5,246 of the 7,015 hospitals identified by the AHA were accredited by JCAH (American Hospital Association, 1979).

The JCAH accreditation standards have begun to include requirements that the hospital conduct evaluations of the process and outcomes of care. However, they remain primarily concerned with structural factors. The accreditation standards include references to the physical plant; the structure and operation of the governing body and administration; organization of the medical staff; and the conduct of various services such as nursing, anesthesia, outpatient department, medical records, laboratory, radiology, etc. Hospitals desiring JCAH accreditation are inspected at triennial intervals by review teams consisting of JCAH staff and health professionals from other institutions.

In an attempt to include additional process and outcome quality control measures in the accreditation process, the JCAH since 1979 has required that hospitals have an organized program designed "to enhance patient care through the ongoing objective assessment of important aspects of patient care and the correction of identified problems" (JCAH, 1980). This quality assurance standard seeks to assure that appropriate internal quality control programs are in place as a prerequisite to achieving accredited status.

Similar accreditation programs are operated by the American Osteopathic Association for osteopathic hospitals and by the JCAH for long-term care facilities, psychiatric hospitals, community mental health centers, and a few other categories of health care facilities.

PROCESS AND OUTCOME POLICIES

The JCAH Quality Assurance Standard

Although the JCAH is not a public agency and its accreditation requirements have no force of law, its influence on the hospital industry has become so pervasive that its standards have much the same impact as those of a public regulatory body. Hospital accreditation has been given a quasi-public status by the provisions of the Medicare law that deem accredited facilities to have met the conditions of participation in that program.

The Joint Commission's efforts to develop stronger programs for evaluating the process and outcome of health care in hospitals stand as a major component of "public" policy in the United States. The roots of the transition from a strict reliance on structural quality control measures to one emphasizing process and outcome may be traced to the landmark decision of the Illinois Supreme Court in 1965 in the case of *Darling v. Charleston Community Memorial Hospital* (1965). This decision (discussed in detail later) reversed previous judicial theory that had held that the acts of the medical staff of a voluntary hospital were outside the facility's control. The *Darling* ruling found that the institution, as a corporate entity, did in fact have a responsibility for assuring that the quality of professional services provided by all individuals allowed to practice within its walls, whether employed or not, met acceptable standards of quality. In essence, this decision placed the hospital in a position of corporate responsibility for the processes and outcomes of care provided by physicians, regardless of their employment or agency relationship with the hospital. Subsequently, this concept has been embraced by courts in many other jurisdictions throughout the United States.

In response, the Joint Commission in 1973 developed a new standard requiring that the hospital medical staff conduct outcome-oriented medical audits. Although a variety of approaches to quality assessment using process and outcome criteria had been developed before that date, the JCAH effort marked the first time that a quasi-regulatory body had specifically required that such procedures be conducted in health care institutions. The approach developed by the JCAH, and taught in its Trustee-Administrator-Physician (TAP) Institutes, focused on measurement of outcomes as indicators of adverse results, then examining the process of care in cases that had an unexpected or adverse result.

The original medical audit standard was strengthened further in 1976 by requiring certain numbers of such studies to be conducted annually. This represented an incremental effort by the JCAH to assure that hospitals had in place mechanisms for evaluating the process and outcome of services provided by the medical staff, primarily as a means of protecting the institution against potential corporate liability for malpractice.

Unfortunately, industrywide reaction to the medical audit requirements generally was negative. Medical staffs, predictably in response to an obvious power strategy for change, resisted the numerical requirements and often resorted to a process of paper compliance (doing the required criteria setting, data collection, etc., on paper, but not looking for significant problems, or taking action to resolve them) rather than engaging in meaningful self-assessment and evaluation. As a consequence, the Joint Commission began to reevaluate its approach to quality assurance and, in 1979, developed a revised hospitalwide standard for quality assurance, replacing the old medical staff requirements for patient care audit.

This new standard, which became effective for hospital surveys conducted subsequent to January 1981, required that there be "evidence of a well-defined, organized program designed to enhance patient care through the ongoing objective assessment of important aspects of patient care and the correction of identified problems." In essence, the new quality assurance standard required that hospitals establish programs for the continuous monitoring of a variety of aspects of services, assessment of potential problems, and actions that could be demonstrated to have resulted in sound clinical performance and improved patient care quality.

The standard did not specify what approach the institution must use to achieve these objectives other than to require that it must include explicit written criteria on essential and critical aspects of patient care that were generally acceptable to the clinical staffs to assess problems and measure compliance with achievable goals. This gave institutions considerable latitude and encouraged innovation in approaches to hospital quality assurance. The evolution of the Joint Commission's efforts in process and outcome quality assurance is a classic example of the evolution of a program of social change from a power strategy to one of facilitation as the means of solidifying a shift well under way in most institutions.

The PSRO Program

The professional standards review organization (PSRO) program was a landmark in public policy. It marked the singular attempt by government to encourage professional self-regulation as a matter of public policy through the provision of tax monies to operate programs of peer review. No precedent for such sweeping authority over federal expenditures as was granted to PSROs existed before enactment of the legislation (Section 249(f) of P.L. 92-603, the Social Security Amendments of 1972). Although evaluations of the success of this experiment were mixed, an analysis of its social and political history offers important lessons for future public policy activities intended to control both the utilization of health services financed by public funds and the quality of the services so funded.

The PSRO legislation was introduced by Senator Wallace Bennett, the senior Republican from Utah and then chairman of the Senate Finance Committee. An earlier proposal, included in the AMA's Medicredit Plan (*Congressional Record,* 1970), called for a national system of peer review organizations (PROs) based on the model that had been established in Utah by the Utah State Medical Association (USMA). There, in response to a request from the state Medicaid program for assistance in controlling hospital utilization, the USMA had established the Utah Professional Review Organization (UPRO), which developed and implemented a program for onsite concurrent hospital utilization review (OSCHUR).

This program, which employed registered nurses to screen the necessity for admission and continued stay in the hospital, using explicit written criteria developed by physicians, was quite successful in reducing utilization in Utah facilities. In addition, the review coordinators became a formidable resource for identifying quality of care issues that could be studied later in greater depth.

The original intent of the PSRO amendment was primarily to assist in reducing unnecessary or inappropriate utilization of hospital services under Medicare and Medicaid. However, questions of the quality of services being purchased with public funds also were a major concern of the drafters of this legislation. In implementation of the law, a conscious decision was made by the Department of Health, Education, and Welfare to emphasize the quality control aspects over the utilization control component in an attempt to gain more widespread professional support.

Nonetheless, opposition to the concept of PSROs emerged from a variety of professional groups. Although the AMA originally was supportive, the Bennett amendment as eventually introduced had deleted the group's proposal for direct association of PSROs with state medical societies. The official AMA position then became substantially less enthusiastic.

Two very conservative physician groups (The Association of American Physicians and Surgeons and The Council of Medical Staffs of the United States) participated in an unsuccessful judicial attempt to halt implementation of the legislation (*AAPS v. Weinberger,* 1975). Their argument that the legislation violated the Social Security Act's prohibition against interference in the practice of medicine and denied constitutional guarantees of due process and equality was rejected by the federal district and appeals courts.

In addition, a tremendous controversy arose over the process by which 203 geographic regions were identified and designated as PSRO areas. In one instance, the Texas Medical Association won a suit to halt the splitting of that state into nine PSRO areas on the ground that such division was "arbitrary and capricious" and that the action of DHHS in making that regulatory decision had been unduly influenced by congressional staff, in violation of the separation of powers (*Texas Medical Association v. Mathews,* 1976).

Compounding this lack of professional support and, in some instances, active opposition, was substantial bureaucratic infighting among the various agencies of the Department of Health, Education, and Welfare that had responsibility for the program. At the time the legislation was enacted in 1972, the Bureau of Health Insurance in the Social Security Administration was responsible for Medicare administration; the Medical Services Administration of the Social and Rehabilitation Service for administering the Medicaid program; and a new Bureau of Quality Assurance in the U.S. Public Health Service for implementing the new PSRO law.

The struggle for control over the implementation of the program was a major obstacle to its progress during its early years. In addition, Congress provided sufficient funds for only 14 PSROs during the program's first year and for only 60 the next year. This delay in starting the program allowed the opposition forces to gather strength and lent substantial credence to critics who indicated that professional self-regulation such as proposed by the PSRO amendment was not feasible.

Despite these formidable obstacles, the program eventually was implemented in most of the 203 areas. Unfortunately, many physician groups that formed PSROs maintained a posture of only token compliance with the letter of the law. As a result, substantial public funds were expended on review activities that had little or no impact on either utilization or quality of services.

A 1978 evaluation of the national PSRO program by the Health Care Financing Administration indicated that, in utilization terms, a saving of $1.10 in federal funds was effectuated for each $1.00 expended on PSRO review (HCFA, 1979). Perhaps more importantly, the evaluation of the impact of the quality assurance review components indicated a significant number of instances in which marked improvements in compliance with critical process criteria or outcome criteria could be demonstrated following PSRO medical care evaluation studies. Although it was extremely difficult to estimate the dollar saving from such quality improvements, the evaluation offered one of the few evidences that programs of professional peer review could, in fact, lead to changes in medical practice so as to influence the quality of services favorably.

Although the PSRO program was earmarked for early phase-out by the Reagan administration, an effective lobbying effort by the program's proponents produced the Peer Review Improvement Act of 1982 in its place (P.L. 97-248). This act replaced PSROs with Utilization and Quality Control Peer Review Organizations (PROs), which may be either nonprofit or for-profit entities that are able to review the pattern of quality of care in a defined geographic area. The previous PSRO areas were redefined; generally, each state then constituted a separate area. Existing PSROs were continued until such time as the Secretary of DHHS could consolidate them into new areas. Thus, the PSRO program metamorphosed into a new, streamlined program of Peer Review Organizations, launching a new chapter in public sector involvement in quality assurance.

The lessons learned regarding the value of communitywide programs for evaluation of medical practices, and the comparison of data from a variety of health care facilities that permitted interinstitutional analysis of differences in performance, proved extremely valuable. Regardless of its organizational form, future public policy should build upon the effective components of the PSRO experiment in developing programs to assure that public funds are expended only to purchase health care services of acceptable quality.

The Medical Liability System

The system of tort law or civil laws has become a major motivating force in efforts to improve the quality of health services in the United States. To the extent that public policy is expressed through judicial opinion and precedent, the medical liability system has become a major factor shaping that policy toward the quality of health services.

During the early part of the 20th century, the prevailing judicial theory held that hospitals were merely convenient locations in which physicians and other health workers provided services. Responsibility for any injuries to patients resulting from either the direct acts of the physician or of other health workers operating under the doctor's direction was solely the physician's responsibility and not that of the institution (*Schloendorff v. Society of New York Hospital,* 1914).

It was not until 1957 that this concept of strict separation of medical responsibility, as the exclusive province of the physician, and administrative responsibility, as the province of the hospital, began to erode. In *Bing v. Thunig* (1957), the New York Supreme Court held that the hospital was liable for the acts of a physician who acted as an agent of the institution, either through direct employment by it or through an appearance of an employment relationship presented to the patient ("implied agency"). During the next several years, a host of cases revolved around the question whether or not physicians in hospitals could be perceived as acting as the agents of the institution. However, the issue was resolved in 1965 with the Illinois Supreme Court *Darling* ruling (noted earlier), which held that the hospital was responsible for the quality of services provided within its walls, regardless of the physician's employment or agency relationship with the institution.

This corporate responsibility for quality of services was extended further in the 1973 unpublished ruling of the Superior Court for Sacramento County, California, in *Gonzales v. Nork and Mercy Hospital*. The presiding judge held that the hospital was liable for the malpractice acts committed by Dr. Nork because it "should have known" that such deeds were occurring if it had had in place even basic procedures for reviewing the quality of services being provided. As a result of this gradual change in judicial theory, substantial pressure has been placed on hospitals as corporate entities to examine the quality of services provided within their walls.

As indicated, the *Darling* decision was a major stimulus to the hospital industry's subsequent efforts to improve quality assurance activities. The medical audit standard enacted by the Joint Commission on Accreditation of Hospitals in 1973, and subsequent amendments to that standard in 1976 and 1979, can be traced in large part to the evolution of judicial theory clarifying the responsibility of the hospital for the quality of all services provided to its patients. At the same time, some malpractice insurers participated in this pressure on hospitals as institutions by offering premium reductions to those that operated effective risk management and quality control programs.

During the early 1970s, substantial public attention was devoted to the rapid spiral in the frequency of malpractice claims and the cost of malpractice insurance. This culminated in physician strikes and the withdrawal of commercial malpractice insurance carriers from several states in 1974 and 1975. As a result, tort reforms were enacted in many states and alternative approaches to risk management and quality control became commonplace. However, these efforts had minimal impact on the underlying problems that led to large numbers of malpractice claims and substantial financial losses.

Industry statistics indicate that the malpractice loss ratio (the ratio of total losses and adjustment expenses to total premium income) exceeded 148 percent for the malpractice industry in the United States in 1981 (Medical Liability Advisory Service, 1982). Under such circumstances, further increases in premium or withdrawal of insurers from the marketplace were inevitable. Until the problem of rapidly increasing patient injury is addressed, it is likely that the malpractice liability system will exert even greater pressures on the health care industry to deal with quality of care.

FUTURE DIRECTIONS

The future of public policy to affect quality of health services obviously is speculative at best, particularly in an era in which the role of government in financing such care is not well-defined. If all Americans eventually are encompassed by some form of publicly financed health insurance or health care program, incorporation of quality controls into such an approach would be mandatory.

One possibility for the future is the amalgamation of certain aspects of the PSRO program with the health systems agency (HSA) concept. Under this proposal, the PSRO's quality and utilization control functions would be performed by a quasi-public agency in which consumers would constitute the dominant force. In addition, approval of certificates of need for capital expenditures would be based on considerations of the quality of services being provided by the institutions making such applications.

This concept of linking quality/utilization control with regulatory programs designed to limit capital construction offers substantial appeal as a potential mechanism for controlling both quality and cost. However, the introduction of such substantial consumer control over quality review raises questions of how candid health professionals participating in such activities would be. Clearly, the public cannot make informed judgments on the quality of services without cooperation from professional groups. Until the health professions engage in more open and candid self-criticism, it is unlikely that this concept will come to pass.

Another concept that received substantial attention (Bureau of Health Manpower, 1977) was relicensure of physicians based on demonstrated competence. A model state act to provide for mandatory relicensure was developed by the Georgetown University (D.C.) Health Policy Center in 1976 (Bureau of Health Manpower, 1977) and circulated to the state legislatures. Difficulties in arriving at a consensus on how to assess competence prevented implementation of this concept by any state. It generally was felt that cognitive testing could measure only one aspect of competence (knowledge). Evaluation of patient care processes and outcomes, through such mechanisms as medical audit, would be preferable, but could not be applied on any large-scale basis within the state of the art of health care review methods.

In any consideration of possible future directions, cost effectiveness of the quality control program itself must be a prime consideration. The death knell of the PSRO program as originally constituted was the estimated cost of more than $350 million annually to operate a fully implemented review program for hospital care alone. When the costs of reviewing long-term and ambulatory care services were added, this sum substantially exceeded the willingness of the public to pay for quality and utilization control in an era of increasing resource limitation.

The exact trade-off between the cost of effective quality control and of continued lack of such systems is an issue for open debate and better definition in the arena of public policy in the coming years.

REFERENCES

American College of Surgeons. *Manual of hospital standardization.* Chicago: Author, 1946, p. 8.

American Hospital Association. *Hospital statistics, 1979.* Chicago: Author, 1979.

Association of American Physicians and Surgeons v. Weinberger, 395 F. Supp. 125 (1975) (N.D. Ill. 1975).

Bing v. Thunig, 2 N.Y. 2d 656; 163 N.Y.S. 2d 3; 143 N.E. 2d 3. (1957)

Bowman, J.G. Hospital standardization series, general hospitals of 100 or more beds: Report for 1919. *Bulletin of the American College of Surgeons,* 1920, *4,* 3–36.

Brook, R.H., & Appel, F.A. Quality-of-care assessment: Choosing a method for peer review. *New England Journal of Medicine, 1973, 288*(25), 1323–1329.

Brook, R.H., & Williams, K.N. Quality of health care for the disadvantaged. *Journal of Community Health,* 1975, *1,* 132–156.

Brown, C.R., & Uhl, H.S.M. Mandatory continuing education: Sense or nonsense? *Journal of the American Medical Association,* 1970, *213,* 1660–1668.

Bureau of Health Manpower. *Competence in the medical professions: A strategy for change.* (Department of Health, Education, and Welfare, Health Resources Administration, Publication No. (HRA) 77-35). Washington, D.C.: U.S. Government Printing Office, 1977.

Bureau of Health Planning. *Characteristics of state health facility licensing practices.* (Department of Health, Education, and Welfare, Health Resources Administration, Publication No. (HRA) 231-77-0084). Washington, D.C.: U.S. Government Printing Office, 1977.

Codman, E.A. *A study in hospital efficiency: The first five years.* Boston: Thomas Todd Co., 1916.

Committee on Standardization of Hospitals. Clinical Congress of Surgeons of North America: Suggested end result system. *Surgery, Gynecology, and Obstetrics,* 1914, *18* (supplement), 9–12.

Congressional Record, House, July 23, 1970.

Darling v. Charleston Community Memorial Hospital 211 N.E. 2d 253 (1965), 14 A.L.R. 3d 860 (Ill. 1965).

Derbyshire, R.C. Personal communication, cited in S. Jonas, *Health care delivery in the United States* (2nd ed.) New York: Springer Publishing Company, 1980, p. 405.

Donabedian, A. Evaluating the quality of medical care. *Milbank Memorial Fund Quarterly/ Health and Society,* 1966, *44*(2), 166–203.

Donabedian, A. *The definition of quality and approaches to its assessment,* Vol. 1 in *Explorations in quality assessment and monitoring.* Ann Arbor, Mich.: Health Administration Press, 1980.

Enthoven, A.C. *Health plan: The only practical solution to the soaring cost of medical care.* Reading, Mass.: Addison-Wesley Publishing Company, Inc., 1980.

Felch, W.C., Jessee, W.F., Mangun, C., Jr., Mason, H., Stern, T., & Wildgen, J. Continuing education: The portent for CME is mandatory. *Patient Care,* January 15, 1976, pp. 124–131.

Flexner, A. *Medical education in the United States and Canada.* The Carnegie Foundation for the Advancement of Teaching, 1910. Reprinted Washington, D.C.: Science and Health Publications, 1960.

Gonzales v. Nork and Mercy Hosp., No. 228556 (Super. Ct., Sacramento County, Calif., 1973).

Havighurst, C.C. Controlling health care costs: Strengthening the private sector's hand. *Journal of Health Politics, Policy and Law*, Winter 1977, *1*(4), 471– 498.

Health Care Financing Administration. *Professional standards review organization 1978 program evaluation*. (Department of Health, Education, and Welfare, Publication No. HCFA-03000). Washington, D.C.: U.S. Government Printing Office, 1979.

Jessee, W.F. Physician competence and compulsory continuing education: Are they compatible? *Journal of Community Health*, 1977, *2*, 291–295. (a)

Jessee, W.F. Quality assurance systems: Why aren't there any? *Quality Review Bulletin*, 1977, *3*(11), 16–26. (b)

Jessee, W.F. An integrated quality assurance system for the hospital. *Journal of Quality Assurance*, 1979, *1*(2), 11–14.

Jessee, W.F. Approaches to improving the quality of health care: Organizational change. *Quality Review Bulletin*, 1981, *7*(7), 13–18.

Jessee, W.F. *Identifying health care quality problems: A practical manual for PSROs and hospitals*. Monograph No. 8. Chapel Hill, N.C.: University of North Carolina, Department of Health Administration, 1982. (a)

Jessee, W.F. Improving patient care by changing physician behavior. *Hospital Medical Staff*, 1982, *11*(1), 2–8. (b)

Joint Commission on Accreditation of Hospitals. *Accreditation manual for hospitals*. Chicago: Author, 1980.

Lembke, P.A. Evolution of the medical audit. *Journal of the American Medical Association*, 1967, *199*, 543–550.

Libby, G.N., Weinswig, M.H., & Kirk, K.W. Help stamp out mandatory continuing medical education. *Journal of the American Medical Association*, 1975, *233*, 797–799.

McLamb, J.T., & Huntley, R.R. The hazards of hospitalization. *Southern Medical Journal*, 1967, *60*, 469–472.

Medical Liability Advisory Service. *Insurance industry malpractice underwriting losses generally up sharply in 1981*. May, 1982, *7*(5), p. 2.

Miller, G.R. Continuing education for what? *Journal of Medical Education*, 1967, *42*, 320–326.

Schimmel, E.M. The hazards of hospitalization. *Annals of Internal Medicine*, 1964, *60*, 100–110.

Schloendorff v. Society of New York Hospital, 211 N.Y. 125, 105 N.E. 92 (1914).

Steel, K., Gertman, P.M., Crescenzi, C., & Anderson, J. Iatrogenic illness on a general medical service at a university hospital. *New England Journal of Medicine*, 1981, *304*(11), 638–642.

Stein, L.S. Mandatory CME: 'Green Stamps' or competence? *Quality Review Bulletin*, 1976, *2*(7), 4, 30.

Texas Medical Ass'n v. Mathews. 408 F. Supp. 303 (1976).

U.S. Health Resources Administration. *State regulation of health manpower*. (Department of Health, Education, and Welfare, Publication No. (HRA) 77-49). Washington, D.C.: U.S. Government Printing Office, 1977.

Wetherill, H.G. A plea for higher hospital efficiency and standardization. *Surgery, Gynecology, Obstetrics*, 1915, *20*, 705–707.

Chapter 4

Shifting Federal Policy and Its Impact on Minorities' Access to Health Services

George M. Neely and Nancy L. Tigar

During the 1960s, the United States rediscovered poverty. Congress proceeded to pass new legislation to fund various kinds of human services, mainly for the poor. These programs were intended to change the way care was delivered, provide new kinds of services, and increase the participation of the poor and minorities in decision-making processes in the country. This success was judged in a new way. Up to this point, a program was deemed successful if it was being implemented; now, however, it became necessary to look also at the outputs and to measure the results of government spending. A new consciousness of the limits of federal resources also emerged.

MacRae and Wilde (1979) defined a policy as a "chosen course of action significantly affecting large numbers of people." If that course of action is chosen by the federal government, it is a "public policy." The criteria used by the federal government to develop health service policy during the 1960s, 70s, and 80s changed as the years progressed. Basic to many federal actions in the 60s was an attempt by the policy makers to provide more equity in the health care delivery system: equity in terms of removing financial and other barriers to services so they would be available to all groups of citizens, particularly those who were, and are, disenfranchised—the poor, the elderly, and minorities.

However, equity considerations were joined in recent years by the quest for efficiency. With health care expenditures increasing at an alarming rate (approximately 4 percent of the gross national product in the 1950s and 9 percent by 1980), the federal government, as well as state and local jurisdictions, began a search for alternative policies that would contain costs and generally slow the outpouring of money in this area.

Decisions based on efficiency usually entail a review of both the costs and benefits of specific programs or projects. With the Reagan Adminis-

95

tration's strong emphasis on the cost portion of the equation, it was entirely possible that benefits, both short-term and long-term, would be ignored. Indeed, a great deal of the progress made during the 1960s and 1970s toward better health services for minority groups and others could be negated in the flurry to see who can trim the most money from their budgets.

SELECTED HEALTH INDEXES

The Office of Program Planning and Evaluation of the National Institutes of Health, in a report on the health of America's nonwhite population in 1971, made two important points:

1. Except for genetic disorders such as the sickling trait, there is no fatal disease that characterizes one race from another.
2. The higher disease incidence, prevalence, morbidity, and mortality among nonwhites and the poor in many instances reflects the consequences of their underprivileged status.

A major problem is institutional racism (defined as an interrelated system of policies, practices, and procedures that limits group decision-making power to one racial group; imposes one cultural set of values (ethnocentrism); and is characterized by a disproportionate share of resources in the hands of one racial group). Because of this institutional racism, many minorities find it difficult to become participants, whether as clients or providers, in a health care system developed by and maintained primarily for white middle-class society. Those differences are mirrored in various health statistics.

Health indexes for the nation's population generally have improved in recent years; however, discrepancies between racial groups still exist. In 1977, the age-adjusted death rate for whites was 6.8 per 1,000 population per year; for blacks, 10.4; and for American Indian-Alaskan natives, 8.2. The infant mortality rate has declined steadily since 1950: in 1977, the rate for whites was 12.3 deaths per 1,000 live births, blacks 23.6, and American Indian-Alaskan natives 15.6. Mortality rates for blacks generally are higher for most major diseases. Incidence rates also are higher.

Many of the data used by policy makers and others to plan for health services are generated by the Health Interview Survey (HIS) conducted by the National Center for Health Statistics. (Approximately 50 percent of all requests for this information come from federal, state, and local government agencies.) Before 1978, race and ethnicity of household members were recorded as white, black, and other; in 1978 respondents were classified for the first time into five categories: black not Hispanic, Hispanic, Native American or Alaskan Native, Asian or Pacific Islander, white not Hispanic origin. This classification system permits the collection of data concerning specific ethnic/cultural groups.

However, problems with the HIS remain. The number of minority persons sampled is small; heterogeneous populations (such as Spanish-speaking individuals) are aggregated into a bloc containing subgroups with very different needs and problems, and groups such as migrant workers and young urban black males may be missed or their number underestimated since they do not live in settled households. Salber and Beza (1980) make an important point:

> [It is] the poorest and the most needy people with the least resources and those with the most illness we need to know about and help. The National Health Survey tells a lot about the majority of the population but not enough about those who need health and social programs the most. [It is] for this group that government makes policy and allocates money, but it is precisely here that information is lacking. (p. 325)

The needs for health services and their eventual conversion into demand by client groups is a function of many separate elements. Demographic and cultural characteristics; current health status; and considerations such as the cost of service, transportation, and insurance coverage all influence this element. Other important variables that have much to do with whether or not health resources eventually are utilized are clients' awareness of services, their accessibility, and their acceptability by client groups (Palmer, 1975). Convenience, high quality, and reasonable prices are what people look for in a health care system. These three factors seem to be particularly elusive for minority groups and certain rural populations. Barriers to access to health care have existed for some time and continue to be prevalent.

DEFINITION OF ACCESS

The term "access" to health care has been used frequently by legislators, planners, researchers, providers, and others to describe phenomena that underlie many of the health policy decisions made in this country beginning in the 1960s. Penchansky and Thomas (1981) tested the validity of a taxonomic definition of "access" that attempted to describe the general dimensions of this concept more precisely. These authors defined "access" generally as "the degree of 'fit' between the client and the system." They described the five "As"—five specific dimensions—as comprising the general concept of access:

1. *Availability:* The relationship of the volume and type of existing services (and resources) to volume and type of clients' needs. It includes the adequacy of health personnel, facilities, and specialized programs.
2. *Accessibility:* The relationship between location of supply and location of clients. This includes client transportation resources, travel time, distance, and travel cost.
3. *Accommodation:* The relationship between the way services are organized to accept clients, their ability to accommodate to these factors, and their perception of whether services are appropriate.
4. *Affordability:* The relationship of prices of services to clients' income, ability to pay, and the type and extent of their existing health insurance.
5. *Acceptability:* The relationship of the clients' and providers' attitudes about the personal and practice characteristics of each other.

From this definition it can be seen that access involves more than just developing health care resources in a community. It includes the ways in which these resources are perceived by the client groups and their subsequent utilization of these services. However, in discussing strategies for developing personal health services in rural communities, Sheps and Bachar (1981) made the point that the availability of a given type of care really was a precondition to access.

They saw structural availability of service as "the controlling variable that makes possible the degree and nature of utilization of the services" and the ultimate effect these resources would have on the target population. Perhaps for this very reason, Penchansky and Thomas discussed availability as their first dimension of access.

PUBLIC POLICY INFLUENCES ON ACCESS

For a number of years the federal government has been involved in developing and implementing policies, programs, and projects that have impacted on the health care system. These initiatives reflected the underlying issues prevalent during particular time periods. As noted previously, the basic criteria used to make specific decisions shifted from attempts to provide equity in the system to judgments made on the basis of the efficient use of scarce resources. The federal presence was felt in the areas of health care financing, health planning, service delivery, and personnel development.

Federal interventions have been imposed at the macro level of the health care system while equity and access problems frequently occur at the micro levels. As a result, initiatives to increase access to health care must depend on changes in the larger system, shifts that often are slow in coming or are circumvented before they reach the service delivery level. In addition, policies in one area frequently interact negatively with the purpose, process, and/or content of policies in another area. A review of federal activities in health financing, planning, service delivery, and personnel development illustrates many of these basic issues.

Health Financing

A strong case was made in the early 1960s for a federal role in the financing of medical care. As Rivlin (1977) pointed out in a retrospective analysis, access to good quality medical care was regarded as a basic right, essential to an individual's well-being. The result was the 1965 enactment of Medicare (Title XVIII of the Social Security Act) and Medicaid (Title XIX). Massive amounts of federal funds were funneled into the health care industry to help pay the bills of the nation's elderly and poor.

A study by Davis and Reynolds (1975) based on 1969 data found that fewer blacks than whites were receiving service under Medicare. They concluded that at that point the program had failed to eliminate the major racial and income-related inequities in the use of medical services by the elderly.

A later study by Link, Long, and Settle (1980a) found that these inequities had largely disappeared by the mid-1970s. While Medicare had increased the access of the low income elderly to health care, it still presented a problem to eligible persons in the high and middle income brackets. Deductible and coinsurance payments frequently represented more money than retired persons on small fixed incomes could afford.

Medicaid is the most important source of medical coverage for the poor in the United States. Since this is a shared program with the states, the latter define eligibility criteria—most specifically, the income levels that determine the "medically needy." Most urban blacks have some form of publicly subsidized insurance. However, about 25 percent of the Spanish-speaking are without such coverage (Aday, 1980). It is estimated that approximately 22 million individuals (mostly poor) have no health insurance whatsoever and another 20 million have inadequate coverage. These figures do not include almost 5 million undocumented aliens in the country (Foley, 1980).

In a second study evaluating access to medical care under Medicaid, Link, Long, and Settle (1980b) found significantly lower access to ambulatory care services for blacks in 1976. They estimated that the program had failed to provide equal access to these benefits to 60 percent of all blacks.

While Medicare and Medicaid relieved the worry about medical cost for many, these programs also created problems. The sheer size of, and the tremendous increase in, their cost underlined the need for controls. Cost containment was permeating the entire health care system but perhaps the hardest hit were the public hospitals, public clinics, and services and programs particularly needed and utilized most often by the poor and minorities (i.e., treatment centers for alcoholism, community mental health programs, long-term services, etc.).

Blacks were less likely to have a single family physician and more likely to use hospital emergency rooms and outpatient departments for their health care. Four percent of all blacks and 5 percent of Mexican-Americans utilized public clinics, while less than 1 percent of the white population did (Aday, 1980). The closure or merging of a significant number of public hospitals and the curtailment of services by others and by some public providers forced these users to seek other modes of health care. These alternatives frequently were some distance away and in neighborhoods unfamiliar to the potential clients.

A specific problem exacerbated by Medicare and Medicaid was the amount of paper work involved. Physicians frequently chose not to be involved with a federal program rather than expend their time and energies complying with regulations for which, in their view, they were not compensated adequately. This situation further complicated problems regarding the availability of both facilities and providers.

Following World War II, Congress passed the 1946 Hill-Burton Act (Title VI of the Public Health Services Act), which provided funds to hospitals to increase their capacity to care for people. Between 1946 and 1979, approximately $4 billion in grants and loans for construction and modernization were given to 7,000 hospitals, nursing homes, and other health care facilities (*Health, U.S.*, 1980). As part of the requirement for receiving these monies, hospitals assumed a "free care" obligation to provide services to a small percentage of patients. While the obligation seemed to have been overshadowed (or overlooked, in some instances), hospital bed capacity increased at a rapid rate with a resulting upsurge in the costs associated with institutional care.

Hospitals are the core of this country's health delivery system. Unfortunately, in many instances there is a dual track system, with public hospitals serving the indigent (including a large population of minorities) while private hospitals are receiving private paying patients, mostly whites. The government's emphasis on cost containment contributed inadvertently to relocation and closure problems for many public hospitals. These older, inner-city facilities were among the first targeted for extinction because they were chronically understaffed, overcrowded, and operated in aging buildings with poor and/or inadequate equipment.

Blatant discriminatory practices, such as separate hospitals or departments for minorities, the denial of staff privileges to minority physicians, requirements for cash deposits before a patient could be admitted (especially for Hispanics), the referral of Indians to Indian Health Service (IHS) hospitals for care (although they might be a great distance away), led to the Community Services Amendments (Title VI of the Civil Rights Act of 1964, P.L. 88-352) (Office of Civil Rights, n.d.).

These amendments, through the threat of withdrawal of funds (Institute of Medicine, 1981), have helped correct many of the injustices and discriminatory practices characteristic of health services institutions. However, enforcement of the amendments was subject to question. Monitoring compliance was under the authority of the Office of Civil Rights in the Department of Health and Human Services, and a substantial number of staff positions in the five federal agencies responsible for enforcing the civil rights laws faced elimination ("Civil Rights Advocates," 1981).

Health Planning

In April 1980, Henry A. Foley, Administrator of the Health Resources Administration (HRA), in testimony before the U.S. Civil Rights Commission, stressed the point that institutions such as public hospitals, which served as the primary sources of health care in underserved areas, either had to be kept viable or else acceptable alternative care centers needed to be developed (Foley, 1980). He reviewed several ways in which financially troubled hospitals could be assisted.

Section 1610 of the Public Health Services Act of 1974, P.L. 93-641, authorized financial grants to institutions for construction and modernization to correct safety hazards and other violations of existing codes. While many public hospitals could qualify for these grants, no money was appropriated for this purpose after 1977. Similarly, under Section 242, the Guaranteed Loan Program of the Federal Housing Administration, institutions could borrow money for capital improvements. However, only financially sound facilities could qualify for these funds. This requirement eliminated most inner city hospitals that, if they were financially sound, probably would not seek government assistance in the first place.

The certificate of need (CON) requirements in the Health Planning and Resource Development Amendments of 1979, Section 117 of P.L. 96-79, stipulated that the effects of closures and conversions on access to health care be considered by health systems agencies (HSAs) when making decisions affecting local health services. Foley indicated that HRA's policy should require that alternative services be in place prior to the closure of any institution serving the poor and minorities. Just how this policy could be implemented was not discussed. Proper planning and coordination between local HSAs and state health planning agencies was presented as one of the ways in which some control could be exercised in these situations.

Health planning, as embodied in the 1979 amendments, did have some positive aspects. The requirement that consumers be involved in HSAs and that the community be broadly represented on their boards presented opportunities for some minorities and poor to have input into decisions concerning the health system as it directly affected them. These efforts had mixed results.

Health planning efforts were to be directed at containing cost while improving access to quality health care. These need not be mutually exclusive goals; however, in the United States health care delivery system as it was operating in the early 1980s, they were seen for the most part as distinctly different and conflicting entities. HSAs were charged with the responsibility for reducing the number of excess acute beds in their specific areas while promoting an appropriate mix of ambulatory services to adequately meet the needs of the population. Many health planning agencies frequently were out of favor in their communities for the decisions they made. By the end of 1982, the entire health planning effort was being questioned at the federal level. Specifically, community input as a necessary component of the process was being challenged. Whether or not health planning would continue in its then-existing form was doubtful.

Service Delivery

The federal government for many years has provided funding for programs and services aimed at increasing the availability and accessibility of health care to the population. The Neighborhood Health Center (NHC) concept had its origin in the Office of Economic Opportunity (OEO) in 1964. NHCs were both accessible and acceptable to their populations and offered consumers a voice in policy making (*Vital and Health Statistics,* 1979). By 1975, there were 154 neighborhood health centers in existence.

In 1972, the Health Services Administration (HSA) fostered the development of Family Health Centers (FHCs) in rural areas. From 1972 to 1975, efforts were made by both HSA and OEO to bring these types of organizations under one federal administration.

The Special Health Revenue Sharing Act of 1975, P.L. 94-63, authorized the use of grant money to modernize existing health centers. This act facilitated the planning and development of new and existing community health centers (CHCs). These centers were required to provide the basic scope of primary medical services necessary to meet the needs of their specific population groups (Beraducci, 1978). CHCs provided services almost exclusively to poor and minority populations. The expectation was that these centers would become financially independent by collecting fees from third party reimbursers. This did not happen and community health centers remained very dependent on federal funding.

Community health centers were an integral part of the federal initiatives from 1975 to 1978. Beginning in 1975, the Rural Health Initiative (RHI) attempted to coordinate the many categorical grants for health programs and services in rural areas and to provide technical assistance to local communities to help them develop their own health programs. At the same time, the parallel Urban Health Strategies were encouraging the expansion and development of community health centers into sites for the delivery of primary care. The Rural Health Initiative and the Urban Health Strategies finally were merged into one entity, the Primary Care Initiative, in 1977.

Federal budget cutting could have a serious impact on community health centers. Many feared that if funding for these centers became part of a block grant to be administered by the states, the centers would not be considered priority items and their money ultimately would be curtailed. As it was proposed, however, the primary care block grant would be composed only of the community health centers program. For 1982, these centers remained under federal control but states had the option of assuming responsibility for them if they so desired. The federal government, however, retained the right to approve any proposed closure of these centers (Sorian, 1981). Whether ambulatory health services delivered to the underserved through these urban and rural centers would continue to grow and develop was not known.

The plight of migrant workers has long been a concern of the federal government. The 1962 Migrant Health Act authorized grants to state and local governments to provide services for this population group. After several amendments, the act was completely revised in 1975. The 1983 federal budget proposed that the Migrant Health Program retain its categorical status at least for the next three years.

Many of the programs and services so vital to minorities and the poor (such as alcohol abuse, drug abuse, mental health, and maternal and child health programs) were federally funded. Since the budget proposed an $8.5 billion reduction in health care through 1985, this certainly would have an impact on what services would be available to those in need, and in what quantity.

Professionals and Other Personnel

While there were inherent structural problems in the health delivery system that created barriers to access to care for minorities and the poor, the lack of health professionals available to provide these services was an increasing concern. Minority physicians historically have served primarily minority patients. The Health Careers Opportunity Program of the National Institutes of Health estimated that 85 percent of the visits made to black physicians were by black patients. Yet in 1975, only 5.7 percent of all medical students were black and only 2.8 percent were Hispanic (Foley, 1980).

Atencio (1972), in discussing access to medical training for minorities, noted that many minorities were disadvantaged because of inadequate primary and secondary schooling and they then had problems with the recruitment, selection and enrollment process of many medical schools. Financing medical education was a major problem. In some cases, minority students were unwilling for the most part to incur a large debt for their education and little other funding was available to help them once they had been admitted to medical schools.

For many years, the federal government helped increase the number of health professionals through programs developed to assist with the financing of medical and nursing education. The number of active physicians increased at a rate greater than the population growth during the decade of the 70s. Even so, there still were some 1,000 primary care shortage areas in the country—75 percent in rural settings, 25 percent in urban areas (representing 50 percent of the total population in all primary health care personnel shortage areas) (*Health, U.S.,* 1980; Foley, 1980).

In order to correct some of these geographic maldistribution problems, the government offered some remedies. The Emergency Health Personnel Act of 1970 (P.L. 91-623) created the National Health Service Corps (NHSC), a cadre of health providers who were federal employees assigned to give direct service to population groups in specifically identified areas of critical shortage.

Recruitment and retention of professional personnel became a major problem after the demise of the military draft. Physicians no longer regarded NHSC positions as an attractive alternative to serving two years in the military. To counteract this situation and to further entice people into underserved areas, a scholarship program was initiated. Both this effort and the National Health Service Corps have thus far survived the budget cuts.

In his Annual Message on Health in 1971, President Nixon endorsed the concepts of nurse practitioner and physician assistant. These nonphysician health providers were trained (at less cost and in a shorter time) to perform some services traditionally done by physicians. The hope was that they would move more readily into physician-shortage areas. The 1976 Health Professions Educational Assistance Act, P.L. 94-484, amended by the Health Services Extension Act of 1977, P.L. 95-83, provided funds specifically for programs preparing nurse practitioners for underserved areas.

Two issues that constrained the use of nurse practitioners were the legal restrictions imposed by state laws through practice acts and the difficulties in payment encountered because of restrictive reimbursement policies, particularly those of Medicare and Medicaid (*Health, U.S., 1980*). In spite of these difficulties, a 1979 study indicated that 23 percent of all nurse practitioners were in service in inner-city areas, 60 percent in other ambulatory care settings, 10 percent in health departments or home health agencies and 7 percent in other areas (Foley, 1980).

Area Health Education Centers (AHECs) were created in 1972 as another mechanism to improve access and health professional distribution in underserved areas. Established primarily in rural areas, they were designed specifically to provide decentralized training, education, and experience for health professionals in an effort to lessen the isolation they might otherwise experience. In addition, the AHECs were charged with increasing primary care training and encouraging more efficient utilization of such personnel. The FY 1983 federal budget gave AHECs at least three more years of life.

TODAY AND TOMORROW

Past federal policies have had an effect on the problems of access to health care by minorities and the poor. However, the shift in the basic approach from that of a concern for equity in the system to an emphasis on cost containment and organization may foretell a lessening of government involvement with these underserved populations. Thus far, the government has tried to intervene by providing some financial assistance to the poor and the elderly, offering specific programs, assisting with the development of ambulatory care services, increasing personnel generally and in underserved areas specifically, and trying to right some of the inequities in the system through the Community Service Amendments and the Civil Rights Commission. The likelihood of these efforts' continuing was speculative.

Other barriers to access fall into the categories of accommodation and acceptability in the Penchansky and Thomas proposed definition of "access."

Frequently, the health care agencies themselves, because of their organization and structure, create barriers in certain groups. Such factors as the location of the facility, hours of operation, clients' reception by the staff, waiting time, and the amount of time spent with the professionals, all have an impact on whether or not people seek and use health services appropriately. In addition, Christmas (1979) wrote: "Services provided to minorities are frequently inferior in quality . . . caused by overt or subtle discrimination, lack of cultural empathy, lack of a second language. . . ."

How health services are delivered by providers and how they are perceived by clients greatly influence how readily the public will accept assistance, and thus, ultimately, the extent to which the system answers their needs.

As the responsibility for providing the policy framework for determining methods to overcome barriers to access to care shifts to the states, counties, and cities, distinctions in quality of availability become clearer. These new arenas of struggle over increasingly shrinking resources are characterized by dynamic political activity. Coordination and collaboration between agencies providing care must increase because of this lack of resources and the need to meet clients' demands. Paradoxically, while this requirement was becoming stronger, these same providers found themselves in an adversary position as they began to compete for scarce resources.

Health services are considered a right by many. This right may dwindle and the services again may become a privilege of monied and informed consumers. Advocacy for the disenfranchised may or may not be taken up by the traditional activist organizations. Pressure tactics focused on hospital boards, city councils, county commissioners, and others in elected or appointed leadership positions could be expected to increase. Skill preparation for these predicted conflicts may be found deficient and the resulting frustration could form an additional barrier to care.

Problem-solving skills and willingness to include clients as legitimate participants with an interest in the process will be the focus of the future. Additional rounds of federal budget cuts could reduce the level of services and experiments to provide care even further. The costs in terms of potential urban rebellion and conflict, and the ambiguity over funds and over scarce resources, are problems. A lack of investment and equity in the health care system can create a critical situation.

Demands on professionals and the systems they operate will not go away because a president says, "It's time for government to get off the back of people" or because of less regulation. How will the holes be filled at the local level? Local and state coffers do not hold more than the federal purse. Creative solutions are few. Research utilization will receive less encouragement and support; evaluation work will be relied on less and less. Priorities will vary by locality, thereby decreasing the opportunity for institutional collaboration. This is not a good picture.

REFERENCES

Aday, L. *Achieving equity of access to the American health care system: An empirical look at the target groups*. Prepared for the U.S. Civil Rights Commission, April 1980. (Unpublished speech)

Atencio, A.C. *Access to medical training for minorities*. Paper presented at the American Association for the Advancement of Science, Washington, D.C., December 1972.

Berarducci, A.A. The federal government's role in ambulatory service development: A management perspective. *Journal of Ambulatory Care Management*, April 1978, pp. 1–12.

Christmas, J.J. How our health system fails minorities. *Health Pathways*, October 1979, *2*, 8.

Civil rights advocates angry. *The Chronicle of Higher Education*, July 27, 1981, *22*, 3.

Davis, K., & Reynolds, R. Medicare and the utilization of health care services by the elderly. *The Journal of Human Resources*, Summer 1975, *10*(3), 361–377.

Foley, H.A. *Civil rights issues in health care delivery*. Prepared for the U.S. Civil Rights Commission, Washington, D.C., April 1980. (Unpublished speech)

Health resources statistics, 1976–1977. Rockville, Md.: Department of Health, Education, and Welfare, National Center for Health Statistics, 1979, pp. 365–370.

Health, United States—1979. (Department of Health, Education, and Welfare, U.S. Public Health Service, Publication No. (PHS) 80-1232). Washington, D.C.: U.S. Government Printing Office, 1980, pp. 45–56.

Institute of Medicine. *Health care in the context of civil rights*. Washington, D.C.: National Academy Press, 1981.

Link, C.R., Long, S., & Settle, R. *Equality and the utilization of health services by the Medicare elderly*. Chicago: University of Chicago Graduate School of Business, Center for Health Administration Studies, 1980 (a) (Unpublished study).

Link, C.R., Long, S., & Settle, R. *Access to medical care under Medicaid: Differentials by race*. Chicago: University of Chicago Graduate School of Business, Center for Health Administration Studies, 1980 (b) (Unpublished study).

MacRae, D., Jr., & Wilde, J.A. *Policy analysis for public decisions*. North Scituate, Mass.: Duxbury Press, 1979, p. 3.

Office of Civil Rights. *Health care and civil rights*. Washington, D.C.: U.S. Department of Health, Education, and Welfare, Office of the Secretary, n. d. (Working paper)

Office of Program Planning and Evaluation. *The health of America's nonwhite population: Status report and future plans for dealing with diseases more prevalent or severe in nonwhites*. Rockville, Md.: U.S. Department of Health, Education, and Welfare, National Institutes of Health, November 11, 1971, p. 65 (mimeographed).

Palmer, P. Models in planning and operating health services. In S. Glass & R. Session (Eds.), *A guide to models: Governmental planning and operations*. Potomac, Md.: Sauger Books, 1975, p. 352.

Penchansky, P., & Thomas, T.W. The concept of access: Definition and relationship to consumer satisfaction. *Medical Care*, February 1981. *19*(2), 127–140.

Rivlin, A.M. Social policy: Alternative strategies for the federal government. In R.H. Haveman & J. Margolis (Eds.), *Public expenditures and policy analysis* (2nd ed.). Chicago: Rand McNally College Publishing Company, 1977, pp. 357–384.

Salber, E., & Beza, A.G. The health interview survey and minority health. *Medical Care*, March 1980, *18*(3), 319–326.

Sheps, C.G., & Bachar, M. Rural areas and personal health services: Current strategies. *American Journal of Public Health*, January 1981 (Supplement), pp. 71–82.

Sorian, R. Most programs cut: Some retain identity. *The Nation's Health*, American Public Health Association, September 1981, *11*(9), 1, 16.

Vital and health statistics series, 1962–1979. Data from the Health Interview Survey, series 10 (128), 1975, 53 pp. Rockville, Md.: Department of Health, Education, and Welfare, National Center for Health Statistics, April 1975.

Chapter 5

The Role of Health Planning in the Delivery of Personal Health Services

Harry T. Phillips

This chapter assesses the role of planning in the delivery of personal health services by means of a historical summary of the evolution of the structure, functions, and outcomes of such planning in recent years; a review of selected related major issues; and consideration of possible future directions.

There are many definitions of planning, the simplest of which is "advance thinking as a basis of doing" (Sigmond, 1967). Another is that planning is "scientific problem solving" consisting of the rational process of problem definition, analysis, establishment of goals, projection of implementation, and evaluation (Moore, 1973). However, in the context in which planning for personal health services occurs, there is a mix of both the rational and advocacy. The rational approach assumes that there is a best, most efficient, logical solution to the problem that can be developed by expert planners. The advocacy model assumes that the alternative solutions involve choosing among the value preferences of competing interest groups, which is a political process (Browne, 1981).

Health planning has been seen in recent years as a mechanism for solving problems and resolving issues in the delivery of services. In the context of this chapter, the term refers only to personal health services and excludes the very large number of interventions on a public or personal basis that affect the environment, group behavior, and many other aspects of society that influence the health of the population. Planning for personal health services is of special importance because of the disproportionate inflation in the cost of medical care and the deep involvement of government in the delivery system; it is important also because most of this is paid for, through complex fiscal mechanisms, by bodies accountable to taxpayers or subscribers to health insurance programs.

While planning for the delivery of services obviously has been a function of public and community health agencies for many years, only recently has the process been made explicit, and so labeled and promoted. Every budget of a public agency is a reflection, conscious or unconscious, of projected action for an ensuing period. In this chapter, however, the focus is on freestanding agencies established with the express purpose of planning for personal health services, and not merely units of governmental agencies that develop plans for the agencies as a staff function.

Political expectations of the capability of this planning strategy gradually escalated in the decades after World War II, reached a peak in the mid-1970s, and have declined since. In the 1980s, the health planning program, together with numerous other social and political efforts developed in the two preceding decades, was undergoing severe modification and faced possible extinction.

PRECURSORS TO PLANNING

In the broadest sense of the term "health services," large-scale planning has gone on in the United States since the very earliest days of the founding of the nation. As an example, when the United States Public Health Service Marine Hospitals were established in 1798 in response to the needs of merchant ships' crews, plans for the delivery of personal health services were of a nature very similar to those in use today in prepaid group practice: beneficiaries were required to pay weekly sums of money in advance to obtain medical care, when the need arose, through an organized series of facilities and services.

An early model for the rational planning of health services was provided by the *Interim Report on the Future Provision of Medical and Allied Services,* commonly referred to as the "Dawson Report" after the chairman of the reporting body, Lord Dawson. This document (Dawson, 1920), published in England, had much appeal to would-be reformers in both the United States and Britain because it projected a regional and rational approach to the organization of facilities and personnel. However, it took a disastrous economic depression, a Second World War, and 26 years to reorganize the delivery of health services in Britain along the lines of this report. Although some degree of regionalization is called for in the planning goals in the United States as well, very little progress has been made in that direction in this country.

Probably every review of the health care situation in the United States for 50 years has recommended a plan or projection of some kind for improved organization and delivery of services. However, the earliest proposal for establishing planning agencies with responsibility to assess needs for local populations and to develop rational responses to those needs was contained in the report of the Committee on the Cost of Medical Care (CCMC) published in 1932. This committee was sponsored and/or supported by a wide range of private foundations, professional associations and governmental agencies. It recommended that:

> In each community, permanent, local agencies should be established to evaluate and coordinate the existing preventive and curative medical services, to eliminate services not needed, and to stimulate the provision of additional services which are needed. Such agencies should make a continuing study of the problems of organization and payment and should prepare a plan for progressive development. They should include representatives of the public, the medical professions, the health agencies, the hospitals, and the social agencies. They may well grow out of existing health and hospital councils or public health councils. Sufficient funds should be provided for executive and secretarial service. Funds or services may be provided by community chests, chambers of commerce, and local governmental or voluntary agencies. (p. 135)

The CCMC also proposed the establishment of similar coordinating agencies for states, which in addition could regionalize their activities by dividing states into several districts. The economic circumstances of the Depression undoubtedly stimulated these proposals.

In the years following World War II the idea of planning for the organization and delivery of personal health services on a systems basis grew steadily, largely the result of burgeoning medical technology, growth of specialization, and a concomitant rise in costs and government involvement.

PLANNING FOR HEALTH CARE—1946–1974

The first nationally supported program in which planning was promoted in a deliberate way was the Hospital Survey and Construction Act of 1946, P.L. 79-725, the Hill-Burton Act. Its essential features were:

1. Each state was to designate a single state agency to implement the act.
2. The agency was to conduct a periodic survey of hospital beds within the state.

3. The state agency was to make a projection of needs based upon numerical standards, using population growth and past utilization of services, and was to make allowances for such factors as the rurality of the population.
4. Each agency was to establish priorities for construction in the substate regions based upon the survey findings and the estimated needs.
5. The state agency was to apply established standards for acceptability and for construction.
6. The federal government was to provide funds to match other monies for hospital construction and modernization.

In subsequent years, numerous amendments and initiatives broadened the scope of the act:

1954: Amendments included nursing homes, diagnostic and treatment centers, rehabilitation facilities, and chronic disease facilities. (P.L. 83-482, Amendments to Hospital Survey and Constitution Act)

1959 to 1962: Hill-Burton program officials were involved in a series of ad hoc joint committees, some of which were cosponsored by the American Hospital Association, to develop areawide planning principles.

1961: Demonstration grants were given for areawide planning. (P.L. 87-395, Community Health Services and Facilities Act of 1961)

1964: The Hill-Harris amendments authorized project grants for comprehensive health planning at metropolitan and areawide levels. (P.L. 88-443, Hospital and Medical Facilities Amendments of 1964). These funds gave additional support for preexisting hospital planning efforts in several metropolitan areas such as Rochester, New York City, Detroit, Chicago, and elsewhere.

For more than a quarter of a century the Hill-Burton program was instrumental in channeling large sums of money into all of the states and in stimulating the growth of many small and large hospitals and other facilities for the delivery of health services. It also was instrumental in stimulating the early growth of areawide planning for health care. (Hill-Burton as an entity died when it and other measures were folded into the new National Health Planning and Resources Development Act of 1974, P.L. 93-641, discussed in detail later. In retrospect, however, Hill-Burton was criticized on the grounds that it stimulated the construction of too many small, inefficient facilities and that it had little or no effect on the coordination of the various components of the delivery system.)

Community Health Services

Simultaneously with these developments, voluntary and governmental agencies began to express the need for improving the organization of health services. To this end a National Commission on Community Health Services was established in 1962, sponsored jointly by the American Public Health Association and the National Health Council and supported by contributions from private foundations, industry, government, and business. The Commission reported on various aspects of community health care and, among other recommendations, proposed the establishment of mechanisms for action planning in health that "should be communitywide in area, continuous in nature, comprehensive in scope, all-inclusive in design, coordinative in function, and adequately staffed" (National Commission, 1966). This idealistic statement is a reflection of the utopianism of the times. The commission had a major influence on the rapid acceptance of the health planning legislation that was adopted shortly after the publication of its reports.

Regional Medical Programs

Another thrust in a similar direction was mounted in the form of the Commission on Heart Disease, Cancer, and Stroke established in 1963 by President Kennedy. It reported in 1965, recommending ways to improve the effective application of the fruits of medical research. This report resulted in the passage of the Heart Disease, Cancer, and Stroke Amendments to the Public Health Service Act of 1965, P.L. 89-239, generally referred to as The Regional Medical Programs Act. The structural outcome of this act was the establishment of 56 regional medical programs (RMPs) covering the whole country, with the purpose of developing cooperative arrangements built around the medical centers. RMPs were required first to assess health care needs in their areas and then to respond by generating plans for improving the delivery of services through such methods as training of personnel and dissemination of new developments in the field. The law prohibited interference with the private practice of medicine.

Regional plans were reviewed and, if approved, funded by the federal government. With the passing of the years, however, the federal priorities and goals were changed in response to political pressures. The RMP program terminated with the passing of P.L. 93-641, the National Health Planning and Resources Development Act of 1974. Regionalization of health services was one of the goals of the new legislation.

Comprehensive Health Planning Agencies

In 1966 the first legislation to establish separate free-standing agencies for systems planning was passed in the form of the Comprehensive Health Planning and Public Services Amendments Act, P.L. 89-749. This law promoted the concept of a partnership between governmental and voluntary agencies in planning for health services. As in the regional medical programs law, an important stipulation was that there be no interference with existing patterns of professional practice. The act required each state to establish a state health planning agency and provided federal funds for the establishment of substate comprehensive health planning agencies (CHPAs). The substate agencies were not required but could be funded if suitable applications were made to the federal government by a range of nonprofit organizations. At both the state and local levels the organizations were to be advised by boards having a majority of "consumers" of health services, "consumers" being defined as nonproviders.

The CHPAs had limited power, small budgets, and often covered areas too small to sustain significant plans or service delivery systems. Moreover, by the end of their existence, when they, too, were merged into P.L. 93-641, they covered only 70 percent of the country's geographic area and were poorly supported by federal initiatives. For example, regulations governing the planning agencies still were labeled "provisional" six years after passage of the law. Most of the CHP entities were successors to preexisting health and welfare councils or health facility planning agencies, established by Hill-Burton funds; on the whole, these latter continued to function in the ways to which they had been accustomed in their previous coordinating roles.

It was generally agreed that the health planning that came out of the CHPAs was not effective. The major benefits were the lessons learned from the experience, such as that voluntary planning was ineffective, health planning without teeth was futile, the science and art of planning were primitive, expectations needed to be made explicit, and planning had to be more structured organizationally and functionally. If planning was to be more effective, a stronger law must be enacted.

P.L. 93-641—PLANNING WITH TEETH

The next step in the legislative evolution of comprehensive health planning was the passage of the National Health Planning and Resources Development Act of 1974, P.L. 93-641 (U.S. Congress, 1975). This replaced the functions of three existing laws—the Hill-Burton Act, the Regional

Medical Programs Act, and the Comprehensive Health Planning Act. The major justification for its passage was that the laws it replaced had accomplished their purpose or had been unsuccessful and therefore no longer were required. Moreover, there was a need to have some strong planning capacity in the country to prepare the way for the then apparently imminent national health insurance program.

The preamble to the act stated in effect that the achievement of equal access to quality health care at a reasonable cost was a priority of the federal government; that the massive infusion of federal funds had contributed to inflation in the cost of health care; and that the many and increasing responses by the public and private sectors had not resulted in a rational approach to solving the problems of access, maldistribution of services, and increasing cost of care. A major assumption in the law was that health planning was the solution or logical approach to resolving these problems. In reaction to the vagueness of the preceding comprehensive health planning act, the new one spelled out many details and laid down a rigorous timetable for implementation of the various parts.

Provisions of the Act

Briefly, the major provisions of the law were as follows:

Primary and final responsibility for implementing the act was vested in the Secretary of the Department of Health, Education, and Welfare (DHEW) (now the Department of Health and Human Services). The secretary was to establish by regulation guidelines for a national health planning policy, including standards for the appropriate supply, distribution, and organization of health resources. The law established ten priorities to be considered by the planning agencies in developing health system plans for their areas, addressing the needs for:

1. primary care for the underserved
2. coordination of health services
3. development of medical group practices
4. use of physician extenders
5. sharing of support services
6. improvement in the quality of care
7. assurance that patients were receiving appropriate levels of care
8. disease prevention measures
9. uniform reporting systems
10. health education of the public.

Amendments in 1979, P.L. 96-79, added additional priorities that addressed the need for: (1) promotion of competition where appropriate, (2) adoption of policies to contain costs through technology and more appropriate use of resources, and (3) more efficient use and improvement of mental health services.

DHEW was to establish a national advisory council on health planning to advise, consult with, and make recommendations to the secretary on the development of national guidelines, implementation and administration of the act, and evaluation of the implications of new medical technology for the distribution of health care services.

Each governor was to establish geographic regions appropriate for the effective planning and development of health services. These areas were to cover a population of between half a million and 3 million people and were to include at least one medical center for highly specialized health services. (Exceptions could be made under special circumstances because of population size.) In each area a health systems agency (HSA) was to be established to serve as the planning body at the local substate level. The HSA legally could be one of several kinds of organization, including an extension of local government. However, in effect, the vast majority turned out to be nonprofit private corporations.

The size of an HSA's governing body and its composition were described in some detail, but the method by which members were to be appointed, selected, or elected was not specified. A majority of the governing body, but not more than 60 percent, were to be consumers, that is, individuals who had no financial connection with the delivery of health services either directly or through members of their immediate family. The consumers were to be broadly representative of the various subgroups of the population in the area with respect to social, economic, linguistic, racial, and geographic characteristics. The rest of the members were to be health care providers and were to include a specified proportion of direct providers such as physicians, dentists, and nurses. Also to be included as either consumers or providers were publicly elected officials and other members of units of general-purpose local government.

The governing body was to have responsibility for maintaining the HSA's internal affairs and for approving its actions with regard to its regulatory functions. HSAs also were responsible for developing and maintaining health systems plans and annual implementation plans for their service areas. These were to be based on reviews of the needs and resources of the population and region served. Plans were to be reviewed periodically and updated, and the HSA was to implement them by assisting individuals in public and private entities to develop services, giving technical assistance when necessary, and assisting in the planning and development of projects and programs with Area Health Services Development Funds. (These funds never were made available to the HSAs.) HSAs also were to coordinate their efforts with other planning agencies and entities in the area.

The HSAs were to review proposals for new services or changes in existing ones—in some cases to approve or disapprove them, in other instances to recommend approval or disapproval to the state planning agency or to the federal government. HSAs also were to review periodically certain existing services in the area and to make recommendations to the state agency regarding their appropriateness. They were to review and make recommendations to the state planning agencies as to the need for new institutional health services and the appropriateness of existing services in its area.

HSAs were to be reviewed by the federal government on a recurring basis on the extent to which the health of residents of the area had improved; the accessibility, continuity, and quality of health services had advanced; increases in the cost of providing health services had been restrained; unnecessary duplication of health resources had been prevented; and resources that met identified needs had been promoted and developed.

The secretary in each fiscal year was to make a grant to each HSA, the amount to be determined by the population size of the area, with a basic minimum for the smallest area.

The governor of each state was to designate a state health planning and development agency (SHPDA) for administering the state's program developed in accordance with federal regulations and guidelines. The SHPDA was to serve as staff to a statewide health coordinating council (SHCC), with a majority of members drawn from the governing bodies of HSAs, together with others appointed by the governor. The function of the SHCC was to advise the state planning agency. Each state agency was to administer a certificate-of-need program (CON) that conformed to federal regulations. (These regulations were modified in both 1979 and 1981—Health Planning and Resources Development Amendments of 1979 (P.L. 96-79), and Omnibus Budget Reconciliation Act of 1981 (P.L. 97-35)). The SHCC also was to review the appropriateness of all institutional health services within the state not less often than every five years and to act on the recommendations of the HSAs on laws and regulations requiring action by the HSAs.

SHCCs were to review and coordinate annually the plans of the HSAs and assist in the development of integrated state health plans. Based on the HSAs' plans, the SHCC also was required to review annually the budget of each agency and to recommend approval or disapproval of the state plans and applications submitted under various sections of the act. Final approval of the state plan was the prerogative of the governor. (This listing is abbreviated and simplified. Full information can be found in the original law, amendments, and regulations.)

As in the case of the HSAs, the federal government was to provide financial support for the state planning agencies. In Title XVI of P.L. 93-641, Health Resources Development, states were to administer a much reduced Hill-Burton function, mainly for modernizing existing health facilities and assisting in removing safety hazards.

Implementation and Evaluation of P.L. 93-641

From the preamble, it is evident that the authors of the legislation were most ambitious. However, a number of major implicit assumptions were made by Congress, the most important of which were:

- Health planning can alleviate the problems of access, costs, and quality of care.
- Health planning will lead to regional arrangements that can increase efficiency of care delivery.
- Community needs in the health care system can be quantified.
- The increase in the cost of care can be contained through control of capital expenditures.
- Voluntary nonprofit planning bodies with little or no connection with local government can be effective instruments for implementing the goals of a national planning policy.
- Plans for health service delivery in these areas can be implemented without strong regulatory and/or financial control.
- The numerical superiority of consumers of health care in decision-making bodies in health planning agencies will overcome the dominance of providers.
- The federal government and its executive branch can carry out efficiently the long list of tasks assigned to it by the law.

The expectations of the federal agency (Department of Health, Education, and Welfare) were extensive. To quote one critic, Congress expected

> The Secretary to: designate health service areas; design a system for judiciously considering applications from potential health system agencies; effectively discriminate among different kinds of HSAs to weed out poor performance; establish national goals and standards for health system improvement; specify essential characteristics of an effective state certificate-of-need program; provide technical assistance to all health planning agencies in

need thereof; follow the federal government's fundamental dictate to ensure quality (if necessary, at the expense of efficiency) by forcing adequate representation of all consumer interests in all the decision-making processes; continually monitor and reevaluate the performance of every component in this complex system to ensure that each was performing its set of tasks effectively; and if possible, carry out all these tasks with full sensitivity to the needs of state and local governments. Incredibly enough, that is an understated simplification of what the planning law actually requires on the part of the federal government. (Cain, 1981)

P.L. 93-64 was not the epitome of health planning. However, it was the most ambitious development in the evolution of health planning as a national program aimed at solving or reducing the problems surrounding the delivery of health services. It was hoped that it would be the instrument for solving the problem of unequal access, inefficiency, and rapidly expanding health services public budgets.

While almost all the literature on the health planning law has given it mixed reviews, some have been more positive, optimistic, or perhaps sympathetic (Rosenfeld & Rosenfeld, 1975; Werlin, 1976; Klarman, 1978; Institute of Medicine, 1981), while others have exhibited various levels of negativism (Vladeck, 1977; Kinzer, n.d.; Havighurst, 1980; Brown, 1981; Browne, 1981). It is evident that health planning in the 1970s was not seen as an unqualified success.

Supporters claimed that HSAs justified their existence through applying the certificate-of-need laws, improving the health care system, and promoting community and professional education (American Health Planning Association, 1979). These claims are not easy to substantiate or measure, and it probably is true that "making impact evaluations of health planning is very difficult and may not produce clear evidence concerning the successes or shortcomings of health planning organizations" (U.S. Comptroller General, 1981).

Whatever the arguments on either side, the Reagan Administration took the view that health planning, as conducted under P.L. 93-641, should be phased out.

No matter which way resources for health care are allocated in the future, it would be wasteful if the performance of the planning efforts of the past were not examined and evaluated.

Performance under the act can be evaluated on at least three levels—the structure for planning, the process of planning, and the outcomes of the process.

More than 50 state planning agencies (SHPDAs) were established in the states, territories, and the District of Columbia with programs based on perceived deficiencies and aimed at controlling changes or growth in health facilities and services. More than 200 areawide planning agencies (HSAs), covering the whole country, were established with the aim of applying rational approaches to systems planning at the regional level. As a consequence of the formation of these structures, 50,000 persons across the country became involved in reviewing the development of systems plans for their areas (Foley, 1981). To accomplish this, the staffs of the agencies, consumers, and providers serving on the governing boards and committees that were reviewing proposals were brought together for discussion, negotiation, and decision making. The areas' perceived needs and resources were made explicit; in many cases, efforts to rationalize the development and deployment of services were effective, which usually meant slowing down the expansion of resources.

Health planning was given a forward thrust by P.L. 93-641. In satisfying the requirements for certificate-of-need approval, proponents of new programs were compelled to demonstrate that they conformed to certain criteria that related to an overall system plan. Although many slippages occurred in the process, it was inevitable that many agencies and institutions for the first time were forced to think in terms of the total delivery system for the area rather than in simply promoting institutional ambitions.

As noted earlier, developing health system plans (HSPs) for the health service area was a function of the HSAs. These documents are important starting points for the process of planning.

According to a review of approved HSPs by the U.S. General Accounting Office in 1979, these plans were inadequate in a number of ways: goals often were not measurable, recommended actions poorly developed, and resource requirements unspecified. According to the report, some of these and other criticisms were rejected by the Bureau of Health Planning and the American Health Planning Association (Comptroller General, 1981). Nevertheless, an important step was taken in initiating a democratic process for choice among alternative modes of personal health services.

Guidelines for planning also were products of the law. When these guidelines eventually were developed, they provoked major criticisms from both opponents and proponents of the act and its regulatory responsibilities. Both locally and nationally important initiatives were taken, and lessons learned that are discussed more fully next.

Interest in the effect of the certificate-of-need laws, the main regulatory instrument available to health planners, preceded the passage of P.L. 93-641. In a number of states such laws had been in place for several years. Salkever and Bice (1976) and Lewin and associates (1975) reported that the certificate-of-need laws had not controlled the overall costs of care. However, their data were based on events before 1974, when the national planning act was enacted. Subsequent studies reported that regulation under certificates of need had been effective in reducing unnecessary investment in medical care (American Health Planning Association, 1979).

MAJOR ISSUES RAISED BY P.L. 93-641

Even during its developmental period, the act stimulated controversy. Its authors were determined to avoid what they perceived as the weakness of past laws and to profit from the lessons learned from problems of implementation. The final version of the act gave the federal government little flexibility as it sought to avoid repetition of the previous vagueness in structure and of delays in carrying out the functions of the planning agencies. The law also favored the establishment of nonprofit private planning agencies, independent of existing state and local governmental units, thereby expressing the legislators' distrust of political processes at these levels (Raab, 1981).

Several interest groups were perturbed by the act, during both its genesis and its implementation. Foremost among these were organized medicine and the state and local governments (Raab, 1981). These groups exercised their influence in the writing of the 1974 law, in the preparation of regulations in subsequent years, in amending the law in 1979, and in effectively lobbying the Reagan administration thereafter, with the result that federal appropriations for health planning were greatly reduced.

Controversy centered on three broad areas:

1. The structure of the planning units, particularly at the local level. This was criticized from two directions:
   a. Local and state governments felt they had been largely bypassed by the law. These criticisms were softened by the amendments enacted in 1979 (P.L. 96-79), which gave greater recognition to the existing political structures at the lower levels.
   b. Consumers' effectiveness in influencing the law was questioned by many of their groups. Dissatisfaction was manifested in numerous criticisms questioning the way the law was written and implemented. In a number of instances, issues were taken to court for decision. An example is *Texas ACORN et al. v. Texas Area V Health Systems Agency, et al.* (C.A. No. 5-76-102-CA). Here, the issue was whether it was legal for the 41 consumer representatives to include only those whose incomes were below the median for

the area ($10,000) (Marmor and Morone, 1979). As a consequence of this and similar cases, federal regulations regarding board composition were modified so that membership became broadly rather than precisely representative of the population served.

2. The role of voluntary, nonprofit agencies in the regulatory process. This also was viewed from two directions:

    a. Existing public agencies objected on the ground that the HSAs were not "accountable" to the public and therefore should not be given regulatory powers.

    b. The agencies that were subject to the regulatory process, such as hospitals, objected to the linkage of planning with regulation. (These regulatory issues are reviewed later.)

3. The expected outcomes of the planning process. For a variety of reasons, the expectations raised by politicians, the federal government, and others were not satisfied. (This is also discussed later.)

SOME CONTROVERSIAL AREAS

During the writing of the law (1974) and in amending it (1979), there was considerable feeling on the part of local governments that their powers as elected political entities were being undermined by voluntary agencies. Moreover, they felt they were not being represented adequately in the governing bodies of the nonprofit voluntary agency boards. The National Association of Counties adopted a policy statement that criticized the way many of the HSA boards were constituted and were made self-perpetuating by their own nominating committees. This was corrected in the 1979 amendments, which stipulated that not less than half of the planning agency board members were to represent bodies unconnected with the HSA itself, thereby reducing their self-perpetuating nature.

The National Governors' Conference (in 1979 the National Governors' Conference changed its name to the National Governors' Association) also was critical of the original act. Governors felt they were being bypassed in many areas by decisions that went directly from HSAs to the federal government. Again, much of this dissatisfaction was eliminated in the 1979 amendments, which increased the powers of the governors in several directions. Because funding and control came essentially from Washington to the SHPDAs and HSAs, they thus were accountable largely to the federal government. Although much of the responsibility for deciding whether the state agencies and HSAs were conforming was delegated to the ten regional offices of DHHS, the central office (the Bureau of Health Planning) had a continuing responsibility to monitor the subordinate agencies.

This kind of arrangement was bound to produce tensions between the different layers of government. A proportion of the regulatory decisions was made at the state level, and it was inevitable that when they were disliked by influential proponents of certificate-of-need programs, political pressure would be brought to bear upon the state government. In at least one state, Massachusetts, disgruntled proponents were able to use the legislature to pass laws that applied to their particular situation in order to reverse a state planning agency decision.

Relations between the state planning agencies and the HSAs varied considerably among the states. Problems arose particularly where states had single HSAs and the roles of the two agencies tended to overlap. In some of these cases (e.g., Rhode Island) the state agency assumed all the functions of the HSA, which then was eliminated.

HSAs were required to develop health system plans that would be amenable to coordination with the state's other health systems plans so that a single statewide program could be developed. This was not easy for the state planning agencies since many HSAs had difficulty in complying with the standards or formats used by the former.

A continuing problem in some states was that some HSAs were more competent (or thought they were) than the SHPDAs. This tended to occur in very large HSAs with high funding levels and skilled leadership. In part, this was a result of the restrictions on salaries paid in state governments as compared with those in private, nonprofit HSAs.

With the passage of P.L. 93-641, planning and regulation were integrated, a step considered desirable by some (Somers & Somers, 1977; Klarman, 1978) and undesirable by others (Havighurst, 1980). The regulatory function of the health planning system provoked the opposition of many powerful parties, which probably was the main reason for the decision by the Reagan Administration to weaken if not dismantle the law.

THE ROLE OF REGULATION

The role of regulation in the planning process needs to be clarified. Regulation has become an abomination in the minds of many, even among those who profess to approve of areawide planning. Foremost among the latter are representatives of hospitals who advocate planning without regulation.

"Planning" under P.L. 93-641 was supposed to consist basically of assessing the health status of the population, reviewing the resources available, developing health status or health system goals, considering alternative objectives, selecting feasible strategies for achieving the goals, promoting methods for implementation of the strategies, and monitoring the effects of these interventions. All of these were to be achieved through negotiation and discussion among the consumers, providers, and staffs of agencies.

Regulation in the HSAs and state planning agencies related mainly to the certificate-of-need laws enacted by the states and to Section 1122 of the Social Security Act Amendments of 1972, a federal law with similar purposes and procedures. P.L. 93-641 required all the states to adopt certificate-of-need laws that conformed to certain basic federal standards by a specified date. Both the federal and the state laws aimed to restrain "unnecessary" investment in health services.

In addition, HSAs and state planning agencies were given roles in the regulation of proposed use of federal funds for delivery of a variety of health programs and in reviewing and making recommendations on the appropriateness of existing services within their geographical areas of responsibility.

Regulation under the law had multiple functions. Many of the federal regulations related only to the establishment, structure, and functioning of the SHPDAs and HSAs and affected the delivery of services only indirectly. Other regulations, such as the Standards Respecting the Appropriate Supply, Distribution and Organization of Health Resources, had a direct impact on the delivery system. Similarly, the state regulations for certificate-of-need implementation had a direct bearing on service providers. These kinds of regulations raised the resistance, if not the anger, of a large proportion of the provider groups.

While the planning function is generally prospective and proactive, regulation has a reactive function. However, regulations affecting this delivery system could not be written without implicit or explicit planning goals or objectives in mind; approved areawide plans provided the legal basis for reviewing proposals for change. Theoretically, the individual proposal was like a piece in a jigsaw puzzle that might fit into a broader picture—the health systems plan.

If it is assumed that plans are made to be implemented, the limited powers given to the HSAs to actually execute the plans they develop was a major deficiency in the law. Regulation is only one of several instruments to promote implementation. Potential tactics included cooperation between the providers or controllers of resources and the HSA in developing the plan, the provision of technical assistance by the HSA, education and logical persuasion, and public involvement. Although regulation mainly had the negative thrust of constraint, it also could be an educational instrument in that proponents of review programs were required to prepare structured proposals that conformed to accepted criteria and standards.

This process encouraged negotiation between the parties at the local level and could have a beneficial effect (Fein, 1977).

It thus can be seen that planning and regulation had complementary functions. Without regulatory support, implementation would follow plan development only infrequently unless other powerful incentives, such as financial rewards, existed.

Critics of the health planning system included such influential provider groups as the American Medical Association, whose governing body recommended that P.L. 93-641 be repealed because of what it regarded as its excessive regulation and centralization. Individuals in many other provider groups felt that if there was to be planning, it should be on a voluntary basis, with regulatory powers limited or eliminated; their sentiment was that local groups knew what was best for their areas and should be given freedom to act independently of any federal interference.

This point of view was represented primarily by Havighurst, who contended that if health planning were to be efficient it would have to be more centralized and, of necessity, arbitrary. This efficiency could be brought about only at the expense of such important values as individual freedom of choice (Havighurst, 1980).

The extent to which regulation by government was resented and resisted was illustrated by the outpouring of 55,000 letters of protest when the proposed national guidelines for health planning were published in 1978. These guidelines were to include standards on the appropriate supply, distribution, and organization of health resources—for example, ratios for hospital beds per 1,000 population; desirable occupancy rates; and utilization rates for obstetrical, pediatric, and other specialized services such as open-heart surgery, radiation therapy, and hemodialysis. It should be emphasized that these proposed standards were not mandated and could be adjusted for an area if justified by certain conditions. The national guidelines, together with the standards established by state certificate-of-need laws, were the most controversial of the components of health planning legislation. The proposed guidelines subsequently were modified and promulgated (*National Guidelines,* 1978).

Regulation in health planning also was faulted because it failed to achieve the major purpose of the law as perceived by the bureaucrats and politicians—the containment of costs of medical care. HSAs generally were faced with the task of approving or recommending approval or disapproval of projects under review. However, since their boards and staffs reflected the interests of individuals more concerned with access and quality, containment of costs was rarely the overriding consideration.

It is impossible to assess the effect of health planning and regulation on the costs of care. All that is known is that these expenditures inflated at a rate higher than the Consumer Price Index. What would have happened in the absence of P.L. 93-641 can only be guessed.

A comprehensive review of the performance of the agencies under P.L. 93-641 was provided by the Committee on Health Planning Goals and Standards established by the Institute of Medicine. Among the recommendations of this body was the following:

> That the limitations of HSAs in reducing health care expenditures be recognized, because unrealistic expectations are likely to lead to the conclusion that the program has not succeeded. The Committee recommends that the planning agencies be judged according to a broad set of measures including measures of improvement in access, quality, and equity, not only cost moderation. The broad strategy is more suited to the statutory mandate. . . .

> The intermediate measures of effectiveness should include: whether the HSA provides a useful forum for public policy discussion; whether it serves as a source of information about local health care problems and steps being taken to deal with them; whether it has credibility in the community; whether appropriate data and analytical methods are being employed as a basis for conclusions; whether the HSA is serving as an effective agency in helping to improve the health services received by the public and promoting health care for the area's residents at an acceptable level of cost; whether health care consumers and providers are being involved in improving the system; and whether the HSA is catalyzing problems of the underserved or underrepresented . . . . (Institute of Medicine, 1980, p. 57)

These recommendations were made and published at a time when the support for health planning as prescribed by P.L. 93-641 was already fading.

RESIDUAL QUESTIONS ON HEALTH PLANNING

A number of philosophical, political, and administrative questions need to be addressed.

Was P.L. 93-641 Really Given an Adequate Trial?

Health planning is an example of collectivism, a strategy that runs counter to the high value this country places on individualism. The real lack of enthusiasm demonstrated by Congress was that at the highest level of funding the planning effort never reached above 75 cents per capita while expenditures for delivering personal health services approached $1,000 per capita. The ratio spent on planning for the system was less than 0.1 percent of the cost of operating it. No rational enterprise would devote so little when the ultimate product was costing so much.

This should not suggest that money per se would have made health planning more effective. But the science and art of planning still are rudimentary and exceedingly difficult in the pluralistic shopping mall that constitutes the health care system. Far more should have been invested in developing the science and art of health planning and in providing assistance to agencies whose limited competence had little influence on improving the delivery and efficiency of health care. A simple illustration of the impact of limited funding was the constant drain of effective staff members from planning agencies into regulated entities such as hospitals, hospital associations, and other major deliverers of health care.

Another example of the lack of support was Congress' decision not to appropriate funds authorized in P.L. 93-641 for the Area Health Services Development Fund intended to support the planning and developing projects and programs. These funds should have been provided to initiate the planning and implementation process and would have been one of the few instruments that HSAs could have used to implement the programs they had developed.

A major limitation for successful health planning is the enormous number of independent decision makers in the system. Among the decision makers who affect the delivery of health care are more than 300,000 practicing physicians, 6,000 hospitals, and 20,000 nursing homes, to name only a few. When powerful groups come together, it becomes very difficult to impose restraints or to promote alternatives for delivering care if the planners and the government lack strong legal authority and influence. The national unwillingness to push planning further is a result of the high value the public places on individual freedom and the lesser value placed on efficiency. The latter can be enhanced only by reducing the ability of individual care providers to act on their own. It also is an unpleasant fact of life that the outcomes of social planning in the United States seldom have been what was hoped for, even when the plans were strongly supported at the outset (Pressman & Wildavsky, 1973).

Is Health Planning Possible or Desirable?

This question is raised by those who would like to define health planning in terms of economics, social engineering, rational responses to epidemiological findings, predictive value, and similar objective and scientific measures. These questioners (Anderson, 1971; Wildavsky, 1976) emphasized that regional or community health planning—if defined as a scientific, rational economic process—was not possible in the context of the United States today with its emphasis on free choice, competition, political action, organized pressure groups, and pluralism.

The goals of health planning often are competitive, if not contradictory, and very frequently are utopian, as can be seen in the expectations set before the agencies implementing P.L. 93-641. On the other hand, if health planning, American style, is seen as a democratic process depending largely on input from consumers, providers, and staff at the local level, reconciling political and technological aspects of health care, and leading up to a consensus on what is acceptable at that level, then the system can be considered feasible.

One of the problems faced by all industrialized countries is that the cost of health care is rising rapidly and there are no objective standards for what is an appropriate expenditure. Is 8 percent of the GNP appropriate? Or 9 percent? Or 10 percent? Or what is the "right" figure? As a result of the Medicare and Medicaid laws passed in the 1960s, which bear the major blame for the inordinate rise in costs of care, a large number of disadvantaged persons who had not previously received health services now were receiving them.

Considering the growth of the population, and particularly of the older segments, the need for judicious use of new medical technology, for modernization, and, in many facilities, for the removal of safety hazards (not to mention general inflation), it is not surprising that the total national cost of health care escalated in the last few decades. In the final analysis, the amount of health care the nation believes it can afford is basically a value judgment and a matter of political decision. It also is a matter of how willing the country is to transfer wealth from the affluent to the poor in the form of government-supported health care programs.

Whether or not to have a national health planning system has become an issue because such a large proportion of the total expenditures on health care—40 percent—is now in the public domain. If spending money on health services were like spending on the acquisition of television sets (which has risen far more rapidly in the last 20 years) there would be no controversy. Since today's culture demands that needed health care be provided whether or not individuals can afford to pay the costs, at least some part of this process must be made a public matter.

The nation is concerned mainly because the public portion of the health bill has been rising so rapidly. How this issue is resolved is a political process. Health planning was only one of several strategies suggested or used to restrain inflation of the health bill. (President Carter supported a cap on expenditures, and a voluntary effort was supported by the American Hospital Association, but none of these worked.)

Is Health Planning Desirable or Feasible?

Apart from the feasibility of planning, is the investment in planning cost effective? Is it worth the trouble? One reason for doing away with health planning is that in the short term it could save the taxpayers, not to mention health care providers, a few hundred million dollars annually. It could be argued that in the long run taxpayers and consumers might have to pay more for the delivery of services if health planning agencies were abolished. However, many politicians wanted to reduce the federal budget as soon as possible, which could well be a good reason in the short run for getting rid of the planning structures.

However, there also are strong philosophical reasons for not having a planning system such as that established under P.L. 93-641. Even though the law allowed for a great deal of action at the local level, it provided for the establishment of national guidelines and standards that were to be applied to the local situation in some way. This kind of regulation sits very badly with many people, whether they are affected directly as providers who wish to change or extend their programs or merely are onlookers who feel that government interference should be as limited as possible.

Nevertheless, even strong opponents of intervention would agree that there are areas in which government must lay down certain standards to protect the public. What should be the role of government and its appendages? How is it possible to justify imposing limits to freedom on enterprise? In any event, how effective is government regulation in achieving the objectives of equity, compassion, and similar social values? These all are important political questions that cannot be explored here.

A major complicating element in addressing these questions is the demonstrated weakness of the classical market model in controlling the delivery of personal health services. Factors that make it very difficult to restrain the growth of health services through consumer choice or marketplace economics include the following:

- The consumer lacks full knowledge on which to base choices.
- The physician is both expert provider and prescriber of treatment but often is unaware of the costs of what is prescribed.
- The patient really does not have the time or ability to shop around for health care.

- The purchasing of services is largely in the hands of third parties and even when there are choices for the consumer, they often are very limited.
- The expectations of medical care and technology are inflated and easily heightened by a desire to avoid pain, suffering, disease, and death.
- The willingness and ability of providers to do more for the patient than already has been done are questionable.

Even where programs introducing competition in the purchase of service packages are proposed, it is essential that there be extensive regulation to protect the consumer against tricky and unscrupulous insurance systems (Caper, 1981).

Society has other reasons for mandating government interventions because there always will be vulnerable groups in the population who need special attention for meeting their health needs. These include the poor, the chronically ill, the elderly, veterans, and minority groups for whom society considers it has a moral obligation to provide assistance. How far this support should go is the subject of much political debate and, again, is beyond the scope of this review.

A ROLE FOR GOVERNMENT—BUT WHAT IS IT?

It is evident that even the most conservative of politicians and practitioners agree that there is a role for government in health care. The question is, how far it should go. Where does the nation draw the line between centralization and government intervention, freedom of choice and private enterprise, providing support or being paternalistic?

There are a number of alternatives for dealing with the questions that health planning is expected to address. However, the alternatives selected must depend on the goals that are set before Congress or other decision-making bodies. These alternatives revolve around the question of the role of government, specifically in the delivery of health care. At one end of the spectrum, it could be argued that government has no role to play at all; at the other extreme, it could be said that the delivery of health care, like defense, should be entirely in the hands of government. Somewhere in the middle of the spectrum lies education, where government plays a significant role at all three political levels. Accordingly, whatever alternative is promoted would depend entirely upon what the national policy for health care is determined to be.

There are few enterprises in the country that are not assisted by the federal government in some way. This help may take the form of a policy that indirectly promotes the well-being of a particular industry, such as the development of a national highway system, which in turn encourages the development of the automobile industry; or more directly in the form of subsidies to such activities as education and the arts. It may take the form of developing resources, such as for research and education in medicine; or of direct payment for care, as in social and/or medical services for certain groups. It may take the form of fairly direct operation, such as the postal service or the military establishment. How much or how little planning is done of the kind seen since 1974, and how the relationship between government and the private sector is shaped, depends on which of these models health care is to follow.

Another aspect of this issue is the degree to which central, as opposed to state, government takes responsibility for ordering the priorities in health care. With the relative financial strengths of the federal vis-à-vis the state governments, it would be very difficult politically to pass on to the states all the health care services that were subsidized or paid for by the federal government without the transfer of the necessary funds. Indeed, much of the process of allocation of resources, establishing of policies, delivery of services, and regulation is being passed on to the states in the form of block grants, but at a lower level of funding than in the past. A model already in place is Title XX of the Social Security Act—social services. The criteria for which the funds could be used could vary, depending upon the mood of Congress and the impact of interest groups.

Should this take place, the states either could take responsibility for allocating and dividing up the block grants themselves or they could pass this task down to the counties and municipalities. Whoever had responsibility for allocating resources and establishing priorities, whether at the state or substate level, would be subjected to pressure from various groups. Unless some mechanism existed for protecting the rights of those who wielded little political influence, such as the poor, minorities, and migrant farm workers, much of the good effects of social legislation enacted since the 1930s could be reversed.

The existence of a cap on spending, however, could have a positive effect in that planning and other decision-making bodies inevitably would have to make "either-or" rather than "yes-or-no" decisions and in this way a better use of resources could be developed if there were a judicious mix of technical and advocacy planning.

If the nation wishes to ensure more efficient application of resources, it must continue to strive for better methods of decision making. Whether these methods are called planning or something else, they must integrate projected actions with the allocation of funds. If this is not done, there will be no assurance that the plans ever will materialize because in today's pluralistic system of delivery, the provider groups will serve their own interests unless they find it profitable to comply with the overall plans and decisions. This policy must apply to both capital and operating finances, otherwise planning will continue to fail to contain costs (Klein, 1981). The need to link planning and financing is a major lesson derived from experience in the United States and abroad (Marmor & Bridges, 1980; Rodwin, 1981).

COMPETITION AND ALTERNATIVES

Much has been said about the need for promoting competition in the health field. Enthoven (1978) proposed a competition model providing greater freedom of choice for the purchasers of services, whether they be groups or individuals, an idea that found favor in many quarters. However, even if this competitive element were introduced into the allocation of health resources it would not be completely laissez faire since there would be a great need to lay down rules to protect the consumer against unscrupulous vendors of health care (Caper, 1981) and to ensure that competition was fair.

Considering the growing resistance to and resentment over the cost of medical care, it is unlikely that the country will go back to the free market situation that prevailed prior to health planning. The increasing number of physicians who are unwilling to accept the "usual, customary, and reasonable" fees prescribed for services they provide to Medicare patients is an indication of what happens if there is no limit on fees. Sooner or later the public and politicians are going to hear the cries of consumers who are stung by increasing health care charges and who want relief (Roe, 1981).

Another alternative to the current health planning structure is the establishment of private voluntary groups that include providers, business people, health insurers, and consumers in varying numbers. Proponents of this idea feel that there is a need to have some local discussion and planning—without regulation. They hope that with pressure from business and industry to hold down costs, accommodations will be made to achieve the goal of cost containment. Unfortunately, the history of voluntary health planning in the country does not lend optimism to this approach.

Another potential approach to health planning is complete decentralization, as is the case in education, where elected school boards or committees have the power to establish facilities, employ staffs, and raise money to carry out the programs they have developed. Under this approach, patients who did not wish to use public facilities still could rely on private doctors or hospitals if they could afford to do so. A local area health authority could hire physicians, nurses, and other health personnel and put them to work meeting the needs of poor people who are covered by the law. The program would have to involve hospitals, too, because that is where the largest proportion of health care money is spent. Since the federal government pays about 40 percent of the money being spent on personal health services, at least some of this could go directly to the local area health authority.

Although this alternative has certain attractions, it has some major obstacles that need to be considered:

1. It would not be easy to employ physicians on salary at a time when the incomes of doctors in practice were very high, and tax money would be needed in order to raise the necessary revenue.
2. Evidence of a trend away from the policy of paying for services through the tax mechanism is seen in the large number of public hospitals being closed or taken over by for-profit hospital chains.
3. An important political consideration at both state and national levels is that the country is in no mood to raise funds through increased taxation for public enterprises. This is not to say that at some point in the future the mood might not change, but it may require a national crisis to prepare the public mind.

EPILOGUE

It is inevitable that some more vigorous form of rationing of personal health services will be used. There is no way of satisfying the human appetite for care to prolong life, stave off death or disease, or reduce pain and discomfort.

For moral reasons, society rejects the simplest form of rationing—rationing by the simple ability to pay for services. But it also hesitates to adopt the policy of ensuring that each receives according to individual needs. Apart from the difficulty in defining what is meant by "needs" or how it is measured, society has to face the implication that such an egalitarian policy would mean increased national involvement in health care. For many years the idea of a national health insurance program has been bandied about. That concept is dead for now, largely because of the inflation of health care costs. But something must be done.

The decisions that will be made will be political compromises that will not please everyone. Rationing will be acceptable to the public to the degree that it is perceived as necessary and fair.

REFERENCES

American Health Planning Association. *Second report on 1978 survey of health planning agencies*. Washington, D.C.: American Health Planning Association, 1979.

Anderson, O.W. Styles of planning health services: The United States, Sweden and England. *International Journal of Health Services,* 1971, *1*(2), 106–120.

Brown, L.D. Some structural issues in the health planning program. In *Health planning in the U.S.: Selected policy issues* (Vol. 2) Papers. Washington, D.C.: *National Academy of Science, Institute of Medicine,* 1981, pp. 1– 45.

Browne, B.E. Rational planning and responsiveness: The case of the HSAs. *Public Administration Review,* July/August 1981, pp. 437– 444.

Cain, H.P. Health planning in the U.S.: The 1980s—A Protagonist's View. *Journal of Health Politics, Policy, and Law,* Spring 1981, *6*(1), 159–171.

Caper, P. Competition and health care—Caveat emptor. *The New England Journal of Medicine,* May 21, 1981, *304*(21), 1296–1299.

Committee on the Costs of Medical Care. *Final report: Medical care for the American people*. Adopted October 31, 1932. (Reprinted by the Department of Health, Education, and Welfare, 1970.)

Dawson, Lord. *Interim report on the future provision of medical and allied services*. London: His Majesty's Stationery Office, 1920.

Enthoven, A.C. Consumer-choice health plan (Part 1). *The New England Journal of Medicine,* March 23, 1978, *298*(12), 650–658. (a)

Enthoven, A.C. Consumer-choice health plan (Part 2). *The New England Journal of Medicine,* March 30, 1978, *298*(13), 709–720. (b)

Fein, R. Financial support mechanisms. In E. Ginzberg (Ed.), *Regionalization and health policy*. (U.S. Department of Health, Education, and Welfare, Health Resources Administration, DHEW Publication No. (HRA) 77-623). Washington, D.C.: U.S. Government Printing Office, 1977.

Foley, H.A. Health planning—Demise or reformation. *The New England Journal of Medicine,* April 16, 1981, *304*(16), 969–972.

Havighurst, C.C. Statement—Appendix A. In *Health planning in the U.S.: Issues in guideline development*. Washington, D.C.: National Academy of Sciences, Institute of Medicine, 1980.

Institute of Medicine, Committee on Health Planning Goals and Standards, R. Fein (Chair). *Health planning in the U.S.: Issues in guideline development: Report of a study*. Washington, D.C.: National Academy of Sciences, 1980.

Institute of Medicine, Committee on Health Planning Goals and Standards, R. Fein (Chair). *Health planning in the U.S.: Selected policy issues, Report of a study* (Vol. 1). Washington, D.C.: National Academy Press, 1981.

Kinzer, D. *Health controls out of control*. Chicago: Teach'em, Inc., n.d.

Klarman, H.E. Health planning: Progress, prospects and issues. *Milbank Memorial Fund Quarterly/Health and Society,* 1978, *56*(1), 78–112.

Klein, R. Reflections on the American health care condition. *Journal of Health Politics, Policy, and Law,* Summer 1981, *6*(2), 188–204.

Lewin & Associates, Inc. An analysis of state and regional health regulation. (NTIS No. 1975) (Quoted in Institute of Medicine. *Health planning in the U.S.: Issues in guideline development.* Washington, D.C.: National Academy of Sciences, 1980.)

Marmor, T.R., & Bridges, A. American health planning and the lessons of comparative policy analysis. *Journal of Health Politics, Policy and Law,* Fall 1980, *5*(3), 419–430.

Marmor, T.R., & Morone, J.A. HSAs and the representation of consumer interests: Conceptual issues and litigation problems. *Health Law Project Library Bulletin.* April 1979, IV(4), 117–128.

Moore, J.R. A normative definition of the process of areawide health services planning. *Health Services Reports,* April 1973, *88*(4), 305–315.

National Commission on Community Health Services. *Health is a community affair.* Cambridge, Mass.: Harvard University Press, 1966.

National guidelines for health planning. (Department of Health, Education, and Welfare, Health Resources Administration, Publication No. (HRA) 78-643). Washington, D.C.: U.S. Government Printing Office, 1978.

Pressman, J.L., & Wildavsky, A.B. *Implementation.* Berkeley, Calif.: University of California Press, 1973.

Raab, G.G. National state local relationships in health planning: Interest group reaction and lobbying. In *Health planning in the U.S.: Selected policy issues* (Vol. 2/Papers). Washington, D.C.: National Academy of Sciences, Institute of Medicine, 1981, 105–129.

Rodwin, V.G. On the separation of health planning and provider reimbursement. *Inquiry,* Summary 1981, *18*, 139–150.

Roe, B. The UCR boondoggle: A death knell for private practice? *The New England Journal of Medicine,* July 2, 1981, *305*(1), 41–45.

Rosenfeld, L.S., & Rosenfeld, I. National health planning in the United States. *International Journal of Health Services,* 1975, *5*(3), 441–453.

Salkever, D., & Bice, T. The impact of certificate-of-need controls on hospital investment. *Milbank Memorial Fund Quarterly, Health and Society,* Spring 1976, *54*(1), 185–214.

Sigmond, R.M. Health planning. *Medical Care,* May–June 1967, *5*, 117–128.

Somers, A.R., & Somers, H.M. A proposed framework for health and health care policies. *Inquiry,* June 1977, *14*(2), 115–170.

U.S. Comptroller General. *Health systems plans: A poor framework for promoting health care improvements.* Washington, D.C.: U.S. General Accounting Office, HRD-81-93, 1981.

U.S. Congress. *National health planning and resources development act of 1974.* P.L. 93-641. Passed December 20, 1974, signed by President Ford, January 4, 1975.

Vladeck, B.C. Interest group representation and the HSAs: Health planning and political theory. *American Journal of Public Health,* January 1977, *67*(1), 23–28.

Werlin, S.H., Walcott, A., & Joroff, M. Implementing formative health planning under P.L. 93-641. *The New England Journal of Medicine,* September 23, 1976, *295*(13), 698–703.

Wildavsky, A. *Can health be planned?* Chicago: University of Chicago, The Center for Health Administrative Studies, 1976.

Chapter 6

Public Participation in Planning for Personal Health Services

Nancy Milio

The 1980s may see a dismantling of the federally mandated means by which Americans have had a voice in planning personal health services since the 1960s. In order to assess the role of the public in this area and the prospects for its role in the years ahead, this chapter reviews the rationale, extent, and consequences of citizen participation in public decision making.

It begins with a discussion of the purposes and concepts that underlie public involvement and describes the differences between ideal notions and the organizational realities revealed in survey data and consumer group studies in health-related agencies. These studies expose the problems and suggest solutions to strengthen the role of the public to enhance the effectiveness of health care decision making. The recommended changes are juxtaposed with the new federal policy directions of fiscal austerity and withdrawal from health and social programs, suggesting what effects these can have on citizen participation and on health planning goals.

WHY PUBLIC INVOLVEMENT?

Extensive public participation in decision making has had the aim of enhancing the democratic process as an end in itself and, of equal importance, helping ensure that governmental decisions have the desired results.

For a half century, advisory groups have issued calls for public participation in state and local health care planning (*Medical Care,* 1932; National Council on Health Planning and Development, 1980). By the end of the 1970s, more than 50,000 volunteers—consumers and providers—were involved on the boards, councils, and committees created under the National Health Planning and Resources Development Act of 1974, P.L. 93-641

(National Council, 1980). This was just one of 20 pieces of federal legislative or regulatory action requiring citizen participation in health care activities, almost all of which developed in the 1970s. This mandate was part of a larger effort, encompassing more than 150 federal agencies, to involve citizens in the governance of federally funded programs (Advisory Commission, 1980).

Citizen participation in community affairs outside the electoral process certainly is not a modern phenomenon in the United States. In the mid-1970s, there were 6 million voluntary associations and 8,000 action- or issue-oriented neighborhood groups (Perlman, 1978).

The purpose of extensive participation presumably is to assure accountability of programs to the public interest or to the general interests of the consumers they affect. However, neither the aims of public participation nor means to achieve them are set forth clearly and consistently in the legal mandates (Koseki & Hayakawa, 1977).

In practice, the generally accepted intent of public participation is twofold. According to a study for Congress by the Advisory Commission on Intergovernmental Regulations, the dual aim is to (1) ensure the right of citizens to enter the decision-making process and (2) assure their right to a beneficial and fair outcome from program decisions (Advisory Commission, 1980).

This joint purpose, focusing on both process and outcomes, also appears in the performance standards for evaluating health systems agencies. The standards relate to how effectively the community participates in the agency's decisions and how successful those decisions are in improving the health and health services of the community (Bureau of Health Planning, 1980).

Although not written into the 1974 National Health Planning and Resources Development Act, the intent of Congress concerning citizen involvement is spelled out in a House committee analysis three years later. It said that a health system that served and was paid for by the public should be controlled by that public and that the planned system ought to (1) promote the health and (2) improve the services of the community (U.S. Congress, 1977). The underlying assumption was that citizen involvement in planning would contribute to decision making in the public interest.

The Public Interest

The lexicon of citizen participation in public decision making contains several terms and underlying concepts that are not always used with clarity. These include "the public interest," "the public," "consumer," "participation," "accountability," and "representation." The following discussion briefly explores these concepts and defines how they are used here.

A decision taken in the public interest is one that a majority of the public would choose if:

1. people were aware of its full costs and benefits—the economic and noneconomic, the short-term and the long-term
2. its costs would be shared according to ability to pay
3. its benefits were shared according to people's needs

The distributional aspects of the public interest are as important as overall benefits because continuing maldistribution tears away the social fabric that is essential to the well-being of both the majority and the minorities in the population.

This view implies that majority decisions neither guarantee that the public interest will be served, nor, on the other hand, that a minority decision will act against it (Moyar, 1980). However, the American democratic belief holds that a decision representing majority views is more likely to enhance the public interest than one that represents a minority, even one that claims to act in the best interests of the public.

The health interests of the public, for example, may not be best served by an expert minority of well-intentioned medical professionals or scientists. There are several reasons for this. As with any specialized group, scientists' interests influence the questions they ask and how they interpret their data. But the use of their technologies involves far broader issues than scientific fact; it includes competing values that can be balanced and negotiated only in a public process.

For medical scientists, there often are technological and economic incentives toward introducing new techniques that provide short-term benefits. An alternative view, however, would be more cautious about adopting new technologies because of possible long-term, unpredictable risks. Correlaries to this view are that technical fixes may create worse problems than the ones they are intended to solve; that natural, nonintrusive technologies are preferable; that products should be proved safe before use; and that the cost of being overcautious is less than that of being too precipitous in accepting new technology (Mitchell, 1978; Skoie, 1979; Stewart, 1975; Weisbrod, Handler, & Komesar, 1978).

In practical terms, serving the public interest in this planning must include improving health and the prospects for it as well as providing adequate quality and equitable distribution of services. An additional aspect is the containment of costs in relation to need, since the effects of health care expenditures (nearly 10 percent of the gross national product) spill over into all major areas of the economy, crowding out other options that might in fact be more health promoting than personal care services alone (Milio, 1981).

The role of the public is especially important in arriving at answers to the questions that underlie health planning:

1. What should be the criteria for defining health problems? Should the problems be defined, for example, as diagnostic entities, personal risk factors, environmental risks, or some interrelated combination?
2. What should be the criteria to judge the priority of problems? Should those most amenable to medical technology receive more attention, or those that are most preventable; the acute problems, or the chronic?
3. What criteria should decide the means to "solve" the problems; what range of strategies should be considered; over what time span should their potential effectiveness be seen, and what range of untoward effects should be acceptable?

Quite clearly, judgments about these criteria, most of which are implicit, will differ between the public and the health care providers, as well as within each group, as suggested later.

The public interest also should be distinguished from public accountability. Accountability implies openness of the deliberative processes of policy making and public information about the decisions that are reached. It includes the ability of the public to recall or replace its representatives if it does not find them effective. Thus accountability may exist but in itself does not ensure that the public interest will be served.

Who Is the Public and What Is Participation?

The "public" referred to in this chapter is a more inclusive term than "consumer." One definition of a consumer of health care is a person, group purchaser, or insuree of health services, one for whom an employer or the government pays the full costs. This definition thus excludes many who have an interest in health care but do not buy, pay out of pocket, or have a third party payer to underwrite their use of services. Consumer also may mean a user of services, regardless of who pays the bill (or whether the bill is paid at all). This label also excludes some 25 percent of the population who do not use health care in any given year (Milio, 1977; Reeder, 1972; van der Heuvel, 1980). Finally, there are those who neither buy nor use health care in any given year and yet as citizens are affected by it indirectly if only through its impact on the national economy, related effects on monetary and fiscal policy, and a variety of consumer prices (Milio, 1981).

Thus there is a general public interest in personal health services apart from the more immediate, particular interests of purchasers and patients. The "public" then is the total population, including economic consumers and users of services. Evidence that the public and consumers or users of health services are different populations is suggested in two new studies, discussed later.

Two recent efforts have been made to tap the public's preferences and view of health—as distinguished from consumers' or patients' attitudes—as criteria for planning personal health care. Among other things, these innovative surveys found patients to be a special interest group whose views, if taken as representative of the general public, would distort the direction of planning toward developing excessive treatment capacity (Sackett & Torrance, 1978). This would not best serve either the health care needs nor economic interests of the public.

In other words, the view of the general public concerning the agenda for health planning is based on a longer term perspective than that of currently ill people. This longer orientation suggests the need for a greater emphasis on preventive strategies in health planning, which indeed are among the stated priorities of the National Health Planning and Resources Development Act of 1974.

"Participation" is another term often used with different meanings. It sometimes means taking the viewpoint of the public or of a particular patient or consumer into account indirectly, through inference or the use of aggregate survey data (Milio, 1975). This is done in consumer protection regulations at the Food and Drug Administration, or in informed consent and other patients' rights requirements (Institute of Society, 1972). Consumer education and information, encouraging access to health literature, or patients' access to their medical records are other variations, as are consumer advocacy programs employing ombudsmen (Shenkin & Warner, 1973).

Another form of citizen involvement widely used by planning agencies and individual provider institutions is the consumer satisfaction survey (Hulka, Zyranski, Cassell, & Thompson, 1971; Korsch, Gozzi, & Francis, 1968; Lebow, 1974; Tessler & Mechanic, 1975). These surveys can be misleading as guides to planning, however, if they do not take into account the demographic backgrounds, social and health status, and health care experiences of respondents, as well as the fact that patients' "satisfaction" often has little to do with the outcome of health care. Furthermore, the surveys tend to be disregarded because providers do not consider consumers competent to judge the quality of care (Kelman, 1976).

Although these indirect methods of involving the public may be useful in some degree in health planning, more direct forms of participation are the focus here. These include membership on boards and committees of planning or health service agencies; they also involve independently organized groups engaged in review and comment, lobbying, public education, or litigation.

Direct participation is essential to ensure the public interest in health planning, if only because the views of special interests so clearly diverge from those of the broader general public. Numerous studies show, for example, that providers are far less interested than is the public in making changes in health care. Providers also prefer to rely on professional judgments rather than on community needs as guides for action, and their priorities differ from those of the public concerning the problems most needing attention (Bradbury, 1972; Brook & Appel, 1973; Fleming & Andersen, 1975; Goldman, 1974; Milio, 1974; Olendski, 1973; Riska & Taylor, 1978; Sanazaro & Williamson, 1970; Strickland, 1973).

Although business corporations are part of the public and are large buyers of health services, their viewpoint also differs from what might best serve the health interests of the public. Research on corporate attitudes toward health care costs illustrates the point (Sapolsky, 1980). Almost 70 major firms employing more than 6 million workers showed a consistent and definite reluctance to alter their health insurance benefits, improve claims control procedures, or promote health maintenance organizations for fear of appearing to jeopardize current programs highly popular among employees. Management felt that worker satisfaction with such programs would avoid unionization. The tendency has been to expand insurance benefits competitively among firms in order to attract and retain employees.

Furthermore, few firms wished to become directly involved in local health planning activities. This was partly because their workers were not concentrated in a single area and partly because local involvement would waste political influence; they preferred to save their "bargaining capital" for larger issues. While they recognized a need for containing health care outlays, and for trying to limit their own insurance expenditures as a cost of doing business, they chose to use traditional corporate methods of controlling their production costs, such as substituting cheaper materials and laying off workers.

The "public," even apart from corporate or institutional consumers, is of course not a single entity. The separate interests and views of its subgroups arise from and reinforce social and economic characteristics, including the likelihood of belonging to special interests groups (Marmor & Bridges, 1980; Milio, 1975).

In 1981 about one in four Americans were involved in special interest groups through membership, donations, or both. These people more often were men, younger than 50 years, likely to have a college education, and earn more that $25,000 a year (Gallup, 1981). Similarly, federally funded programs mandating broad-based citizen involvement drew mainly male, middle- and upper middle-class participants who had the time and resources to commit to such activities (Advisory Commission, 1980).

"Representativeness" of the public also is an unsolved issue in planning entities, notably the health systems agencies (HSAs). The leadership positions in their governing structures, although consumers were in the majority, were almost 75 percent male and college educated; 84 percent were white, and almost six in ten earned more than $25,000 (Health Resources Administration, 1980). By contrast, the public members on the less influential subarea councils had a larger share of women (38 percent) and minorities (24 percent) (National Council, 1980).

Organizations and the Public Interest

In any area of decision making, the public interest is rarely if ever made explicit and its achievement cannot be taken for granted. It must result from public dialogue and is a continuing creation of social discourse. However, in the American pluralist tradition, the main dialogue occurs among particular parties. The public interest then is assumed to be served as a result of the negotiation and balancing among organized special interests. In reality, however, this results in a balance of power among competing interests—and not necessarily the public interest (Blum, 1981).

Because of this political fact of life, it has been necessary for citizens to find other ways to influence decisions in the public interest. This need was suggested in public opinion polls of the 1970s that showed a decline of public confidence in big government and large-scale industry. That decade also saw an increase in organized public interest groups attempting to bring new and broader perspectives into the arenas of decision making in legislatures, public bureaucracies, and the courts. Public interest groups defined themselves as seeking "a collective good," one that would not materially or solely benefit its members or leaders (Berry, 1977). This definition represents criteria by which to evaluate the groups' claims to act in the public interest. The public also can use the same criteria to judge the activities and decisions of other groups, whether producer associations, single interest groups, medical scientists, or health care providers and suppliers.

Public interest groups, as one avenue of wider participation in health issues, usually engage in a broad set of concerns, some of which directly affect care. This is in contrast to more traditional disease-specific organizations such as the American Heart Association that have not engaged primarily in legislative or legal action. Some of the most active public interest groups in recent years, however, are longtime organizations that are rooted in local and state chapters. These include Common Cause, the League of Women Voters, the National Council of Churches, the Parent-Teacher Association, and the Sierra Club. The agendas of these nonhealth groups include public access to information and the right to affect decision making without undue competition from special interests; national health insurance; access of disadvantaged people to health care; school health education; and gaining public support for environmental protection (*Success Stories,* 1980).

Somewhat more specific organized efforts to represent citizens' health needs are the public interest law groups. These groups have used the courts and administrative proceedings to represent the public view on health and services issues. Organizations such as the Health Research Group, Critical Mass Energy Project, Congress Watch, and the Litigation Group challenged—often successfully—regulatory decisions and special interests on issues involving health services access, and food, drug, worksite, environmental, and consumer product safety. They also have dealt with public participation issues such as access to health planning information and service evaluation data (*Public Citizen Annual Report 1980,* 1981).

THE RESULTS OF PARTICIPATION

A first generation of evaluations of public participation was done in the early 1970s based on the experience of the War on Poverty and neighborhood health center programs begun in the 1960s (Bellin, Kaveler, & Schwarz, 1972; Campbell, 1971; Chamberlin & Radebaugh, 1976; Danaceau, 1975; Douglass, 1973; New & Hessler, 1972; Notkin & Notkin, 1970; Partridge, 1973; Sparer, Dines, & Smith, 1970; Stokes, Banta, & Putnam, 1972; Ulrich, 1969; Young, 1975). The findings on citizen involvement in health services and the conditions under which it could be effective were essentially repeated in other studies of public activity within health systems agencies and other federal programs. The studies continued to show the dominance of provider over consumer interests and of special interests over the general public interest (Public Health Service, 1976; Jonas, 1978; Navarro, 1975a, 1975b; Parkum & Parkum, 1973; Rayack, 1967).

Much of this dominance was not in numerical representation but rather was in organizational resources (Koseki & Hayakawa, 1977; Zwick, 1978). It is providers who, after all, receive program funds and who have a full-time, paid commitment to planning and program activities (Falkson, 1976; Greer, 1976). Just as importantly, health professionals, in contrast to public participants, have networks that supply timely and relevant information in familiar "languages," including assessments of political realities, without which planning strategies cannot be effective (Consumer Commission, 1975; *Consumer Health Perspectives*, 1978; Diamond, 1978; Knox, 1978).

As a result of this provider-public imbalance in the planning process, participation comes at a higher cost to citizens. These costs include the difficulty, complexity, and inconvenience of the process, and the real economic losses they face when absent from work or when they have to travel long distances to attend meetings (Cooper, 1979; Marmor & Bridges, 1980; National Council, 1980; Paap, 1978).

Partly because of this difference in organizational strength, most evaluations showed that the public had little or no influence in the health plans with which it was involved (Douglass, 1975; Ittig, 1976). For example, at the end of the 1970s, 20 out of the 40 existing southeastern health systems agencies were studied to discover whether consumer participation had made any difference in their areawide health plans (Burdine, 1980). Overall, the analysis found that the public had made no difference in either the preventive nature of the plans, the forcefulness of their proposed interventions, or the resources proposed to implement them. However, progressive changes, moving away from traditional medical approaches, were evident in agencies that fostered greater participation through organizational methods. These methods included giving higher priority to plan development than to other agency activities when allocating staff resources— providing more board and staff training—and creating a larger network of standing committees and subarea councils, thus providing more opportunities for participation.

Another study in six cities showed that local citizen groups, including health-oriented ones, had created more than 600 innovative changes but they had had little impact on agency programs because 99 percent of their steps involved only cosmetic shifts in agency procedures (Warren, 1974). The report showed that the most important feature of an effective grassroots group was its ability to hire a full-time professional staff. This in turn allowed more continuous and sophisticated use of skills in organizing, information gathering, planning, monitoring, negotiating, lobbying, and coalition building. Second in importance was a support network of allied groups, newsletters, and organizer training schools (Perlman, 1978).

Nonetheless, even when the public had no measurable impact on plan documents, other effects that could enhance the health care goals of planning occurred because of citizens' work. Notably, these included community education, improving the planners' credibility, and increasing the agency's community contacts that become essential to implementation. These contacts were especially important with private physicians who might be more willing to cooperate locally through citizen representatives in order to avoid greater control from outside, more remote agencies (Arthur D. Little, Inc., 1979).

There also was evidence to suggest that opportunities for the public discussion of planning issues, created through participatory channels and led by citizen representatives, clarified what the public interest was in matters of health and health care (Arthur D. Little, Inc., 1979; Blue Ribbon Commission, 1979). Such findings suggested that if participation were enhanced and sustained, it might result in more effective planning and improved community health in the long term.

ESSENTIALS FOR EFFECTIVE INVOLVEMENT

Under what conditions can public participation be effective both as a process that allows citizens to influence planning decisions and as an achievement that contributes to the health and service goals of health systems and other planning agencies? In short, if the public interest in democratic processes and in improved health and health care outcomes is to be served, what changes are needed in the extent or methods of citizen involvement in health planning?

Most assessments described in the next section conclude that improvements should be made in the selection of public participants and in reducing the disparity in resources between provider and public representatives.

Selection of Representation

Many health systems agencies created governing boards that became self-perpetuating. These continued through nominating procedures that tended to perpetuate membership of the same individuals and thereby the boards became narrow, individualistic, and perhaps self-serving.

To avoid this, several sources recommended the election or appointment of representatives to governing boards of planning agencies by broad-based community organizations (Kleiman, 1979; Knox, 1978; National Council, 1980). This alternate selection process would improve the participatory process in several ways.

- It would represent the diversity of the public more accurately, rather than relying on the assumption that people who had sex, race, or income characteristics similar to their counterparts in the population clearly knew and represented the interests of that aggregate.

- It also would make possible the presentation to the boards of policy-relevant positions as public constituencies discussed and defined them for their representative.
- It would improve the accountability of the representative board members since they would report back to their constituencies for evaluation there (more readily done with an organized group or coalition than with an open electorate).
- It could enhance the influence of the representatives among other board members because of their relationship to an organized constituency.

The main problems concerning the use of public elections to select public representatives for planning boards are the costs of informing the electorate and of holding the vote. A third potential problem is the elaborate spending and media saturation by provider groups, including large hospital staffs, that have occurred when they are allowed to vote for consumer representatives (Kleiman, 1979).

Election by a "congress" of organizations may be an option if its votes are weighted in proportion to the groups usually underrepresented by public members. These groups include minorities, women, those with low incomes, and rural dwellers (Arthur D. Little, Inc., 1979). The special needs of heavy users of services, such as the chronically disabled, also must be represented (Advisory Commission, 1980).

Organization of Agencies

Most evaluations also agree on some minimal organizational changes to redress part of the imbalance between providers and other board members. For example, planning staff members should be assigned to support public participants to enhance their information capabilities. Timely staff briefings, summaries, analyses, and translations, as well as board and staff training focusing on the needs of public participants, also would help offset the superior information network available to providers (Advisory Commission, 1980; Burdine, 1980; National Council, 1980).

In addition, more channels for organized participation could be developed, including a public caucus plus more subarea councils, task forces, and committees (Arthur D. Little, Inc., 1979; Gerlach, 1971). Public representatives should be reimbursed for their expenses, including travel, telephone, and printing costs.

Greater organized strength could be promoted by closer ties between public representatives and coalitions of consumer-oriented or general interest groups and health planning centers in the community as well as nationally

(Knox, 1978; Lazarsfeld & Reitz, 1975; National Council, 1980). Proponents differed on whether government funds should finance this public
support network (*Health Perspectives,* 1977; National Council, 1980).

Finally, the likelihood that such changes would in fact produce their
intended effects depended on how well they were monitored by units in
the legislative and executive branches of government. The Advisory Commission on Intergovernmental Regulations urged accountable units within
each branch to assure compliance with procedures that ensured effective
public participation. Indicators that could be taken as evidence of effective
citizen involvement in the planning process included the demographic and
group representativeness of participants, public awareness of health issues,
requests for information or collaboration with the agency by local private
and governmental units, initiatives and advocacy of community interests
by the HSA, and changes in traditional patterns of delivery (Advisory
Commission, 1980; Bureau of Health Planning, 1980; Metch & Veney,
1976).

To judge the other major facet of effectiveness of public involvement—
whether the outcomes of planning decisions assisted the agency in reaching
its objectives—the relevant indicators included the community's health
status, access to and use of health services, and the rates of cost inflation
(Bureau of Health Planning, 1980).

Some of the ways recommended to strengthen public participation in
the health systems agencies were included in the 1979 amendments to the
National Health Planning and Resources Development Act. For example,
self-perpetuating boards were disallowed; governing board members' training
was to be improved; staff time was to be allotted to agency members; and
staff members were allowed to support citizen members who sought to
lobby in favor of planning agency views (U.S. Congress, 1979).

PROSPECTS FOR PUBLIC PARTICIPATION

With the advent of the Reagan administration in 1981, and a different
approach to health planning, the prospects for public participation through
the health systems agency structure changed.

In order to project the probable or the possible role of public participation in health services planning, the general political context in which it
would occur must be noted. This context shapes the means that may be
open to the public to influence health services. It also affects such funds
as may be available to support effective participation.

For more than a decade, political party discipline has declined as ideo-
logical or issue-oriented blocs emerged crossing party lines. Thus as a

channel of involvement, political parties have lost their ability to stand effectively for broad interests. People turned increasingly to single interest and special interest groups. These groups, however, were most effective in blocking rather than supporting changes and often opposed progressive change (Broder, 1979). An indication of this fragmentation was the fourfold increase in political action committees (PACs) in the 1970s with corporation committees outstripping those of labor by more than 2 to 1 (North, 1978). PAC campaign spending in support of congressional incumbents, particularly those who headed committees, more than doubled in the late 1970s and early 1980s. The leading PAC was the American Medical Association (Common Cause, 1979).

Another avenue for influencing public policies, organized lobbying, also was dominated by special economic interests and mushroomed in the last decade. Hospitals, physicians, insurers, suppliers, and large corporate users formed new alliances to "preserve the private market in health services" and keep their economic interests protected (Bacheller, 1977; *Washington Report on Medicine and Health,* 1978; Weinberg, 1978).

These circumstances have had a dampening effect on public involvement in political processes, including voting. Only 35 percent of those eligible voted in the 1978 congressional elections; others believe their votes did not matter (Gans, 1978; Hadley, 1978). Moreover, many voters, especially in less advantaged groups, said they had no confidence that the leadership in either major party would act in their interests. At the same time, large segments of Americans believed they personally had less control over the material conditions of their lives, including the adequacy of their medical care (Miller, 1979).

As the public's discouragement grew because of its incapacity to influence policies through traditional means—and since lobbying came at a high dollar premium dominated by narrow, well-organized, and well-financed groups rather than public interests—alternate channels became necessary. At the same time, the outlook for public resources to develop or sustain new participatory channels was dim, in spite of the commitment and mandate written into the 1974 National Health Planning and Resources Development Act and reaffirmed in the 1979 amendments (U.S. Congress, 1974, 1979).

Alongside sharp reductions in federal funds in 1981, the Bureau of Health Planning in the Department of Health and Human Services issued a new policy direction for planning agencies to "accomplish more, sooner, and with fewer resources" (*Health Resources News,* 1981). In pursuit of this goal, HSAs were to concentrate on problems of area health care costs and availability of services, to publicize their success items, and to build local coalitions, most of which turned out to be with business groups. Although

HSAs were expected to meet the public-professional composition requirements for their governing bodies, documentation no longer was necessary,
nor were public hearings on applications for program and capital reviews,
nor was dissemination of health plan documents required. In short, results
were to take priority over process. Thus, tangible output, in dollar terms,
and the perspective of the professional and technical experts responsible
for them were to overshadow public participatory values and citizens'
interest in them.

The Reagan Administration's planned phasing out of health systems
agencies was marked in 1982 by further severe budget reductions and
other statutory changes. This curtailing of scope, activity, and staff meant
that the potential effectiveness of HSAs would be restricted and any hope
of a stronger public role diluted. Furthermore, planning units were permitted to merge or consolidate over wider areas, with the effect of reducing
the opportunities for local community involvement. Agencies were allowed
to accept operating funds from health insurance companies, opening the
door to conflicts of interest and the possibility of drawing planning agencies' attention away from the public interest (*Medicine and Health Perspectives,* 1981).

Changes enacted or proposed concerning other aspects of personal
health care also were likely to have important impacts on HSAs' effectiveness and on public involvement. These include cutbacks in Medicaid
financing and in maternal-child health and preventive and chronic disease
programs. Moreover, proposals for competitive health care financing were
expected to have an important effect. Financing changes and service
cutbacks would reduce access to care and lessen the chances for developing new services in underserved areas. Most explicit in this regard was
a relaxing of the rule that federally financed hospitals under the Hill-Burton
Act provide a certain amount of free care to medically indigent people and
keep their doors open to all persons in their communities (*Medicine and
Health Perspectives,* 1981).

The new policy of loosening regulations and softening enforcement in
other environmental, occupational, and social programs also was likely to
make the planning objectives of improved health, access to care, and public
involvement more difficult to achieve. These "nonhealth care" policy
areas included environmental pollution control; food and drug regulations;
work-related safety and health regulations; and affirmative action programs affecting opportunities for improved education, jobs, housing, and
health care. Clearly, too, budget restrictions on income maintenance and
rent subsidies for poor families, and reductions in food programs for
pregnant women, children, and elders could not help but deter planning
for improved community health.

Public participation in health care, even outside the HSAs themselves, appeared less likely with the introduction of legislation to remove the requirement that a third of health maintenance organization (HMO) board members be consumers (*Consumer Coalition for Health Newsletter*, 1981). A preelection Republican platform promise to reduce consumer participation in administrative programs was to be carried out by rescinding Executive Order 12160 of 1980 that had required a consumer affairs plan and program in every federal government unit (*Federal Register*, 1980).

In short, the prospects in the early 1980s for a federally supported health planning network with significant public participation were dim, as was the likelihood of mandated citizen involvement in many other federal programs.

Nevertheless other nongovernment-supported avenues of participation were expected to continue and perhaps new ones to develop. Continuing public interest, consumer, and other problem-oriented groups, some with general purposes, others with a single interest, were expected to continue to try to influence public health care policy. As in the past, they promoted their aims through public education and information campaigns, lobbying, litigation, and involvement in such administrative decision-making processes as critiques, comments on proposed regulations, presentation of testimony, or petitioning for regulatory action. All of this, however, depended upon their success in raising private funds for these costly tasks.

Public participation through these traditional channels, supported by private monies, also was likely to skew participation toward a continued pattern of middle- and upper middle-class people, dealing mainly with issues most important to those groups. Although other groups could form, they would tend to mobilize around ad hoc issues and be short term, effective sometimes in blocking cutbacks in public programs but not necessarily in sustaining new directions in policy because of lack of funds and organizational strength (Marmor & Bridges, 1980).

CONCLUSION

Whatever the fate of health systems agencies, the public interest in improved health; in equitable, effective, and efficient services; and in a public voice in how these should be pursued, would remain and would be pursued, if only through different channels and formats.

Whatever the difficulties in fostering interest in better personal health services through public participation—whether government supported or privately organized—they are less pronounced than the general promotion of the public interest in health. It continues to be easier to gain support for combating a particular disease or delivering a specific service than for supporting broad-scale healthful living conditions. Unlike planning issues in personal health care, conditions for improved general health are less specific. They are not dramatic and they have many indirect causes that are controversial even, or especially, among experts. They often threaten powerful special interests, and the costs of creating them in the short term may be large.

They also call for extending such traditional values as equity in the distribution of health services to include fairness in the distribution of achieved health status and in the environmental and occupational conditions that are prerequisites to healthful living.

Providers of care are constrained by their interests from finding ways to make persuasive the case for the primary prevention of illness and the promotion of health. If such a reevaluation of health and how to create it is ever to be made, the impetus will have to come from strong, public support, placing the people's interests above particular interests.

This review of the history and widespread exercise of citizen participation in public decision making suggests that this kind of involvement will not disappear even with the withdrawal of federal support. The evidence also shows that if and when organizational resources are available to sustain the process, public participation can enhance democratic goals and also contribute to more effective decision making in the health interests of the public.

REFERENCES

Advisory Commission on Intergovernmental Regulations. *Citizen participation in the American federal system.* Washington, D.C.: U.S. Government Printing Office, 1980.

Arthur D. Little, Inc. *An evaluation of the operation of subarea advisory councils.* Washington, D.C.: Department of Health, Education, and Welfare, Health Resources Administration, Bureau of Health Planning, 1979.

Bacheller, J.M. Lobbyists and the legislative process: The impact of environmental constraints. *American Political Science Review,* 1977, *71,* 252–263.

Bellin, L., Kaveler, F., & Schwarz, A. Phase one of consumer participation in policies of 22 voluntary hospitals in New York City. *American Journal of Public Health,* 1972, *62*(12), 1370–1375.

Berry, J. *Lobbying for the people.* Princeton, N.J.: Princeton University Press, 1977.

Blue Ribbon Commission on Public Health Services. *New directions in public health.* City of Springfield, Mass., 1979.

Blum, H. *Planning for health* (2nd ed.). New York: Human Sciences Press, 1981.

Bradbury, R. A comprehensive health planning board of directors. *Health Services Reports,* 1972, *87*(9), 905–908.

Broder, D. Campaigns, parties and the public purse. *The Washington Post,* April 15, 1979.

Brook, R., & Appel, W. Quality of care assessment. *The New England Journal of Medicine,* 1973, *288*(12), 1323–1329.

Burdine, J. *Determining the impact of consumer participation on health systems plans.* Paper presented at the meeting of the American Public Health Association, Detroit, October 1980. (Mimeographed)

Bureau of Health Planning. *Draft impact performance review system and standards.* Washington, D.C.: Department of Health and Human Services, Health Resources Administration, July 1980.

Campbell, J. Working relationships between providers and consumers in a neighborhood health center. *American Journal of Public Health,* 1971, *61*(1), 97–103.

Chamberlin, R., & Radebaugh, J. Delivery of primary health care—unstyle: A critical review of the Robert F. Kennedy plan for the United Farm Workers. *The New England Journal of Medicine,* 1976, *294,* 541–545.

Consumer Commission on Accreditation of Health Services. Recommendations: National quality controls. *Health Perspectives,* July-August, 1975.

Consumer effectiveness: Now and under NHS. *Consumer Health Perspectives,* 1978, *5*(4), 1–4.

Cooper, T. The hidden price tag: Participation costs and health planning. *American Journal of Public Health,* 1979, *69*(3), 368–374.

Danaceau, P. *Consumer participation in health care: How it's working.* Arlington, Va.: Human Services for Children and Families, Inc., 1975.

Diamond, E. *Good news, bad news.* Cambridge, Mass.: MIT Press, 1978.

Douglass, C.W. Consumer influence in health planning in the urban ghetto. *Inquiry,* 1975, *12*(2), 157–163.

Douglass, C.W. Representation patterns in community health decision-making. *Journal of Health and Social Behavior,* 1973, *14.*

Executive Order 12160. *Federal Register,* February 4, 1980.

Falkson, J. An evaluation of policy-related research of citizen participation in municipal health service systems. *Medical Care Review,* 1976, *33,* 156–209.

Fleming, G., & Andersen, R. *Health beliefs of the U.S. population: Implications for self-care.* Background paper, Conference on Self-Care Programs, National Center for Health Services Research, Rockville, Md., March 25–26, 1975.

Gallup, G. The Gallup poll. *The Chapel Hill Newspaper,* August 17, 1981.

Gans, C. The politics of selfishness: The cause: The empty voting booths. *Washington Monthly,* October 1978, pp. 27–36.

Gerlach, L. Movements of revolutionary change: Some structural characteristics. *American Behavioral Science,* 1971, *4*(6), 812–836.

Goldman, L. Doctors' attitudes toward national health insurance. *Medical Care,* 1974, *12,* 413–423.

Greer, A.L. Training board members for health planning agencies—A review of the literature. *Public Health Reports,* 1976, *91*(1), 56–61.

Hadley, J. Political action committees. *Washington Monthly,* October 1978.

Health Resources Administration. HSA evaluation reported. *Health Resources News,* 1980, *7*(11), 3.

HSAs receive action proposal. *Health Resources News,* 1981, *8*(1), 1.

Hill-Burton: Program with a future? *Medicine and Health Perspectives,* August 24, 1981.

How money talks in Congress. Washington, D.C.: Common Cause, 1979.

Hulka, B.S., Zyranski, S.J., Cassell, J.C. & Thompson, S.J. Scale for the measurement of attitudes towards physicians and medical care. *Medical Care,* 1971, *8,* 429.

Institute of Society, Ethics and the Life Sciences, Research Group on Ethical, Social and Legal Issues in Genetic Counseling and Genetic Engineering. Ethical and social issues in screening for genetic disease. *The New England Journal of Medicine,* 1972, *286*(10), 1129–1132.

Ittig, K.B. *Consumer participation in health planning and service delivery: A selective review and a proposed research agenda.* Rockville, Md.: U.S. Department of Health, Education, and Welfare, U.S. Public Health Service, National Center for Health Statistics Research, 1976 (Mimeographed).

Jonas, S. Limitations of community control of health facilities and services. *American Journal of Public Health,* 1978, *68*(6), 541–543.

Kelman, H. Evaluation of health care by consumers. *International Journal of Health Services,* 1976, *6*(3), 431–441.

Kleiman, M. A consumer analysis of the 1979 Health Planning Act Amendments. *Health Law Project Library Bulletin,* 1979, *4,* 327–336.

Knox, J.J. *The functions of consumers on programs and policymaking of health systems agencies and statewide health coordinating councils.* Memorandum to the National Council for Health Planning and Development, May 5, 1978.

Koseki, L.K., & Hayakawa, J.M. *Consumer participation and community organization practice: Implications of national health legislation.* Paper presented at the Annual Meeting of the American Public Health Association, Washington, D.C., November 2, 1977.

Kosch, B., Gozzi, E., & Francis, V. Gaps in doctor-patient communication—I: Doctor-patient interaction and patient satisfaction. *Pediatrics,* 1968, *42,* 855.

Lazarsfeld, P., & Reitz, J. *An introduction to applied sociology.* New York: Elsevier Scientific Publication Co., 1975.

Lebow, J.L. Consumer assessments of the quality of medical care. *Medical Care,* 1974, *12*(3), 328.

Marmor, T., & Bridges, A. American health planning and the lessons of comparative policy analysis. *Journal of Health Politics, Policy & Law,* 1980, *5*(3), 419–429.

Medical care for the American people: Final report. The Committee on the Costs of Medical Care (adopted October 31, 1932). Washington, D.C.: Department of Health, Education, and Welfare, U.S. Public Health Service. (Reprinted 1970)

Medicine & Health Perspectives, August 31, 1981.

Metch, J., & Veney, J.E. Consumer participation and social accountability. *Medical Care,* 1976, *14*(2), 283–293.

Milio, N. Dimensions of consumer participation and national health legislation. *American Journal of Public Health,* 1974, *64*(4), 357–363.

Milio, N. *The care of health in communities: Access for outcasts.* New York: Macmillan Publishing Company, Inc., 1975.

Milio, N. *Consumer participation with the consumer in view and involved.* Cincinnati: University of Cincinnati College of Community Health Services, Graduate Program in Health Administration, 1977.

Milio, N. *Promoting health through public policy.* Philadelphia: F.A. Davis Company, 1981.

Miller, A. Analysis of 1976 American national election survey. *ISR Center for Political Studies Newsletter,* 1979, *7*(1), 3.

Mitchell, R.C. What the public thinks. *Resources,* 1978, *57,* 1–2, 20–21.

Moyar, R. *Social science and institutional change.* Washington, D.C.: U.S. Department of Health, Education, and Welfare, National Institute on Mental Health, 1980.

National Council on Health Planning and Development. *Report on consumer participation in the health planning program* (draft). Washington, D.C.: U.S. Department of Health and Human Services, June 1980.

Navarro, V. The political economy of medical care. *International Journal of Health Services,* 1975, *5,*(1), 1. (a)

Navarro, V. Women in health care. *The New England Journal of Medicine,* 1975, *292*(8), 398–402. (b)

New, P.K., & Hessler, R.M. Neighborhood health centers: Traditional medical care at an outpost? *Inquiry,* 1972, *9*(4), 45–58.

New regulations proposed. *Consumer Coalition for Health Newsletter,* August 1981.

North, J. The effect of PACs: The growth of the special interests. *Washington Monthly,* October 1978.

Notkin, H., & Notkin, M.S. Community participation in health services. *Medical Care Review,* 1970, *27,* 1178.

Olendski, M. *Concerns of the consumer.* Paper presented at the Conference on Redesigning Nursing Education for Public Health, Washington, D.C., Division of Nursing, Department of Health, Education & Welfare, May 22–25, 1973.

Paap, W.R. Consumer-based boards of health centers: Structural problems in achieving effective control. *American Journal of Public Health,* 1978, *68*(5), 578–582.

Parkum, K., & Parkum, V. *Voluntary participation in health planning: A study of health consumer and provider participation in comprehensive health planning in selected areas of Pennsylvania.* Phila.₈ Pa. Department of Health, November 1973.

Partridge, K.B. Community and professional participation in decision-making at a health center. *Health Services Reports,* 1973, *88*(4), 527–534.

Perlman, J. Grass-roots participation from neighborhood to nation. In S. Langston (Ed.), *Citizen participation in America.* Lexington, Mass.: Lexington Books, D.C. Heath and Company, 1978.

Public Citizen Annual Report 1980. Washington, D.C.: Public Citizen, 1981.

Public Health Service. *HRA, HSA, CDC, & ADAMHA: Public advisory committees: Authority structure, functions, members* (U.S. Department of Health, Education, and Welfare, U.S. Public Health Service, 1976). Washington, D.C.: U.S. Government Printing Office, 1976.

Rayack, E. *Professional power and American medicine.* New York: World Publishing, 1967.

Reeder, L. The patient-client as a consumer: Some observations on the changing professional-client relationship. *Journal of Health and Social Behavior,* 1972, *13,* 406–412.

Riska, E. & Taylor, J.A. Consumer attitudes toward health policy and knowledge about health legislation. *Journal of Health Politics, Policy and Law,* 1978, *3*(1), 112–123.

Sackett, D., & Torrance, G. The utility of different health states as perceived by the general public. *Journal of Chronic Disease,* 1978, *31,* 697–704.

Sanazaro, P., & Williamson, J. End results of patient care: A provisional classification based on reports by internists. *Medical Care,* 1970, *6*(2), 123–130.

Sapolsky, H. Corporate attitudes toward health care costs. Executive Summary. Washington, D.C.: Department of Health and Human Services, National Center for Health Services Research, December 1980.

Shenkin & Warner. Giving the patient his medical record: A proposal to improve the system. *The New England Journal of Medicine*, 1973, *289*(7), 688–692.

Skoie, H. (Ed.). *Scientific expertise and the public proceedings: Studies in research and higher education.* Oslo: Norwegian Research Institutes, 1979.

Sparer, G., Dines, G.R., & Smith, D. Consumer participation in OEO-assisted neighborhood health centers. *American Journal of Public Health,* 1970, *60*(6), 1091–1102.

Stewart, R.B. The reformation of American administrative law. *Harvard Law Review,* 1975, *88*(8), 1669–1813.

Stokes, A., Banta, D., & Putnam, S. The Columbia point health association: Evolution of a community health board. *American Journal of Public Health,* 1972, *62*(10), 1129–1134.

Strickland, S. *U.S. health care: What's wrong and what's right about it.* Washington, D.C.: Potomac Associates, 1973.

Success stories in the public interest. *N.C. Insight,* Fall 1980, 26–27.

Tessler, R., & Mechanic, D. Consumer satisfaction with prepaid group practice: a comparative study. *Journal of Health and Social Behavior,* 1975, *16*, 95.

The development of a consumer health network. *Health Perspectives,* 1977, *4*(4,5), 1–12.

Ulrich, R. Tribal community health representatives of the Indian Health Service, *Public Health Reports,* 1969, *84*(1), 11.

U.S. chamber group seeks more funds for study of national health policy. *Washington Report on Medicine and Health,* January 9, 1978.

U.S. Congress, House, Committee on Interstate and Foreign Commerce, *National Health Policy, Planning and Resources Act of 1974,* 93d Cong., 2d sess., 1974, H. Rept.

U.S. Congress, House, Committee on Interstate and Foreign Commerce, *Health Planning and Health Services Research and Statistics Extension Act of 1977,* 95th Congress, 1st sess.

U.S. Congress, House, Committee on Interstate and Foreign Commerce, *Health Planning and Resources Development Amendments of 1979,* 96th Cong., 1st sess., 1979.

U.S. Congress, Senate, Committee on Human Resources, Subcommittee on Health and Scientific Research, Report prepared on *Biomedical Research and the Public,* 95th Cong. 1st sess., 1977.

van den Heuvel, W. Role of the consumer in health policy. *Social Science and Medicine,* 1980, *14a,* 423–426.

Warren, R. *The structure of urban reform.* Lexington, Mass.: Lexington Books, D.C. Heath and Company, 1974.

Weinberg, A.J. The WGBH. *Washington Business Group on Health.* Washington, D.C., 1978.

Weisbrod, B.A., Handler, J.F. & Komesar, N.K. *Public interest law, an economic and institutional analysis.* Berkeley, Calif.: University of California Press, 1978.

Young, T.K. Lay professional conflict in a Canadian community health center: A case report. *Medical Care,* 1975, *13*(11), 897–904.

Zwick, D. Initial development of national guidelines for health planning. *Public Health Reports,* 1978, *93*(5), 407.

Chapter 7

Regional Organization and a National Health Program: A Pipedream?

Leonard S. Rosenfeld

For approximately 70 years, debate on national health insurance has waxed and waned. Despite the growth of a consensus on the need for a more effective system of health care financing, this issue has not been resolved. Factors responsible for failure to achieve agreement are easily identified. They are a function of the American social and political matrix, which is far more complex than in most other countries. Its large size; regional variation; social, cultural, and racial heterogeneity; the three-tier system of government; and strongly held traditions of pluralism, private enterprise, and institutional autonomy magnify difficulties in arriving at a consensus on strategies.

Powerful organizations with their own agendas have emerged as strong political forces. Examining patterns of health care financing among industrialized nations, Brian Able-Smith speculated that the United States' inability to act might be attributable in some measure to delay in formulation of public policy that provided time for special interests to grow and to consolidate their positions (Abel-Smith, 1969).

This analysis (an elaboration of an earlier discussion (Rosenfeld, 1978), provides a perspective on the problems of moving toward a national health program and of potentialities for revising local organization and the system of incentives for providing care. Particular consideration is given to the concept of basing local responsibility within the framework of regional organizations. While inclusion of regional organizations has been a feature of national health plans proposed in the past, discussion of that aspect has been limited. Expanding responsibility of local jurisdictions for planning, organizing, and financing services would bring these functions closer to the population served, offering the public a greater insight into the dynamics of program and costs. This, in turn, could mobilize a higher level of participation in decisions and more responsible use of services than is possible under state or federal administration alone.

It is not expected that this or any other proposal will motivate early legislative action. The premise here is that examination of alternate policy formulations is important for understanding the relative values and limitations of each approach, as well as their social, economic, political, and geographic implications, against the time when the issue of a national health program once again becomes a matter of serious consideration.

The phrase "national health care crisis" has been in common use since the 1960s. However, its meaning has changed over time. At first, the term expressed a widespread preoccupation with equality of access to health care during the rapid expansion of federal commitment in this area, i.e., the now defunct Office of Economic Opportunity and the two 1965 mammoth programs, Medicare and Medicaid.

With the rapidly mounting rate of expenditures, the focus of national concern shifted from equality of opportunity for health care to reduction in costs. Starting in the late 1960s, numerous efforts at cost containment were launched by government agencies at all levels and by voluntary programs. Although many of these strategies were well conceived and based on awareness of factors fueling inflation in health care costs, none seemed to affect the rate of increase significantly.

While the dominant feature of the "crisis" has been the rapidly escalating costs, focus on this aspect of the health care system without considering others constitutes an oversimplification. Indeed, cost experience is a symptom of characteristics rather than the root problem of health services in the United States.

Among the factors responsible for burgeoning costs are:

- the continued uncontrolled trend toward specialization
- the absence of a coherent national policy for adapting health services organization to economic, technologic, and professional trends
- the outmoded methods of payment for services
- the failure to reconcile aspirations for achieving equity in access and improvement in quality with economic and organizational realities.

While expenditures for health care have been increasing in all industrialized nations, comparisons of trends among countries using distinctive approaches to structure and financing suggest that uncontrolled escalation of costs far in advance of economic trends is not inherent in the delivery of health services in general. The rates of increase in both England and

Canada, countries with national health programs, have been significantly lower than that of the United States (Simanis & Coleman, 1980).

COST TRENDS AND RESPONSIBLE FACTORS

The inflation of health care costs is not a phenomenon of recent years alone. Although it was given renewed impetus with the initiation of the Medicare and Medicaid programs, serious concern had been expressed about mounting costs in the 1950s. Then, rapid expansion of coverage under voluntary insurance resulted from the attention given to health and welfare benefits in collective bargaining. This had been ushered in by the Office of Economic Stabilization regulation in 1943 to exempt such benefits from the wartime wage-price freeze (Office of Economic Stabilization, 1943) and the concurrent policy of allowing corporate income tax deductions of expenditures for such benefits. Table 7-1 provides a perspective on the relative rates of increase in national health expenditures and as percent of gross national product for selected years.

The factors responsible for increasing costs are complex, and although a number of them have been identified, their individual impact is difficult to measure objectively. The Health Care Financing Administration (HCFA), in estimating the relative importance of major factors stimulating growth in personal health care expenditures from 1972 to 1977, found that price accounted for 66 percent of the increase. Population growth was responsible for 7 percent and "intensity," reflecting changes in quantity and/or composition of goods and services, for some 28 percent of the increase

---

Table 7-1 Increases in National Health Expenditures

Year	National Health Expenditures	% of GNP
1929	$3.6	3.5
1940	4.0	4.0
1950	12.7	4.4
1960	26.9	5.3
1970	132.1	8.6
1980	247.0	9.4

Source: Reprinted from "National Health Expenditures, 1980," by Robert M. Gibson and D.R. Waldo, *Health Care Financing Review,* 1981, *3*(1), p. 18.

(Gibson, 1980). Such an analysis is useful in studying trends but it is of limited value in gaining insights into mechanisms that power the growth in expenditures. A number of plausible reasons have been suggested to explain price and intensity, two of the major factors identified by HCFA.

The Impact of Price

Among the forces contributing to escalation in prices are:

1. general inflation
2. payments to providers on the basis of units of service, combined with prepayment
3. the strong influence of hospital medical staffs on institutional policy, utilization, and acquisition of sophisticated equipment
4. similar elements in nursing homes, plus the need to stimulate investment in them
5. multiple sources of financing

As to the first of those points, inflation—spurred in part by soaring health care costs—obviously is a major factor. This has produced almost a "Catch-22" situation: inflation raising all costs (including those for health care), the industry reaching and often passing the new levels, the rest of the economy again catching up or moving ahead, and so on in a seemingly never-ending spiral.

On the second point, with the advent of third party payment, many physicians raised their fees. This trend was augmented by the growth of major medical insurance in the 1950s (Somers & Somers, 1961).

On the third point, some of the dysfunctional trends in hospital development may be traced to the powerful role of medical staffs. Visiting physicians, who constitute the majority of the staffs, in many cases have only limited understanding of (or are unwilling to accept) the economics of hospital care. They have little, if any, responsibility for the hospital's financial welfare or appreciation of how this relates to the public good. Under the prevailing payment system, the hospital administrator and board of directors are in a poor position to resist medical staff pressures to acquire expensive equipment, regardless of its justification.

As for the fourth point, among nursing homes there has been an increase in utilization, coupled with the cost of operating a for-profit industry supported by human misfortune and suffering. In addition to the expense of maintaining often spartan and substandard services must be counted the costs of providing incentives for investment to guarantee the supply of these beds and, unfortunately, the price of substantial fraud and abuse (Vladeck, 1980).

And finally, the vast expenditures for health care could provide potentially powerful leverage in negotiating more favorable prices. However, this use is precluded by the existence of many payment agencies and private and public programs at national, state, and local levels. Multiple sources of financing also contribute to high administrative costs.

Intensity of Service

Among the significant elements in the other major factor, "intensity," that are motivating ever-increasing expenditures are:

1. utilization
2. third party responsibility for payment
3. patients' demands that "something be done"
4. malpractice suits
5. incentives to expand treatment and utilization
6. the lack of a national health personnel policy

As to utilization, improving access to achieve equity in availability of needed services, regardless of race, ethnic origin, or ability to pay, has been one of the national goals enunciated for some decades, with the considerable impetus from President Johnson's Great Society program of the 1960s. This has been only partially successful. There is evidence that the amount of service provided among some groups, depending on their eligibility under voluntary insurance or public programs, exceeds needs, but among others, available service falls short. Deviation from need in either direction is undesirable in terms of health and economy.

On the second point, the advent of third party responsibility for payment removes a deterrent to demand. It reduces constraints on the provider, when recommending services, to assess critically the potential values of intervention for the patient.

This, coupled with the patient's often unsophisticated demand that "something be done"—the third point—frequently leads to decisions on modes of therapy that may be costly and, while not contraindicated, may be of marginal value for the individual's health and welfare.

The desire that something be done is reinforced by the fourth point—growth of malpractice suits.

As to the fifth point, leaving aside the moral issue of intervention to increase provider income, there are strong incentives to pursue a regimen of care that may impress the patient with the provider's concern and skill rather than relying on less dramatic but often more effective forms of management such as advice and guidance and administration of preventive measures. The effects of incentives inherent in different systems of organization and financing of services are evident on comparing utilization in different settings. The significantly lower rates of surgery in the United Kingdom, and of both hospital utilization and surgery in group practice prepayment plans in the United States as compared with populations covered under forms of health insurance traditional in this country, have been well documented (Bunker, 1970; Luft, 1980; Perrott, 1971).

The final factor is the continuing absence of a national health manpower policy. The number of medical graduates doubled in the 1970s. Projection of this trend indicates that the supply is outstripping reasonable demand and is likely to suppress effective use of less costly new health practitioners such as nurse practitioners and physician's assistants. At the same time, not enough is being done to balance the distribution of physicians either among the medical specialties or geographically (Report to Secretary of HHS, 1981). It is estimated that each physician, whether or not essential to adequate service, adds more than $350,000 annually to health care expenditures.

Technology and the Technological Imperative

Closely related to this is the impact of rapidly burgeoning technology. New technologies often reach the market before there has been an opportunity to assess their values and limitations through clinical trials. This, combined with the highly developed marketing and promotional skills of producers, often results in the substitution of more expensive forms of diagnosis and therapy for previously established methods, without the clear assurance that they are superior. Once new technology is available, there are strong pressures for its acquisition, even though it may be underutilized.

For example, the DeBakey Commission reported in the early 1960s that 30 percent of 770 hospitals equipped for open-heart surgery had not performed procedures in the year under study and 87 percent of those with cases had performed less than one operation a week (President's Commission, 1964). The situation was no different in 1967 when 31 percent of hospitals with open-heart surgical units had not used the facilities within a year (McCarthy, 1981). There is, furthermore, evidence that case fatality is inversely proportional to the numbers of procedures done (Luft, Bunker, & Enthoven, 1979).

Lack of Risk Sharing by Providers

Lacking requirements that providers share responsibility for costs, and without the discipline of operating within the framework of a budget, there are few constraints on either providers or consumers in the utilization of services. Even if services are offered in good faith, the multiple decisions involved in managing health needs of large population groups produce high rates of utilization of services, many of which do little to improve outcomes.

Wildavsky (1977) epitomized the effects of the system of incentives in health care on utilization and costs of care in the following:

- the uncertainty principle: "There is always one more thing that might be done;" and,
- the medical money law: "Medical costs rise to equal the sum of private insurance and government subsidy," a medical variation of Parkinson's Law.

Effects of Cost Increases

Escalating costs of health care are pervasive. They have affected virtually all health programs and modalities of care, both public and private. They have frustrated the broadly based desire for more effective protection against the often devastating expenses entailed in caring for serious or protracted illness. As a result of the inexorable advances in costs, eligibility for and coverage by Medicaid has been cut back progressively by states across the country. Despite continuing increases in expenditures for Medicare, out-of-pocket expenses by those eligible continue to mount. Basic problems of assuring availability and quality of long-term care remain unresolved.

The continuing growth of the elderly population, particularly in the more advanced ages, poses a growing challenge to the cohorts of younger age groups to provide at least minimum adequate services and facilities for the aged. The visibility of these expenses by virtue of the special entitlement for this group under Medicare invites a political backlash among the members of the working community who contribute support through taxes while carrying the burden of mounting costs for their own medical care. This backlash was manifest in the Reagan program. Delays in the adoption of a national health policy designed to partially relieve all age groups of the burden of direct costs of care have been attributed, in some measure at least, to escalating expenditures for Medicare and Medicaid.

Labor and industry keenly feel the impact of cost escalation: the former by the erosion of benefits achieved through collective bargaining (in lieu of take-home pay) and the latter through the effect on sales and on competitive positions in the world market. Further, public welfare suffers as it vies for governmental financial support with the more glamorous health services that command greater attention from appropriating bodies. Like Laocoön and his sons enmeshed in the coils of the sea serpents, American society seems helpless in fighting the strangulating grip of rising costs of health care.

While the political climate of the early 1980s was not conducive to a basic change in the economic structure of health care in the United States, this could change in the event of a sharp economic recession, an international emergency, or a change in administration. In any case, the public health community must continue to explore alternative strategies for preserving and improving the structure of the health sector of Social Security that has been developed thus far.

SOCIAL CONTROL OF HEALTH CARE

Legislation and regulation are the response of government to social problems. They express the values and goals of the body politic in a democracy, or of the oligarchy in an authoritarian government. In each, they are essential to the functioning of the particular society. While unfettered free choice would be a natural preference, acceptance of a framework of public policy is integral to life in the community. Regulations are designed to restrain price, to prevent abuse, to assure standards of quality, to promote efficiency, and in general to protect the public interest.

In the face of mounting health care costs in recent decades, the rate of adoption of legislation and regulations accelerated. The years since the early 1970s have seen the consideration or adoption by federal and state governments of a wide range of health policies and regulations. Among them are the National Health Planning and Resources Development Act of 1974, P.L. 93-641, and related regulations, certificate-of-need legislation, state rate review procedures, wage and price controls, health maintenance organization (HMO) legislation, utilization review and professional standards review organizations (PSROs), and proposals to establish a cap on revenues of hospitals in order to contain escalating costs.

To protect quality of services, there are policies and regulations governing licensure, there are detailed conditions for participation to be met by various groups that wish to provide services under Medicare and Medicaid, and there are numerous grant programs. Federal and state policies have been designed to control fraud and abuse and regulations have been adopted to assure equality of opportunity under various programs.

Many professional organizations and voluntary agencies are also responsible for maintaining standards of service. They review facilities and programs for accreditation and certify certain categories of professional and technical personnel. The Joint Commission on Accreditation of Hospitals measures compliance of institutional facilities with established norms; the Association of American Medical Colleges and the American Medical Association accredit medical schools; the National League for Nursing performs the same function for schools for nursing, and, in cooperation with the American Public Health Association, accredits home health and community health agencies; and specialty boards conduct examinations for certification of specialists and subspecialists in medicine. The AMA also certifies training programs in the several technical disciplines, including physical therapy and occupational therapy, among others.

Regulatory bodies such as the Federal Trade Commission monitor business practices in the health field as well as in others for evidence of monopoly practice. Finally, the courts are playing an increasingly important role in defining liability for malpractice; in issuing injunctions to postpone activation of regulations that may exceed legislative authority; in adjudicating constitutional issues related to federal, state, and local legislation; and in judging cases of felony. To say that the web of social controls, safeguards, and regulations surrounding the delivery of health care is complex is an understatement. It also is inefficient.

The multiplicity of uncoordinated regulations on the books at the three levels of government is overwhelming. The Hospital Association of New York estimates that the average hospital must file reports with some 160 regulatory agencies. Inconsistencies and overlapping are frequent.

Many of the regulatory agencies are inadequately staffed to carry out mandated functions. In response to public demand and expectations, or bureaucratic ineptitude, government agencies often develop regulations on the basis of inadequate analysis of the need, insufficient perspective on related statutes and regulations, and unrealistic concepts of the feasibility of their administration. Frequently both the formulation and administration of regulations are unduly influenced by powerful interests.

Finally, there is the pervasive human trait of ingenuity that often is used to circumvent the most carefully devised system of regulations. Appeals, injunctions, and other strategies for using and abusing due process protections can cause endless delays in arriving at final decisions. The resulting regulatory system may be not only inefficient but also very costly.

Complicating this elaborate system of health services regulation is the size and heterogeneity of American society. As is true of organizations generally, large size attenuates identity and accountability and the cooperation and communication that are central to effective functioning.

These comments should not be construed as support for the thesis that regulation is not necessary. As suggested earlier, constraints are essential to living in society. Rather, the argument is that many of the regulatory mechanisms are inappropriate and poorly designed. Social organization is not based on rules alone. The very complexity of human relationships makes such an arrangement impossible, even if it were desirable. Interchange among individuals and groups is primarily an outgrowth of mores, preferences, motivations, and incentives.

PUBLIC FINANCING OF HEALTH SERVICES

Until the Great Depression and the social legislation enacted to stem its ravages on the economy, with the exception of the Sheppard-Towner Act of 1921 (Mustard, 1945), what modest public investment in health services that existed emanated from state and local government (Sheppard-Towner was a federal grants-in-aid program to encourage states to develop maternal and infant care programs.) Except for the few functions clearly allocated to the federal government by the constitution, states were responsible for regulation of health care under police powers implicit in the Constitution.

With the passage of the Social Security Act and legislation authorizing federal grants-in-aid, federal responsibility for regulation of the health care industry expanded. Increasing recognition of the wide variations in economic potential among the states and of the great inequities in access to basic services motivated adoption of legislation providing for vastly expanded federal commitments to the support of health care.

Categorical grants to states (not including payments to individuals and institutions) increased from $4 million in 1936 to $1.9 billion in 1975. These grants spanned a wide range of health programs encompassing maternal and child services, categorical disease control programs, hospital survey and construction, research facilities, poliomyelitis vaccination, health services planning and development, regional medical services, mental retardation, and others. Each of these programs had its own requirements and regulations. Moreover, state and local government agencies have had little discretion in the use of funds allocated for each category beyond an initial decision whether or not to accept the grant.

Federal health grants-in-aid to state and local governments represented 3.9 percent of the $48.5 billion appropriated for all grants in 1975. This constituted a significant addition of 29 percent to "own source" income of lower government units (Dales, 1976).

Federal financing of health services took a quantum leap in 1965 with the passage of Medicare and Medicaid. As a result, government financing increased from 25 percent of total health care expenditures in 1965 to 40 percent after inauguration of these programs. Federal expenditures in this sector surpassed those of state and local governments combined. Federal intervention and regulation of the health care industry also increased in proportion.

As a result of confusion and controversy over the organization and administration of programs such as those of the Office of Economic Opportunity and of Medicaid, anxiety was expressed concerning the wisdom of continuing the trend of transfer of initiative and responsibility from the local and state level of government to the federal. Moynihan commented on the dangers in the continuation of such trends (Moynihan, 1968).

Viewed from a detached perspective, the failure of programs to achieve their objectives, and of regulations to fulfill expectations, is understandable. Without adaptation of organization and the system of incentives within an expanding matrix of technology, and without revision of the system of financing in response to changes in perception of need and cost trends, it is unrealistic to expect that programs and regulations would fare better than they did. This holds true particularly in a situation in which the multiplicity of uncoordinated regulations is administered by a number of independent agencies, each concerned with only one aspect of the whole.

The progressive transfer of responsibility for financing, program initiative, and regulation of health programs from nonfederal to federal government eroded local responsibility and capability for providing leadership in planning, organization, coordination, and administration of health services.

It cannot be denied that significant progress has been made toward the goal of achieving equity in access to needed services among the various socioeconomic, geographic, and ethnic groups and improving the standards of care in general. Nevertheless, these changes have retarded development of an essential part of the health service structure and reduced its ability to respond to the new demands. Most of the major federal health programs since the mid-1960s circumvented either state or local government. These programs included, among others, Medicare (P.L. 89-97), Regional Medical Programs (P.L. 89-239), the PSRO Amendments of 1972 (P.L. 92-603), and the National Health Planning and Resources Development Act of 1974.

If the nation is truly to address the issue of moderating the inordinate increase in health care costs, a more fundamental approach will be necessary, one in which appropriate incentives are created and an effective system of mutual accountability among the various participants is adopted. If this could be accomplished, the need for detailed regulation would diminish.

To reinstitute balance in the growth of health services within a framework of socially constructive goals, the United States must develop two strategies in tandem, as suggested by the Committee on Costs of Medical Care 50 years ago: the financing of services by social insurance and/or general revenues, and the reorganization of services (CCMC, 1932). While the two issues have been addressed piecemeal, and in part by evolving national policy, the changes have not been sufficient to maintain balance within the system.

The problem has not been in the recognition of needs but in the failure to develop a political consensus and the will necessary for the adoption of changes in public policy.

Two trends affecting organization of services are relevant: (1) scientific and technological advances and associated specialization and costs, and (2) growing appreciation of the significance of the local jurisdiction in organization of public programs. This chapter is particularly concerned with health care but it is hardly necessary to point out that these trends influence virtually all public services. With the increasing share of health service support coming from government sources, trends in organization of public programs have a direct bearing on progress in the field.

Impact of Technological Change

Rapid advances in the basic sciences and technologies, with attendant increases in specialization, have brought both stimulus and stress to health service organization. Meeting the costs of expanding technology demands an expanding population base for support. A population of 2,000 can keep a personal physician efficiently occupied; however, a neurosurgeon, a cardiovascular surgeon, or a neonatologist requires a population base of 100,000 or more. Such specialists depend on teams of supporting personnel and facilities, adding to the costs of maintaining their services. Further, for a variety of reasons (coverage, consultation, training requirements), specialized physicians rarely practice alone.

A large center serving a substantial population is requisite for such care. Although a community hospital of 150 beds staffed by personal physicians and representatives of the basic medical specialties can effectively meet the needs of a population of approximately 50,000, a large teaching hospital may require a population of 1 million to 2 million to make effective use of its highly specialized staff and sophisticated facilities. Indeed, it is difficult to recruit and retain a high calibre of specialists without appropriate facilities and a population large enough to produce a sufficient number of challenging cases.

Similar considerations relate to management. Large programs can justify employment of specialists in various aspects of management, i.e., data processing, management engineering, facilities planning, and the like. Similar principles apply to local health departments. While large city health departments can employ program specialists equipped to bring current knowledge and experience to bear on planning and organization related to their area of expertise, the small county department inevitably is limited in staff resources.

Economies of scale are within the grasp of larger institutions but may be impossible to accomplish in smaller facilities operating in isolation except by means of merger or shared resources through contractual arrangements. Strategies for achieving these ends have been developed by various governmental and private organizations.

In the voluntary sector, the decades of the 1960s and 1970s saw an accelerating growth of multi-institutional arrangements in recognition of increasing interdependence of programs and institutions. A 1978 American Hospital Association survey indicated that 80 percent of all hospitals in the United States shared at least one service (AHA, 1979). The "invisible hand" of the economy has turned to tasks not anticipated by Adam Smith. These arrangements have taken various forms, including formal affiliation, shared or cooperative services, consortia for planning or education, contract management, lease/condominium arrangements, and corporate ownership and management (Mason, 1979).

Shared services cover a wide range, the five most frequent being blood banking, purchasing, data processing, disaster planning, and laboratory staffing (Hepner, 1978).

Numerous values have been ascribed to these systems. Economies of scale loom high, with advantages to both provider and consumer. Advantages in recruitment and retention of specialized clinical and administrative personnel, greater access to capital markets for expansion and for acquisition of equipment, and ability to provide a broader range of services are others. In some cases, benefits may take the form of institutional survival itself (Zuckerman, 1979).

While multi-institutional arrangements have gained wide acceptance, many questions remain unanswered. Zuckerman shows, in an excellent evaluation of research and experience, that the economic benefits of these arrangements are mixed; that there is as yet little understanding of the relationships between organizational form and economic, personnel, or organizational benefits; and that there are serious barriers to development posed by antitrust laws, tax laws, and reimbursement policies. There is need for more research, in both methodology and evaluation.

In forging the National Health Planning and Resources Development Act of 1974, Congress expressed its appreciation of the potentialities of multi-institutional systems, and of the organizational inadequacies of the health care system generally. In its listing of priorities in Section 1502 of the act, it indicated support for the following strategies, among others:

- the development of multi-institutional systems for coordination or consolidation of institutional health services, and for the sharing of support services necessary to all health service institutions
- the development of medical group practice, health maintenance organizations, and other   organized systems for the provision of health care
- the development by health service institutions of the capacity to provide various levels of care on a geographically integrated basis
- the adoption of uniform cost accounting, simplified reimbursement and utilization reporting systems, and improved management procedures for health service institutions

While the program provided was not equal to the task called for in these priorities, the priorities themselves show a clear appreciation of the need. The shortfall in performance may be attributed in part to the fact that the planning structure was not closely integrated with the organization and financing of services.

Intergovernmental Relationships

The last 50 years or more have seen revolutionary changes in the functions and status of local government. Counties, municipalities, school districts, and special purpose authorities are creatures of state government. While municipalities always have enjoyed a range of home rule, counties for the most part have functioned as administrative subdivisions of states for carrying on road maintenance, schools, recording, public health, and fire protection. There always has been wide variation in the range of power accorded to county governments. With advances in the basic economy and in technology, this range gradually increased.

The Great Depression of the 1930s brought about widespread economic distress to local governments. Many defaulted on debt obligations. Supreme Court decisions upholding the welfare legislation of the New Deal opened the way for a rapid increase in federal grants to states and local jurisdictions. The trend begun in the 1930s continued into the 1970s, when the flow of funds decelerated. In 1981, legislative initiatives of the Reagan Administration began reversing the fund flow. Between 1950 and 1975, federal grants increased from $2.2 billion to $48.5 billion. Health funding rose from $4 million in 1937 to $1,892 million, 4 percent of all grants in 1975, not including assistance to institutions and individuals (Dales, 1976). It was observed that relationships among the three levels of government gradually changed from resembling a layer cake to one looking like a marble cake.

Grants were categorical, each with its own goals, conditions, and standards. They continued to proliferate through the 1960s. Between 1941 and 1960, 29 major grant programs were introduced. By 1961, there were some 40 categorical programs. This proliferation was characterized by the late Franz Goldmann as "hardening of the categories." The Great Society legislation of the Johnson years accelerated the trend and by 1969, there were 150. This mélange called forth the description of "spaghetti federalism" (Wright, 1974).

Increasing pressures to expand services in response to public demand and federal policy, and mounting costs of maintaining standards, encouraged cooperation among local governments. By 1972, 61 percent of municipalities had entered into agreements with adjoining jurisdictions for joint administration of programs. Under the "Lakewood Plan" in California, 77 municipalities in Los Angeles County had made arrangements with the county for program administration. Nationally, 21 metropolitan communities had negotiated contracts with counties for a wide range of functions, including water supply, sewage disposal, fire protection, health and hospitals, recreation, and purchasing, among others (Seyler, 1974).

Federal grants policies placed increasing stress on state and local governments. Initially allocating grants among the states on the basis of formulas using population and per capita income to equalize resources, Congress in the 1960s resorted increasingly to matching grants requiring state and local contributions. Attempts to maximize grant revenues by state and local governments became difficult, with the former trying to meet the challenge by allocating larger sums to local governments. Such subvention grew from $7.4 billion in 1957 to $28 billion in 1970. In the latter year, grants to local jurisdictions accounted for 37.3 percent of state expenditures (Seyler, 1974).

Public policy moved toward consolidation of categorical grants and encouragement of district and regional compacts among local units of government to achieve greater coordination and efficiency in use of these monies. The Intergovernmental Cooperation Act was passed in 1968 to promote coordination of policy development and program administration at federal, state, and local levels. In 1969, the Office of Management and Budget issued Circular A-95 urging states to establish planning and development districts as geographic bases of cooperation. States passed enabling legislation. Efforts were made under the PSRO Amendments of 1972 and the National Health Planning and Resources Development Act of 1974 to conform boundaries for federal planning and organization to substate planning and development districts (Hammond, 1978).

These trends were extended in 1972 with the authorization of general revenue sharing and in 1973 by the first block grant program. Under the former, the federal allocations to states and localities were made on a formula basis allowing recipient governments to spend for almost any purpose without matching requirements. These changes were consistent with the philosophy of President Nixon's New Federalism, based on the principle that those closer to the people were better able to solve society's problems in contrast to the philosophy that underlay categorical grants. The New Federalism denoted a transfer of power to state and local governments and delegation of broad discretion for determination of program goals and their implementation.

Revenue sharing represented a small victory for policy generalists over program specialists who favored continuation of categorical grants. As the program evolved, only a modest share of the total federal grant monies were allocated to revenue sharing. Because of anxiety among state and local governments that these funds might not continue, most of what they did receive was spent on capital development rather than on support for program operations. The states feared that if these grants were terminated, their legislatures would be in the vulnerable position of having to raise funds for continuation of basic support programs.

In incremental steps, public policy moved toward delegation of greater discretion to state and local governments and toward development of some form of regional organization for administering grant funds at the local level. Experience in applying the principle of regional organization to the health services is discussed in a subsequent section.

REGIONAL ORGANIZATION IN A NATIONAL PROGRAM

For purposes of discussion, it is assumed that, in keeping with the values and traditions of the United States, a national health program would be financed principally by social insurance, with contributions by employers and employees. The program would be subsidized sufficiently from general revenues to maintain premiums at a level that could be afforded without undue hardship by the majority of the population.

It also is assumed that the entire population, including the indigent and the aging, would be enrolled in the same system. Because of the vast inequities in eligibility and benefits among the states under Medicaid, it is proposed that basic services for the indigent and the medically indigent be federally financed from general revenues. States would have the option of expanding benefits for these groups. For the aging, premiums would be paid from a social insurance fund and from general revenues.

The entire population would be covered for basic hospital, medical, mental health, nursing home, home health care, and day care benefits. Estimates of total funding requirements would be based on projected costs of the benefit package. In the event that these exceeded feasible levels of financing, benefits might be reduced initially. Alternatively, consideration could be given to levying a modest deductible at the time of use for those above the poverty level. This arrangement is used by many group practice prepayment plans to maintain premiums at a competitive level. Experience indicates that such deductibles do not deter early use of services.

It probably would be necessary to limit nursing home benefits initially, to possibly 100 or 120 days in a skilled facility, because such care is expensive. To encourage use of community services in lieu of institutional care, a provision would be adopted similar to that in the Omnibus Budget Reconciliation Act of 1981, which was signed by President Reagan August 13, 1981 (P.L. 97-35). The act authorizes the Secretary of Health and Human Services to waive statutory requirements to enable a state to cover certain home and community-based services for persons who would otherwise require a skilled nursing or intermediate care facility (Washington Report, 1981). This would address in part the problem of rapid escalation of expenditures for nursing home care.

It would not be possible in any national program to make the full range of health services available. The goal should be minimum adequate coverage of essential services with assurance of equity in access and a reasonable method for establishing priorities when the supply of services might not be sufficient to meet all legitimate needs. A system for expansion of facilities where they were insufficient and a mechanism for quality assurance should be provided. The American Public Health Association resolution, "Criteria for Assessing National Health Service Proposals," provides further discussion of such a program's desirable attributes (APHA, 1978).

Within that framework, the rest of this chapter describes a local organization model that could accomplish the desired adequacy, equity, good standards, and efficiency in use of resources. Because of the complexity of issues involved, many of them subject to compromise in the course of political debate, this model, at minimum, serves as an initial agenda for discussion.

DEVELOPMENT OF A MODEL ORGANIZATION

Basic to the success of a national health program are local authorities with responsibility and power to plan, organize, and coordinate services; to monitor the program; and to maintain an effective level of mutual accountability. Roemer and Davis addressed the crucial issue of regionalization as the local organizational unit in a national health program. Roemer (1975) advocated coordinating HMO and regional development. Davis (1977) explored the place of regional organization in various legislative proposals strategies for meeting the needs of medically underserved areas.

The concept of regional organization first articulated in the Dawson Report of 1920 (Consultative Council, 1920) and experience in its application and adaptation in the United States and elsewhere would be useful in examining its potentialities in a national health program.

Regional organization of health services constitutes a system of relationships among medical care and public health facilities and services within a "medical trading area" surrounding a medical center. By articulating generalized services and facilities in the local community with increasingly specialized services at the district and regional levels, it is designed to improve the availability, quality, and efficiency of services throughout the geographic area. The organization may be adapted to the requirements of clinical services for the individual, education and training in the health disciplines, and the development of certain central services that may lend themselves to more economical delivery in this manner.

Geographic Area and Structure

The two essential ingredients are indicated in the phrase "regional organization": a functional geographic area with sufficient population to support the full range of health services, and structure in the form of a system of cooperative relationships and communications among interdependent facilities and services.

This concept has been applied extensively throughout the world, less so in the United States than in other Western nations. While common principles have been applied in the various countries, wide differences in structure and in the scope and degree of organization have emerged. These reflect differences in political philosophy and organization, in traditions relating to institutional and local autonomy, and in geographic and demographic characteristics (Rosenfeld, 1972; McLachlan, 1980).

In comparison with other countries, progress toward regional organization in the United States has been limited. The slower pace of development may be attributed to the complexity of the social and political matrix. Unlike other countries, there is no program for financing universal health services in the United States. Rather, multiple systems of financing prevail, each with its own conditions for reimbursement.

Despite the fact that the United States does not provide fertile soil for regional organization, there have been several significant demonstrations of broad scope and a number of narrower applications of these principles to special aspects of health services. Among the former have been programs of the Bingham Associates Fund, initiated with philanthropic support in 1932, involving hospitals in southern Maine with the New England Medical Center; the Rochester (N.Y.) Regional Hospital Council, organized with support from The Commonwealth Fund, including hospitals in an 11-county area (Rosenfeld & Makover, 1956); and, finally, the program of regionalization in Puerto Rico organized in 1956 with support from the Rockefeller Foundation (Arbona & Ramirez, 1978).

Among the programs of narrower focus supported by federal and state funds and foundation grants are: the hospital survey and construction program based on 1946 legislation (the Hill-Burton Act), providing for federal grants-in-aid to the states for hospital planning and construction on a regional basis; the 1964 Hill-Harris amendments to Hill-Burton, which supported areawide planning of health facilities in metropolitan communities; the 1965 regional medical programs designed initially to support continuing education on management of major chronic diseases; and the program developed under the 1966 Comprehensive Health Planning and Public Health Service Amendments Act. These programs were incorporated into the National Health Planning and Resources Development Act of 1974, which provided for a planning program based on some 200 health service areas (HSAs) into which the country was divided.

The 1972 amendments to the Social Security Act authorized federal expenditures for support of approximately 200 PSRO regions (not all coterminous with the later-organized HSAs) to develop voluntary organizations of physicians to monitor appropriate use of hospitals, nursing homes, and ultimately ambulatory care for beneficiaries of Medicare and Medicaid, and also to assess quality of care. In 1973 the Emergency Medical Services Act authorized grants-in-aid to support the development of regions for planning and operation of ambulance services, the training of emergency medical technicians, and establishment of communication systems in an effort to moderate the rate of increase in mortality and disability from accidents and medical emergencies.

To reduce mortality and morbidity among high-risk infants, many states in the mid-1970s mounted regional perinatal care programs based on the principle of coordinating clinics and hospitals in the local community with more specialized facilities at regional centers (McCormick, 1981).

In 1970 the Carnegie Foundation published a report advocating application of the principle of regional organization to the programs of continuing medical education (Carnegie Commission, 1970). Based largely on this report, federal support for development of area health education centers was authorized by the 1971 Comprehensive Health Manpower Training Act and extended in the Health Professions Education Assistance Act of 1976. With this stimulus, several states established networks of educational programs for the health professions through cooperative arrangements between medical schools and strategically located hospitals. By reducing professional isolation in smaller communities, their supply of physicians and other health professionals was increased. The Veterans Administration and the Department of Defense also applied the principle of institutional coordination and cooperation in utilization of costly specialized service and facilities, and in assuring good standards for care (Miike & Strickland, 1977).

Most of these programs were based on regions composed of functional groupings of local government jurisdictions. Each was designed to achieve the common objectives of improving access to needed services, quality, efficiency, and economy in providing health care. The same was true of the move among many states toward consolidation of health departments into health districts. Further, the marked trend toward multi-institutional arrangements was motivated by the need to achieve economies of scale as a strategy for institutional survival in an environment of constricting economy and increasing standards. In the aggregate, these programs employed an array of strategies to conserve resources and safeguard a wide range of services.

While each of these approaches succeeded to varying degrees in achieving parochial goals, the advances were made at measurable cost. Each of the programs maintained its own organizational structure, administrative and supporting personnel, accounting and monitoring system, facilities and standards, and system of financing. Geographic areas of operation of the programs were not coterminous, forcing each to maintain its own system of demographic and economic intelligence.

These trends were evidence of mounting acceptance of the values of cooperation and of principles of regional organization, whether motivated by instinct for survival and stronger competitive position or a desire to improve standards and access to services. Research and evaluation being conducted on these programs is adding to the store of knowledge of values and limitations of organizational strategies.

It is argued that were it possible to consolidate the various specialized programs within a common framework of regional organization, potential values would emerge that could not be realized through a system of segmental programs. Economies would be possible by eliminating duplication in organization and administration. Technological advances could be exploited more readily because of an enhanced ability to employ highly specialized staff. The regional arrangement probably would assure greater stability than programs could aspire to individually because of the broader base of community support and political leverage that would characterize such general purpose programs. This could replace interprogram competition with mutual support and give greater meaning and effect to health planning.

From the accumulated experience in the United States and abroad, it is possible to project a regional system that would address many of the vexing problems in designing a national health program. This analysis gives first consideration to the functions the regions might be expected to carry out, followed by discussion of the characteristics of regions and their organization to discharge these functions.

Goals and Functions

Organizations provide the framework for cooperation and communication among individuals and groups to achieve defined ends. One of the important functions is control of the system. The purposes to be served by regional organization may be discerned by an examination of problems encountered in past operation of the health care system.

The goal of the health system should be to make good care available at an affordable price. Major problems emanate from the fact that the essential parts of the system are out of phase and out of control—they do not fit together as an operating whole. Following is a brief description of some of the major problems in operation of the health care system in terms of its goals.

Control of Costs

This is concerned with a rate of inflation far in excess of that of the general economy. While there should be allowance for accommodation of useful new technologies, a comparison of the rate of cost increases in the United States with that of other industrialized countries suggests that there are opportunities for economy without sacrificing quality of care. Factors responsible for inflation of health care costs were discussed earlier.

Fragmentation of Service

The trend toward increasing fragmentation of care is given impetus by, among others, the following factors:

- the multiplicity of payment agencies, each with its own policies of reimbursement and widespread disinclination or inability to institute reasonable controls on utilization and costs
- the general failure among health insurance agencies to provide support for preventive services
- the absence of competent coordinating agencies to reduce duplication and promote meaningful patterns of care
- the lack of data systems that would maintain a good level of information concerning patient needs and management among the various services.

Further, the surplus of physicians in many specialties, coupled with the usual practice among payment agencies of reimbursing them for services without regard to discrepancies between patient needs and the doctor's qualifications, places generalists and highly trained specialists in direct competition. The consumer, moreover, is not channeled toward seeking care from the generalist who could coordinate the various modalities of care and provide continuing advice and supervision.

The group practice model of HMOs was designed to change the system of incentives to reduce fragmentation and costs; although it is expanding, it still covers only about 5 percent of the population.

Planning and Regulation

The concern of Congress with prevailing trends and its recognition of some of the underlying problems was evident in the goals enunciated in the National Health Planning and Resources Development Act of 1974. Nevertheless, this program has been only partially effective at best, and continuance of its support is in jeopardy as a consequence of Reagan Administration budget cutting.

In part, the program's failure to help reshape the system may be attributed to the inadequate and unsustained support it mustered, reluctant acceptance by providers, and the fact that the planning process was not closely meshed with the method of payment for services. Despite certificate-of-need legislation, large hospitals persisted in expanding where need for more beds was questionable and the race among institutions for acquisition of ever more sophisticated equipment and services was unabated. Public hospitals in areas of high need were closing while private institutions in areas of marginal needs survived. The need for an effective planning mechanism persists.

Other aspects of the regulatory system are chaotic. As mentioned earlier, multiple agencies at all levels continued to produce regulations in a vain effort to address individual problems, with limited perspective of the whole and little appreciation of how these regulatory efforts related to others. The result was a piling up of regulations of dubious value and of high cost of compliance for health care agencies. This often led to paper compliance to satisfy the requirements and produced unanticipated effects that could be costly and deleterious to health care. Solutions often do not deal with the problems they are designed to solve.

Functions of Regional Organization

Although the proposed functions of the model regional organization must be discussed serially, they are basically interdependent and should be viewed as interacting and mutually reinforcing. In exploring them, an effort is made to draw on the experience thought to demonstrate their feasibility.

Planning and Policy Formulation

The governing body of the region would be responsible for formulating policy within the framework of federal and state legislation and regulations. This body would be expected to determine issues on:

- allocation of responsibility among the various elements of the regional program, including planning, service, and support units
- financing and allocation of resources
- the nature and scope of supplementary benefits and their funding
- financing of any deficits that might be incurred in supplying basic services provided for in the national program

The entity also would be responsible for approval of plans for development and deployment of health facilities, manpower and services.

To discharge these responsibilities effectively would require the services of an adequately staffed planning unit for exploring needs and strategies in the various essential areas. Such a unit would resemble a health systems agency.

The governing body thus would function in part as the board of directors of an HSA but with the additional responsibility for development of the regional program and its financing. Among past limitations in planning was the situation in which " . . . each institution is a separate, relatively autonomous unit" and " . . . more often than not, there is little coordination between the planning of capital expenditures and payment of hospital operating costs in spite of the fact that planning bodies such as health systems agencies were intended to effect such coordination" (Sorenson & Saward, 1978).

Among the functions of the planning unit would be examination of potentialities for sharing and for mergers among institutions as a basis for budget negotiations. It also would be responsible for pinpointing areas of unmet need, for preparation of recommendations on the nature of the program and its facilities in response to those identifications, and for assistance in drawing up proposals for any federal aid available for underserved areas.

Because of the almost chaotic status of medical manpower supply and distribution, federal consideration of relevant training policies should be pursued, building further on the initial work of the Graduate Medical Education Advisory Committee appointed by the Secretary of DHHS. Unplanned proliferation of manpower constitutes a major factor in uncontrollable costs. A system of regional franchising for location of physicians might well serve to equalize distribution and begin to address the problem of bizarre distributions of specialties that characterizes many areas of the country. Continuing development of group practice HMOs could ameliorate the situation in time. The move toward geographic organization would greatly facilitate manpower planning.

Financing

It is assumed that financing of basic medical, hospital, and long-term care services would be provided by the national health program. These funds would be allocated to regions in proportion to population, with adjustments for variations in regional costs and supply of manpower and facilities. In regions or subregions with inadequate facilities and lack of physicians and other staff members to meet minimum standards of availability, consideration should be given to allowing the entity to retain some part of unused service funds. These could be used to expand facilities and offer inducements to attract physicians and to stimulate the development of services according to a program and budget approved by state and federal authorities.

fforts of various medical and social disciplines. Coordination of such a
ange of services generally is not well done in the existing framework of
ealth services.

Although deficiencies in the system may be detected by program evaluation and may be rectified in the process of planning and budgeting, there
must be continuous monitoring and coordination to redirect components
of services into effective channels and, where necessary, to negotiate
changes in relationships.

Institutionalization of primary care, as in the British National Health
Service and in HMOs, is a strategy of potential importance for effective
coordination of personal health services. It conserves resources by assuring appropriate use of specialized services, normally by permitting such
care only on referral by the personal physician. Experience shows that as
much as 85 percent of required service can be given adequately by the
agent of primary care, be it a physician functioning alone or as a member
of a team including midlevel practitioners. Furthermore, this strategy
facilitates the coordination of a wide range of diagnostic and therapeutic
services that may be required in the provision of comprehensive care. The
possibility of designating primary care physicians and specialists should
be explored. Outside of group practice HMOs, specialists, under such an
arrangement, would be eligible to receive payment only for service provided on referral from a primary care physician.

Continuing Education

Insofar as may be practical, regions should be designed to include
sufficient services and facilities within their borders to provide the full
range of health services and educational resources for training essential
professional and ancillary personnel. To the extent that this is not feasible,
contractual arrangements would be made with adjoining regions.

The values of linking educational institutions with regional hospitals and
related facilities have been established by the VA program and by area
health education center programs in the last decade or so. By means of
these networks, programs of continuing education for both rural and urban
areas have been mounted, and a broader range of resources representing
various environments for clinical education in the health disciplines has
been developed. They foster improvement in the professional environment
of smaller communities and exert a measurable effect on recruiting and
stabilizing physicians and other categories of health manpower in these
areas. Such programs also bring new challenges to educational institutions
to assess regional needs for education and to adapt academic programs to
meet them.

It is proposed that a single community budget be drawn up for the entire region, as provided in the Rochester MAXICAP Project (Sorenson & Saward, 1978), with separate allocations for each major service. "Named in part to indicate the notion of maximum allowable revenues and expenses, MAXICAP is an approach to prospective hospital payment that identifies the total sum of dollars that a community is willing to spend during any given period on hospital care " (Sorenson & Saward, 1978, p. 313). If states or regions wanted to expand benefits beyond the basic services provided for in the national program, they would have the option to do so with support from state government and by levying regional taxes. Deficits would be financed in a similar manner. This would establish an incentive for the state and region to administer the program so as to avoid deficits.

The achievement of such budgetary control would entail adoption of strategies for protecting the financial plan. Methods of reimbursement and control would have to be negotiated with the provider groups and organizations, and institutional and program budgets adapted to the regional budget. The latter would have to be sufficiently large to maintain the resources necessary to assure services but carefully administered by regional authorities to avoid overruns. This implies the partial adjustment of resources to available funds and providers' acceptance of their fair share of the risk.

Funds for planning and monitoring standards would be stipulated in regional budget proposals negotiated with federal authorities. With changes in systems of incentives and payment for services, most responsibility for monitoring utilization could be delegated to institutions and medical service agencies. Funds for administration at the regional level also would be included in regional budget proposals. States could assume responsibility for their administrative costs in view of this plan's proposed nationalization of medical care for the indigent. (Suggested regional budgeting procedures are taken up later.)

Coordination of Services

Possibly the most critical requirement in the planning and organization of services is the adaptation of combinations of medical, psychological, and social services to the needs of the individual and the family. Inadequate or inappropriate care or combinations of services that are not coordinated effectively can be dysfunctional, costly, and wasteful. The solution would be to require systems of strategically placed responsibility capable of assessing needs and of assuring the orderly and timely provision of service to address these needs. This is particularly true of the chronically ill and aging. While clearly indicated methods of medical intervention may be sufficient in themselves for acute illness, care of the chronically ill requires efforts of various medical and social disciplines. Coordination of such a range of services generally is not well done in the existing framework of health services.

Although deficiencies in the system may be detected by program evaluation and may be rectified in the process of planning and budgeting, there must be continuous monitoring and coordination to redirect components of services into effective channels and, where necessary, to negotiate changes in relationships.

Institutionalization of primary care, as in the British National Health Service and in HMOs, is a strategy of potential importance for effective coordination of personal health services. It conserves resources by assuring appropriate use of specialized services, normally by permitting such care only on referral by the personal physician. Experience shows that as much as 85 percent of required service can be given adequately by the agent of primary care, be it a physician functioning alone or as a member of a team including midlevel practitioners. Furthermore, this strategy facilitates the coordination of a wide range of diagnostic and therapeutic services that may be required in the provision of comprehensive care. The possibility of designating primary care physicians and specialists should be explored. Outside of group practice HMOs, specialists, under such an arrangement, would be eligible to receive payment only for service provided on referral from a primary care physician.

Continuing Education

Insofar as may be practical, regions should be designed to include sufficient services and facilities within their borders to provide the full range of health services and educational resources for training essential professional and ancillary personnel. To the extent that this is not feasible, contractual arrangements would be made with adjoining regions.

The values of linking educational institutions with regional hospitals and related facilities have been established by the VA program and by area health education center programs in the last decade or so. By means of these networks, programs of continuing education for both rural and urban areas have been mounted, and a broader range of resources representing various environments for clinical education in the health disciplines has been developed. They foster improvement in the professional environment of smaller communities and exert a measurable effect on recruiting and stabilizing physicians and other categories of health manpower in these areas. Such programs also bring new challenges to educational institutions to assess regional needs for education and to adapt academic programs to meet them.

Regions should develop programs of continuing education where they are lacking and should assess manpower and training needs of the area. Existing area health education programs should be accommodated to regional operations.

Consultation

Related to the program of education would be the establishment of consultative services in various aspects of the health field, including clinical and organizational management. While each facility could not expect to retain the full range of specialized disciplines required to keep various clinical services and organizations operating at acceptable standards, it would be feasible to assure their availability in each region. Such arrangements could be particularly valuable in expediting the organization of HMOs as units of service delivery.

Quality Maintenance

Major devices for maintaining adequate standards of care within the present system include federal standards for various types of facilities and services in the form of conditions for program participation, professional standards review organizations, state licensure of facilities and personnel, and certification of personnel qualification and programs by voluntary agencies. Of particular importance are standards and procedures for the selection of medical and supporting personnel by hospitals and other organized programs.

In general, these safeguards should be continued under a system of regionalization, with adaptation to reduce duplication and improve efficiency. State acceptance of national board examinations in place of state boards for professional personnel would facilitate movement between states and could reduce recruitment problems for group practice HMOs. State restrictions often pose barriers to relocation of professionals.

PSRO regions should be adjusted to conform to service area boundaries to facilitate cooperation between the two entities in such efforts as continuing education and adjustment of manpower policies.

Regional Services

Certain services, such as emergency medical and perinatal programs, by their nature would be organized regionally. Others, such as institutional support services, lend themselves to more economical and more productive functioning on a regional basis. Among the services for which regional programs should assume responsibility are:

- blood and tissue banking
- purchasing
- computer services
- special laboratory procedures
- any other services that experience indicates can be provided at a regional or subregional level

While computers are almost indispensable for administration of complex programs, they also are expensive. For lack of sufficient specialized staff and capital to acquire adequate equipment, most institutions do not use their computer facilities efficiently. At the fifth annual Medical Symposium on Computer Applications in Medical Care, the excess expense and doubtful cost-effectiveness of present hospital usage of computers was discussed (AHA, 1980). Technology has advanced to the point that it permits centralization of facilities without the loss of flexibility for meeting the needs of individual programs. Furthermore, strategies have been developed to assure confidentiality of data for each user of a centralized system. Central computer facilities could process data for standard statistical and financial reports more rapidly and cheaply than each institution operating individually.

Approach to Organization

Organization of services and arrangements for financing are fundamental to achievement of the goals of a national health program. Concepts and principles relating to these aspects based on experience in this country and abroad are dealt with next.

Organization

Consideration should be given to changes that may be necessary in state and federal policies to support regional development.

Delineation of Regions

To assure that regions are capable of carrying out an appropriate range of functions, they should be of sufficient size to encompass facilities and manpower for delivering general and most specialized services required by the population. Swedish experience suggests that a self-contained health region should have a population of at least a million. Elling (1975) recommends a range of half a million to 3 million. This is substantially larger than that of most counties. To the extent possible, regions should encompass natural service areas: groups of communities dependent on a center to which they look for specialized services, including education, marketing, and recreation, as well as specialized medical care.

In the delineation of regions it generally is considered vital to maintain the integrity of local governmental jurisdictions to preserve their responsibilities and to assure accountability for expenditures of public funds. Boundaries should be drawn to include whole local governmental jurisdictions rather than be divided along geographic, economic, or social lines. In the hierarchy of values, that of maintaining local government integrity would seem to be overriding.

For instances in which the region would overlap state boundaries, interstate compacts would be necessary, subject to congressional approval. In general the criteria and processes developed in delineating health service areas under the National Health Planning and Resources Development Act of 1974 would appear to be appropriate.

In areas of very low population density, characteristic of many predominantly rural states in the Midwest and the South where, to meet population requirements, regions would be of inordinate geographic size, consideration should be given to developing contractual arrangements among adjoining regions for highly specialized services. Where distance and transportation problems would make effective exchange among communities impossible, incorporation of provisions for transportation by air or water is an alternative, as has been adopted in the Scottish Highlands and Island Service and for services to remote areas in Saskatchewan, to mention just two.

Most regions, particularly sparsely populated ones, should be divided into districts of a size to support one or more secondary inpatient facilities. These, too, should conform to local government boundaries. The cooperation of all health facilities in the district should be promoted. To the extent feasible, local health department jurisdictions should be made coterminous with districts or regions. Distribution of responsibilities between regional and district centers would be adapted to the geographic, social, and economic characteristics of the region.

Size

Clear inferences regarding maximum size are not easily drawn from experience. For effective operation, and in the interest of maintaining human scale and local identity and responsibility, there is danger in designing regions that are too large. One approach would be to divide large metropolitan areas into several regions, as was done in London with the introduction of the National Health Service. Such experiences should be examined as possible models. While maintaining a reasonable size would be desirable, probably no maximum can be established at this time.

Nature of the Jurisdiction

There appear to be three theoretical alternatives concerning the nature of the regional jurisdiction: a subdivision of state government, a special purpose authority, or a reconstituted local government entity. These are discussed briefly in order of feasibility.

The Substate Entity

A substate unit composed of a functional combination of local jurisdictions probably would be the least complicated to develop. Given the political support to act, legislatures could create such subdivisions by statute, specifying their powers and responsibilities and according them taxing authority within specific limits. The legislation would charge health institutions and programs with responsibility for submission of statistics, accounts, and other reports, as required by the regional authority, and establish regional responsibility for submitting corresponding reports to state and federal agencies at specified intervals. There are numerous precedents for similar state action such as the creation of:

- public health districts
- hospital authorities in Michigan and in other states, providing for the levying of district taxes and issuance of bonds for the construction and operation of a hospital to serve the adjoining counties that make up the district
- health planning jurisdictions, first in New York State and later extended to all the states under P.L. 93-641

The Special Purpose Authority

The constituting of special purpose authorities would offer a second option. There is considerable precedence in the United States for establishing authorities of this sort for many purposes. Often they overlap local government and state boundaries. Their realization would require state legislation within the framework of national policy delineating the powers and responsibilities of regional health authorities.

The Reconstituted Local Unit

The third alternative, that of reconstituting local units of government, creating jurisdictions generally larger than counties, probably would encounter the greatest resistance. Because of people's identification with established jurisdictions and established political interests, changes in local government boundaries could generate political problems of major magnitude.

Although many counties are outmoded by changes in communications and technology, and do not provide for changing patterns of interdependence among communities, the political energy required to make changes would seem to preclude this approach.

The Regional Body

The legislation would establish the authority of the region to receive and disburse state and federal funds for personal health services and to establish regional policy within the framework of higher governmental requirements. It would authorize reviews of programs and budgets submitted by health institutions and negotiation of rates of payment to institutions and to other vendors of service subject to approval by the state health authority.

In the event that responsibility for planning of health facilities and services was made part of regional functions, amendment of state laws on planning would be necessary.

In the legislation and regulations, special consideration should be given to the constitution of the regional authority. The governing body probably would best be composed of ex officio representatives of local government, with a majority of members either elected, or appointed by legislative bodies of constituent local jurisdictions. Provision also should be made for creation of appropriate committees to assure effectiveness and continuity of operations. Such committees might represent the major professional interests involved, corresponding to a degree with the organization of governing and advisory functions developed in the Rochester Regional Hospital Council Program (Rosenfeld & Makover, 1956).

Recommended: Group Practice HMOs

The optimal arrangement for providing comprehensive care at reasonable cost would be a system of group practice model HMOs closely related to hospitals and other facilities and services in the region. Incentives should be provided in the financing and administration of regional services in addition to any federal aid in initiating the programs. At the same time, this would exploit the potentialities of this form of organization for economies in delivery of care and would rationalize the use of personal physicians, specialists, and midlevel practitioners in providing continuing health supervision (Luft, 1980).

An emerging potential for group practice HMOs lies in the extension of the concept to development of social health maintenance organizations. A demonstration was initiated in 1981 in New York, with support from a Department of Health and Human Services contract. This program is setting up a network of medical and social agencies to provide comprehensive long-term care for a population of aging and disabled. The network consists of geriatric rehabilitation programs, hospitals, HMOs, nursing facilities, home care, day care, and social services. These services are supported by various categorical programs (Kodner, 1981).

Financing

It is proposed that the program be financed as much as is feasible by social insurance, with contributions from employers and employees. This would make the program less vulnerable to reductions in the course of annual budgeting. However, there should be a substantial contribution from general revenues to prevent the earmarked tax from becoming onerous.

As noted earlier, another source of revenue would be a regional tax, which might be required to pay any deficit if federal fund allocations have been exhausted. Regional authorities would be accountable to the electorate for such deficits. This would ensure a higher level of consumer and provider understanding of reasons for deficits and a greater degree of local responsibility. States might participate in meeting such deficits.

Regional and state funds could be used for benefits broader than those provided under the national program. To that end, at any given level of funding, consideration might be given to levying modest deductibles at the time services are received. Group practice prepayment plans have found that such an arrangement does not act as a deterrent to the use of services and does help to maintain premiums at levels competitive with those of other plans.

It would be desirable that Medicare be incorporated into the basic program. As a categorical program for one age segment of the population, it invites attack from the younger groups that may be resentful of carrying a tax burden for a special cohort. In the unlikely event that benefits under the proposed national program would be narrower than those under Medicare, the broader benefits for the aging and the disabled should be continued with appropriate support from general revenues.

To overcome some of the serious inequities inherent in Medicaid, the program should be nationalized. Wealthier states have had more liberal eligibility standards and have provided broader benefits than have poorer states. Under the matching formula, wealthy states received much larger federal subsidies. As an example, two states, New York and California, received 35 percent of federal Medicaid support although they accounted for only 15 percent of the nation's poor (*Health, United States,* 1978). It has been suggested that one of the effects of these disparities has been to motivate the migration of indigent and medically indigent families to states with more liberal Medicaid programs.

In allocating funds among the states and regions, the simplest and most equitable arrangement probably would be on a per capita basis. However, this would not be appropriate under the circumstances of the early 1980s. The wide differences in the supply of health manpower and facilities among the states and regions demand a formula that takes into account an area's population and health resources. The formula should provide for lower per capita funding of regions with resources below the national average but with additional support to offer incentives for expanding resources toward the national average. Conversely, regions with resources above the national average would receive proportionately greater allocations, but below the national average capitation level, to create incentives for gradual reduction in resources toward a national mean. Such incentives would be particularly important in largely rural states, where there typically are fewer health resources than in urban states.

Similar consideration should be given to adjustment of capitation levels for variations in regions' age composition. Retirement communities with their elderly populations obviously have higher costs per capita than the national average.

A preliminary national budget estimate would be based on computations of the capitation rate for each form of service in a region. These estimates would serve in negotiating regional budgets and be used, in turn, by the regions in their contractual discussions with various provider groups. Institutions would be invited to submit a budget proposal for the next fiscal period, as would group practice HMOs and regional independent practice associations (IPAs).

Physicians who preferred to continue in independent practice would be obliged to join an IPA form of HMO to participate in the national program. They would have the option of not joining either a group practice or an IPA but then would be ineligible for payment under the national program for any private patients they accepted. Persons choosing to receive private care on a fee-for-service basis would not be exempted from any earmarked medical taxes or enjoy tax relief for expenditures for services covered under the national plan. Insurance companies might offer coverage for these individuals.

After completing their budgeting process, regional authorities would negotiate a final reckoning with the state and national funding agencies.

Although regional organizations would be much closer to the service delivery point than state agencies, many regions still would be quite large, so their administrators could not be currently conversant with experience at all community and institutional levels. To ensure that this knowledge becomes part of the decision-making process, it would be desirable that governing bodies be constituted to include representation of community members who utilize the facility, or that community advisory committees be established, or both. The latter should receive copies of the institution's reports to regional authorities and be invited to be present during budget negotiations. Needless to say, the process would be arduous, but it would establish a system of accountability extending from the local to the federal level. Budgets for capital improvement would be arrived at in a similar manner.

Provider Payments

A system of payments for services fair to both providers and consumers would be critical to the program's success. Although the reasons for change are clear enough, gaining acceptance would require careful preparation and a broadly based consensus among legislators to help them withstand the blandishments of special interests that would make themselves heard. The greatly reduced number of independent sources of payment should enable regional authorities to negotiate methods and levels of payment that would support the system of services adequately and moderate the rate of increase in expenditures.

The change from traditional cost-related unit-of-service payments to a prospective reimbursement arrangement for institutional care would be extremely important in restraining regional expenditures. The system should be so devised as to assure the supply of institutional facilities, adequate standards, and containment of costs.

For this purpose, an approach similar to one developed in 1947 by the Province of Saskatchewan in its program of universal hospital insurance should be of interest. It was based on the premise that the province would reimburse the hospitals through contracts negotiated on the basis of stipulated annual budgets (Roth, Myers, Mott, & Rosenfeld, 1953).

Starting in 1948, large institutions were paid a contract rate per diem, based on a budget negotiated with a rate board established by the Department of Public Health. No adjustments were made for deficits. For institutions of intermediate size, the province met 80 percent of the deficit. For the smallest institutions, it met up to 100 percent of the deficit, with the understanding that reasonable supervision by the health department would be accepted.

Because of the incentive to overhospitalize during periods of low occupancy, the system of reimbursement was modified later. Semimonthly payments to hospitals were instituted to cover slightly more than fixed costs. Payment also was made on receipt of individual accounts at per diem rates covering slightly less than the amount of such variable expenses as food, laundry, and drugs, which fluctuate with occupancy. Variable per diem rates were related to hospital size, based on estimated operating costs of each hospital at a projected rate of average occupancy for the year. This reduced incentives to overhospitalize and tended to stabilize expenditures under the insurance plan, which covered virtually the entire population. The system was well accepted by hospitals.

Other Funding Elements

To return to the United States model, additional funds would be kept in reserve for emergencies and unforeseen needs. Such an arrangement would place a significant share of responsibility for expenditures on the hospital and provide a strong incentive for rigorous control.

In regard to capital replacement, funds for depreciation should not be allocated to individual institutions but rather placed in a regional fund for disbursement on the basis of need, as assessed by the regional planning authority.

Similar methods could be used in paying other institutions such as nursing homes, home health agencies, and day care centers. HMO contracts might rely on the capitation principle with an incentive, perhaps in the form of a modest additional sum for each year hospital utilization was kept under a target level. This would be advantageous to group practice HMOs because of their typically lower utilization experience.

For residents of a region who normally would depend on providers in adjoining areas, interregional contracts should be drawn, with rates corresponding to those within those regions. To pay out-of-region claims for emergency services to residents, to cover unanticipated expenses, and to meet deficits of small hospitals, the region should retain a sufficient reserve. Regions should be vested with taxing authority to defray deficits incurred for mandated services or for broader services than those required by federal and state law. They also should have authority to issue bonds for supporting capital improvements.

Statistical and accounting controls would be essential for state and federal supervision to assure maintenance of standards in accordance with policies at both governmental levels.

CONCLUSION

Trends in the economics of health care are narrowing choices in formulation of national policy. While access to care has improved significantly among middle- and low-income groups over the last 40 years, this has been achieved at a very heavy cost. Mounting expenditures place an increasing strain on the economy even as major problems of access to adequate services persist among large segments of the population. It is estimated that some 25 million persons have no protection against the cost of medical care, while among those in a much larger group, what coverage they have patently is inadequate.

There is evidence of much waste in the system, yet at the same time it is not addressing increasingly pressing needs in the social services. The national desire for a more adequate system for financing health services, as expressed in repeated surveys of national opinion, remains frustrated.

The prospect for adoption of almost any national program of health services appears small. Nevertheless, the political climate could change rapidly in the event of a national crisis precipitated by a major downturn in the economy, or by serious deterioration of international relations. Such eventualities brought about the passage of the first compulsory health insurance program in Germany in 1883, the Social Security Act in the United States in 1935, and the adoption of a National Health Service in the United Kingdom in 1948.

Comparison of trends in health expenditures in the United States and abroad indicates that organization of a national health program is not inevitably followed by uncontrollable expenditures. Although costs of care are escalating in all industrialized countries, the rate of increase in the United States is greater than that in most of those with national health programs in place.

Control of expenditures depends primarily on arrangements that provide for

- appropriate methods of payment for services
- ability to screen and channel demand and ration services according to medical indications and urgency
- adaptation of supply of various services to reasonable assessment of need
- ability to budget

A higher level of organization than exists in the United States seems necessary to realize effective use of costly resources. Indeed, experience with Medicare and Medicaid suggests that it would be foolhardy to extend entitlement to personal health services to the population at large without adjustment in the prevailing system of incentives.

A certain degree of regulation is necessary to living in any community. From the very beginnings of civilization, people have relinquished some freedoms for the greater good of living in society. It is true that regulation is essential in developing any effort as complex as a national health program, yet experience indicates that regulation alone is not adequate, and indeed can be counterproductive.

What is needed more is a system of incentives based on appropriate allocation of responsibility and mutual accountability and designed to reduce dependence on elaborate and costly regulation. When new regulations are deemed essential, they should be evaluated within the context of those existing already. A national health policy advisory committee could make valuable contributions through serious deliberations and recommendations.

This analysis has explored the possibility of designing a system of health regions with significant responsibility for planning, organization, administration, and financing of services. It could serve as an important step toward mounting a national health program that would achieve social goals at reasonable economic cost. Perhaps the discussion will enhance understanding of basic issues against the time when the political constellations are right for addressing the adoption of a national program of health services.

REFERENCES

Abel-Smith, B. Major patterns of financing and organization of medical care in countries other than the United States. In *Social Policy for Health Care.* New York: New York Academy of Medicine, 1969, pp. 13–33.

American Hospital Association. Cost effectiveness of existing hospital computer systems questioned. *Hospital Week* 1980, 45(17).

American Hospital Association. *Multihospital arrangements: Public policy implications.* Chicago. AHA, 1979, p. 2.

American Public Health Association. Criteria for assessing national health services proposals. *American Journal of Public Health,* 1978, 68(2), 182–184.

Arbona, G., & Ramirez de Arrellano, A.R. *Regionalization of health services: The Puerto Rican experience.* New York: Oxford University Press, 1978.

Bunker, J.R. Surgical manpower in the United States and in England and Wales. *The New England Journal of Medicine,* 1970, *282*(3), 135–144.

The Carnegie Commission of Higher Education. *Higher education and the nation's health.* New York: McGraw-Hill Book Company, 1970.

Committee on Costs of Medical Care. *Medical care for the American people: The final report of the Committee on costs of medical care.* Chicago: The University of Chicago Press, 1932.

Consultative Council on Medical and Allied Services, Ministry of Health of Great Britain. *Interim report on the future provision of medical and allied services.* London: His Majesty's Stationery Office, 1920.

Dales, S.R. Federal grants to state and local government, fiscal year 1975—A quarter-century review. *Social Security Bulletin,* 1976 *39*(9), 22–33.

Davis, K. Regionalization and national health insurance. In E. Ginzberg (Ed.), *Regionalization and health policy* (U.S. Department of Health, Education, and Welfare, U.S. Public Health Service, Publication (PHS) No. 77–623). Washington, D.C.: U.S. Government Printing Office, 1977.

Elling, R.H. Regionalization of health services: Sociological blocks to an ideal. In S.R. Inzman & A.E. Thomas (Eds.), *Topias and utopias in health.* Chicago: Aldine Publishing Company, 1975.

Gibson, R.M. National health expenditures, 1979. *Health Care Financing Review,* 1980, 2(1), 1–36.

Gibson, R.M., & Waldo, D.R. National health expenditures, 1980. *Health Care Financing Review,* 1981, *3*(1), 1–54.

Hammond, J.R. Substate districts, HSA and PSRO designations. *American Journal of Public Health,* 1978, 68(2), 182–184.

Health, United States, 1978. U.S. Department of Health, Education, and Welfare, U.S. Public Health Service, Publication No. (PHS) 78–1232 . Washington, D.C.: U.S. Government Printing Office, 1978.

Hepner, J.O. Multihospital systems: An overview. In *Health planning for emerging multihospital systems.* St. Louis: The C.V. Mosby Company, 1978.

Kodner, D.L. *The social health maintenance organization: A new option for the care of the elderly.* Presented at the annual meeting of the American Public Health Association, Los Angeles, November 3, 1981.

Luft, H.S. Assessing the evidence on HMO performance. *Milbank Memorial Fund Quarterly/ Health and Society,* 1980, 58(4), 501–536.

Luft, H.S., Bunker, J.P., & Enthoven, A.C. Should operations be regionalized? The empirical relation between surgical volume and mortality. *The New England Journal of Medicine* 1979, *301*(25), 1364–1369.

Mason, S.A. (Ed.) *Multihospital arrangements: Public policy implications.* Chicago: American Hospital Association, 1979.

McCarthy, C. Financing for health care. In S. Jonas (Ed.), *Health care delivery in the United States.* New York: Springer Publishing Co., 1981, p. 301.

McCormick, M.C. The regionalization of perinatal care. *American Journal of Public Health,* 1981, 17(6), 571–572.

McLachlan, G. (Ed.). *The planning of health services: Studies in eight European countries.* Copenhagen: World Health Organization Regional Office for Europe, 1980.

Miike, L., & Strickland, S.P. Closed systems: Department of Defense and Veterans Administrations. In E. Ginzberg, (Ed.), *Regionalization and health policy* (U.S. Department of Health, Education, and Welfare, U.S. Public Health Service, Publication (PHS) No. 77–623). Washington, D.C.: U.S. Government Printing Office, 1977.

Moynihan, D.P. The politics of stability. *ADA World Magazine,* 1968, 3(2), 1 M.-2M.

Mustard, H.S. *Government in public health.* New York: The Commonwealth Fund, 1945, pp. 73–77.

Office of Economic Stabilization, 32 CFR. 1943 Supp. 4001-1 (e.g).

Perrott, G.S. *The federal employees health benefits program: Enrollment and utilization of health services, 1961–1968.* Washington, D.C.: Health Services and Mental Health Administration, 1971.

President's Commission on Heart Disease, Cancer, and Stroke. *A national program to confine heart disease, cancer, and stroke.* Washington, D.C.: U.S. Government Printing Office, 1964.

Report of the graduate medical education national advisory committee to the Secretary, Department of Health and Human Services. Washington, D.C.: U.S. Department of Health Services, Health Resources Administration, 1981.

Roemer, M.I. A realistic system: Health maintenance organizations in a regionalized framework. In R. Roemer, C. Kramer & J.E. Frink. *Planning urban health services: From jungle to system.* New York: Springer Publishing Co., 1975, pp. 253–287.

Rosenfeld, L.S. *Regional organization of health services in the United States: An international perspective.* Presented at the Third International Conference on Social Science and Medicine, Elsinore, Denmark, August 14–18, 1972.

Rosenfeld, L.S. Regional organization in a national health system. *Medical Care Section Newsletter,* American Public Health Organization, Washington, D.C.: 1978.

Rosenfeld, L.S., & Makover, H.B. *The Rochester regional hospital council.* Cambridge, Mass.: Harvard University Press, 1956.

Roth, F.B., Myers, G.W., Mott, F.D., & Rosenfeld, L.S. Payment of costs of hospital care in Saskatchewan. *American Journal of Public Health* 1953, 43(6), 752–756.

Seyler, W.C. Interlocal relations: Cooperation. *Annals of the American Academy of Political and Social Sciences,* 1974, 416, 158–169.

Simanis, J.G., & Coleman, J.R. Health care expenditures in nine industrialized countries, 1960–76. *Social Security Bulletin* 1980, 43(1), 3–8.

Somers, H.M., & A.R. Somers. *Doctors, patients and health insurance,* Washington, D.C.: The Brookings Institution, 1961, pp. 202; 385.

Sorenson, A., & Saward, E.W. An alternate approach to hospital cost control: The Rochester project. *Public Health Reports,* 1978, 93(4), 311–317.

Vladeck, B.C. *Unloving care.* New York: Basic Books, Inc., 1980.

Washington Report on Medicine and Health. *Perspective* (special insert section). 60-day wonders: HHS issues new Medicare and Medicaid rules. October 5, 1981.

Wildavsky, A. Doing better and feeling worse: The political pathology of health policy. *Daedalus,* 1977, *106*(1), 105–124.

Wright, D.S. Intergovernmental relations: An analytical review. *Annals of the American Academy of Political and Social Sciences,* 1974, 416, 1–16.

Zuckerman, H.S. Multi-institutional systems: Promise and performance. *Inquiry,* 1979, 16(4), 291–314.

Chapter 8

Health Risk Appraisal: Accuracy, Prediction, and Policy Implications

David W. Dunlop and
James A. Wiley

There are two principal reasons for social interest in predicting health risks. First, individuals and societies seek to minimize the uncertainty of risk. Second, important indicators of social intervention success are measures of health risk reduction, e.g., infant mortality and death rates.

With respect to the former, the minimization of the uncertainty of risk, many social institutions are based on the predictability of significant life events. In the United States, for example, the life insurance industry was developed to minimize the risk of premature earning loss to families and other dependent persons. The age of retirement is taken as a norm that individuals, families, corporations, and governmental entities consider in their planning for the future, both from financial and life style perspectives. Societies throughout time, and the world over, have developed social insurance mechanisms either in the form of large families or in the form of social institutions to deal with the inevitable changes that occur in the life of each individual as the day of death approaches. The uncertainty of the timing of death and of illnesses that adversely affect health status prior to that point has increasingly affected desired family size and the timing of births.

With respect to changes in health status that are less definitive than death, individuals and social institutions seek to minimize uncertainty in the timing and duration of probabilistic events. There are many instances where additional knowledge about specific health risks alters the behavior of many people. For example, individuals can be observed subjecting themselves to the pain of an immunization injection. Similarly, as more people become aware of on-the-job hazards, the intraoccupational wage differential necessary to employ the same number of individuals in a given type of work increases when health status hazards have been demonstrated (Thaler & Rosen, 1976).

However, individuals differ in the extent to which information alone alters behavior. Mountain climbers still can be seen hanging onto slender ropes and precarious devices, people still work in plants manufacturing possibly hazardous substances, and many still smoke. Nonetheless, as people become more aware of the probable risks of a particular activity, greater precautions are taken, e.g., more workplaces are air-conditioned or otherwise protected, more sophisticated devices are developed for hanging on to exposed mountain faces, and greater tar-reducing filters are devised for cigarettes.

Another public interest in health risk prediction—measuring the impact of social interventions—is involved when the costs of external negative health-related life events are borne by society. At that point, it is in society's collective self-interest to know more about these events, e.g., their frequency, pattern, reasons of occurrence, and characteristics of the population involved. In 1965, the United States made a commitment to fund a substantial share of the medical care costs born by the aged and poor. As medical care inflation subsequently became more pronounced (Feldstein, 1971), federal funding of research was expanded to focus on many aspects of health care behavior, including more thorough analysis of health status and the factors related to it over a life cycle (Dunlop, Revo, & Tychsen, 1980; Belloc & Breslow, 1979; Public Health Service, 1979). Other research findings have determined that perhaps as much as two-thirds of all medical care costs are incurred in the last year of an individual's life (Schwartz, Naierman, & Birnbaum, 1973). Since Medicare and Medicaid pay a significant share of those costs, and since expenditures for these programs are under increasing pressure for political, demographic, and economic reasons, it is important to refine the actuarial basis of these financing mechanisms through improvements in the measurement of health status and of health risk.

Society is faced increasingly with the knowledge that economic progress has not been without increased health risks imposed on certain subsets of the population. For example, cancer has been increasingly linked to specific substances that exist in the workplace or comprise a part of an individual life style (Kneese & Schulze, 1977; Schulze et al., 1979; PHS, 1979; Crocker, 1979). The debate over equity of risk bearing and cost sharing becomes more specific as a consequence of such information. To the extent that the United States continues to aspire to the Declaration of Independence's objective of enhancing all individuals' rights to "Life, Liberty, and the Pursuit of Happiness," it is important to know how the pursuits of one person or of many can benefit others or require them to bear additional costs. To maintain social vigilance and to sharpen the focus of these future debates is reason enough for continued and more specific research regarding health risk prediction.

The remaining sections of this chapter review the conceptual, methodological, and empirical state of the art for predicting health risks. The multiple policy implications of improved predictability are analyzed, and some of the unresolved issues confronting policy makers who use health risk predictions are presented.

HEALTH RISK ESTIMATION IN THEORY AND PRACTICE

Background

Until recently, the most comprehensive and sophisticated estimates of risks associated with health events were based on life-table techniques, e.g., methods of converting the raw material of vital statistics—deaths, morbid events, and populations at risk—into probability estimates. Applied to human mortality and morbidity data, these methods yield quantitative measures of the probability of death or ill health, usually for large aggregates of the population. There is no inherent reason why these methods cannot be applied to more specific subgroups. However, in practice, the data available to actuaries were sufficient only for calculating risks in subgroups defined by age, sex, race, occupation, and residential region.

It generally is acknowledged that currently life tables do not even begin to summarize what is known (or strongly suspected) about the causes of human mortality and morbidity. This fact has motivated a number of attempts to modify life-table predictions by incorporating findings from epidemiological studies of specific diseases or causes of death. The goal of this work is to improve predictions, making it possible to estimate them for even smaller subgroups even down to the level of personalized risk assessment (Robbins and Hall, 1970; Wiley, 1980; and Hall and Zwemer, 1979).

In this discussion, one of the most popular and widely used of the new methods of risk assessment, a class of procedures known collectively as health risk appraisal, is evaluated. One important concern involves the validity of the risk estimates generated by these procedures. The analysis focuses on three questions: (1) How accurate are these estimates? (2) How accurate can they be? and, (3) How accurate do risk estimates have to be in order to be of use to the public and to decision makers?

Standards for Evaluating Risk Estimates

Before analyzing health risk appraisals, risk estimation in general is defined and the principles for evaluating it are reviewed.

There are at least three ways to characterize a risk estimate:

1. the nature of the event in question (e.g., the onset of a chronic disease, changes in functional ability, death from a specific cause)
2. the level of uncertainty of an event or its complement
3. the interval of time in which the event may occur (e.g., within ten years, over the normal life span).

Combining these elements, a risk estimate attempts to specify the likelihood that a given health event will occur in a particular time interval. The likelihood of an event usually is expressed on a probability scale that ranges from 0 (the event will not occur) to 1 (the event will occur). In theory, the midpoint of the scale represents maximum uncertainty.

The most obvious test of the adequacy of a risk estimate would be an assessment of its ability to predict future events. However, the application of such a standard is not straightforward—all outcomes can occur with at least some degree of probability and the occurrence of any one event cannot be the single test of the prediction's accuracy. On the other hand, risk estimates that are completely unrelated to the future occurrence of events are not satisfactory. The expected degree of correspondence depends on the assumed unobserved distribution of risks. Gordon, Kannel, and Halperin (1979) explore this question in the context of predictions of the onset of coronary disease. Making rather general assumptions about the underlying distribution of risks, they derive upper bounds for the predictability of coronary deaths. However, when the distribution of risk is not known in advance—the usual case—it is hard to formulate firm expectations about prediction. Even a correct method of calculating risks may perform poorly as a predictor of events.

The Validity of Health Risk Appraisals

The term health risk appraisal denotes a class of procedures that uses life-table probabilities as the raw material for calculating risk. The basic idea is very simple: to construct a risk estimate for an individual, the average risk of death attributed to a given cause is used. It then is modified up or down in relation to the individual's profile of risk characteristics. Although the actual calculations are tedious, the principles used can be represented in a simple formula:

$$R = \sum_{j=1}^{k} f_j m_j. \tag{8.1}$$

The R in this formula represents an individual's total risk of death from all causes over some interval of time (usually, but not necessarily, ten years). The m_j are average risks for the jth cause for all persons who share the same age, sex, and racial traits as the individual. These are defined on the same time interval as R. (One of the m's is defined as "death rate from all other causes." This is a residual category that carries a constant adjustment factor equal to unity for all persons.) Adjustment of risks to suit individual circumstances is accomplished by multiplying the averages by positive factors (the f_j), whose values depend on a specified set of individual characteristics. By summing the adjusted rates of death from each cause, a total predicted risk of death is obtained.

Accuracy of Estimates

Several methods use Equation 8.1 as the basis for calculating risk of death. The validity of these methods can be established only by prospective studies that compare predicted outcomes with actual ones. The results of a study that evaluates the predictions of the Health Hazard Appraisal (HHA), a method of risk estimates developed by Robbins, are discussed later. The actual procedure used to calculate risk is described in Robbins and Hall (1970).

Two types of data are required for the HHA: (1) 10-year average mortality rates by age, sex, and race for major causes of death, and (2) information (obtained by questionnaire) concerning health history and patterns of behavior to determine how an individual's risk will deviate from the average risk for that person's age, sex, and race.

Wiley (1980) compared the HHA risk estimates with the actual mortality experience of more than 3,300 adults who are part of a continuing longitudinal study of residents of Alameda County, California. These individuals were selected randomly in 1965, completing a self-administered, mailback questionnaire that included items on current health status, medical history, and health practices. These responses were used (some 15 years later) to fill out a standard HHA questionnaire that serves as input data for a computer program that calculates the risk estimates. A more complete account of the validation study is presented in Kramer, Wiley, and Camacho (1980).

A mathematical criterion to measure goodness of fit between risk estimates and actual mortality outcomes is required. A method suggested by McFadden (1973) is appropriate because it provides a scale for comparing observed outcomes with the probabilistic prediction of discrete events. This is the likelihood function, which specifies the probability of the observed distribution of outcomes, given a particular set of risk estimates. The likelihood of the observed outcomes is given below as Equation 8.2, assuming that the events in question (i.e., death or survival) are independent, (this is not strictly true in the Alameda County cohort because households, rather than individuals, were the smallest units sampled, and the death of one member of a household is related to the survival chances of the other members).

$$L = \prod_{i=1}^{N} R_i^{X_i} (1 - R_i)^{1 - X_i}, \qquad (8.2)$$

where R_i is the risk estimate for the ith individual and X_i is a dummy variable that indicates whether the individual survived the period of risk:

$$X_i = \begin{cases} 1 & \text{if the } i\text{th person died, 1965–1974,} \\ 0 & \text{if otherwise.} \end{cases}$$

L has the intuitively appealing interpretation of being a measure of the adequacy of prediction; its value increases toward a maximum of 1 as the R_i approach the X_i. The maximum actually is attained when all R_i are either 0 or 1 and $X_i = 1$ if and only if $R_i = 1$ and $X_i = 0$ if and only if $R_i = 0$ for all i. This represents the case of perfect prediction, i.e., no uncertainty. In practice, the natural logarithm of L is used in place of L to avoid the extremely small decimal values of L that occur in large samples.

The log-likelihood normally is used for testing statistical hypotheses related to sets of risk estimates that are hierarchically ordered. For example, one set of R can be calculated by fitting a logistic function to observed deaths. The log-likelihood associated with this function can be compared with the log-likelihood of a similar function with one or more predictors deleted. This way it is possible to rigorously test the statistical significance of the deleted predictors.

The use of the log-likelihood for validation of a risk instrument is based on its interpretation as an index of the adequacy of prediction rather than on its statistical properties. The predictive validity of any set of risk estimates, however derived or calculated, can be compared with any other set of estimates, using the log-likelihood scale, so long as the sample and outcome events are the same. Although log-likelihoods often are interpreted comparatively, they have an unambiguous interpretation as magnitudes; a log-likelihood is the natural logarithm of the probability of observing the obtained set of outcomes, assuming that the hypothesized risk estimates are correct.

Log-likelihoods for several different probabilistic predictions of deaths in the Alameda County cohort are shown in Table 8-1. These range from a log-likelihood corresponding to maximum error of prediction, to perfect prediction at zero. In general, prediction of outcome events improves as the log-likelihood increases toward zero.

The table shows the log likelihoods corresponding to four levels of prediction that fall between the end-points of the scale. The least satisfac-

Table 8-1 Log-Likelihoods for Probabilistic Predictions of Deaths

Alameda County Cohort

n = 252 deaths
N = 3347 persons at risk[a]

Probabilistic Prediction	Log-Likelihood
1. Maximum Error of Prediction	
R_i = 1 if X_i = 0 R_i = 0 if X_i = 1	$-\infty$
2. Maximum Uncertainty	
R_i = ½, all i	$-2320.0 (= N$ ln½)
3. Mean Risk	
R_i = $^n/_N \cong .075$, all i	-894.0
4. "Actuarial" Risk	
a. R_i = average risk for age, sex, & race (times .95)[b]	-765.4
b. R_i = best-fitting logistic function of age, sex, & race	-729.0
5. Health Risk Appraisal	
a. R_i = HHA risk estimate (times .95)[b]	-718.9
b. R_i = best fitting logistic function of 13 HHA input variables.[c]	-695.1
6. Perfect Prediction	
R_i = 1 if X_i = 1 R_i = 0 if X_i = 0	0

a. This number represents a randomly selected half of the number of persons who were members of the Alameda County cohort in 1965.

b. The mean follow-up period for the Alameda County cohort is approximately 9.5 years whereas the HHA estimates are based on 10-year risks of death. To make the HHA risk estimates commensurate with the follow-up period, each estimate was multiplied by 0.95.

c. The following characteristics were used as predictors for the logistic regression analysis: age in years, sex, race (black vs. other), diabetes history, bronchitis history, diastolic blood pressure, alcohol consumption, physical activity in leisure time, current and past smoking, body mass, socioeconomic status, and depression. The estimated parameter values for the logistic function are given in "Predictive Risk Factors Do Predict Life Events" by J.A. Wiley, in *Proceedings of the 16th Annual Meeting of the Society of Prospective Medicine,* Tucson, Arizona, October 1980, Page 79, Table 3.

Source: James A. Wiley, original analysis.

tory of these is labeled "maximum uncertainty," a prediction of even odds of survival for everyone in the cohort. The next benchmark is "mean" risk, a level of predictability attained by assuming that every member of the cohort has a risk of death equal to the average mortality of the entire cohort. Improved predictions, derived by actuarial methods, yield somewhat larger log-likelihoods. These are followed by the log-likelihoods generated by the Health Hazard Appraisal and a related method of risk assessment.

The figures in Table 8-1 point toward several conclusions. First, as is expected, merely knowing the average level of risk in the cohort significantly improves the log-likelihood scale above the point of even odds. Second, predictions based on age, sex, and race are significantly better than those based on average risks. This finding is no surprise because the cohort includes both young and old and both males and females; age and sex characteristics are known to differentiate risk in all human populations. Most important, the health risk appraisal estimates improve prediction of the mortality outcomes significantly relative to the actuarial estimates.

In the case of the logistic functions (4b and 5b) this statement can be justified by referring to the sampling distribution of the difference between the log-likelihoods with and without HHA's behavioral variables. This shows that the difference between the fit of actuarial and health risk appraisal estimation is statistically significant well beyond conventional significance levels of probability, i.e., 0.05. The likelihood ratio chi-square statistic for this comparison is 67.8 with 13 degrees of freedom.

Thus, these data clearly indicate that the HHA procedure provides risk estimates that are generally superior to those obtained by conventional life-table methods. It also is interesting to note that the HHA fits the observed outcomes nearly as well as a logistic function fitted to the data (compare 5a and 5b of Table 8-1).

Potential Accuracy

How good are the HHA estimates? The answer depends on which standard of comparison is used. The HHA estimates appear to be better than those based on actuarial data but far short of perfect prediction. Moreover, there are several indications that the estimates can be refined to improve the fit between predictions and outcomes.

First, the quality of the input data can be improved. A 1980 study of stability and change in the questionnaire responses used to calculate HHA estimates suggests the presence of a considerable amount of measurement error in the self-reports of life style and medical history (Sacks, Krushat, & Newman, 1980). In addition to the usual problems of response unreliability that plague questionnaire research, there also is a strong possibility of bias. People may be motivated to underreport risk behaviors in a context where accurate reporting may elevate their perceived risk of death. Applications of known methods of improving the quality of self-reported data (through questionnaire design and carefully structured administering of the instruments) should increase the accuracy of risk estimates.

Second, the level of predictive accuracy can be improved by revising the basic formulas for calculating risk by addressing three potential sources of error in the risk estimates: (1) misclassification of deaths by cause (errors in the m_i), (2) overestimation or underestimation of the adjustment factors (errors in the f_i), and (3) problems that arise from competition between risks of death from different causes.

The most important source of error is inadequate estimation of the adjustment factors, f_i. These normally are derived by combining information about the relative risks associated with a given set of traits or behaviors with data on the prevalence of the behaviors. Since the HHA instrument was first constructed, the data base for making such calculations has expanded considerably. The availability of new data may permit the incorporation of new risk characteristics (e.g., exposure to toxic wastes, social and psychological stresses) into the HHA, and encourage refinements in the method of adjusting average rates that take interactions and correlations between risk characteristics into account. In addition, improvements in estimates for high-risk individuals can be accomplished by applying results of mathematical theories of competing risks. Projects designed to improve risk estimates in these ways were conducted in Canada and the United States.

The Center for Disease Control of the United States Public Health Service in 1980/81 funded two Risk Factor Update Projects, one to revise risk estimates for cardiovascular and traumatic death, the other to improve prediction of cancer deaths. During the same period, the Health Promotion Directorate of the Department of Health and Welfare in Canada completed a thorough revision of its Health Hazard Appraisal (Spasoff et al. 1981). Both the United States and Canadian efforts were motivated by the desire to improve the accuracy of prediction through refinements in the method of calculating risks.

There are, then, some grounds for believing that there can be important advances in the ability to predict mortality based on present knowledge.

Policy Use Standards for Accuracy

The HHA was conceived originally as a tool for motivating "healthy" behavior. It is assumed that the gains in reduced risk will be perceived as more valuable than the losses associated with a change in life style, so that "rational" individuals will adopt the course of action linked to lower risks. The strategy is to tell people what their risks are and what they can be if they adopt a healthier life style. The natural desire to live longer will provoke a choice in favor of a low-risk life style. Equation 8.3 can be used to generate the two kinds of risk estimates the individual needs to reach such a decision, one of current risks and another of those that can be achieved if the person adopts a list of recommended behaviors (e.g., stop smoking, reduce alcohol consumption, lose weight, etc.).

Are HHA estimates good enough to serve this purpose? One criterion for evaluating the adequacy of risk estimates is implied by the Hippocratic principle that interventions should do no harm, yielding the formal condition:

$$R_c \geq R_a \text{ if and only if } R_c^* \geq R_a^*, \text{ (ordinal risk scale)} \qquad \textbf{(8.3)}$$

where,

R_c = HHA estimate of current risk,
R_a = HHA estimate of achievable risk,
R_c^* = true current risk, and
R_a^* = true achievable risk given adoption of the recommended behaviors.

That is, there should be no possibility that the recommended course of action will increase the individual's risks.

A second and more stringent condition follows from the requirement that individuals should have enough information to balance benefits against costs: they should be able to compare the utility of diminished risk with the costs of adopting new behaviors or giving up old ones. Something like the following should be true:

$$R_a - R_c = K(R_a^* - R_c^*) + \text{small random error} \qquad \textbf{(8.4)}$$
$$\text{(approximate interval scale of risk),}$$

or

$$R_a = R_a^* + \text{small random error, and}$$
$$R_c = R_c^* + \text{small random error}$$
$$\text{(approximate cardinal scale or risk),} \qquad \cdot$$

where K = positive constant.

It is not possible to say whether either of these two criteria is met by the HHA or by any other method of risk assessment currently available. The data necessary to make such a judgment could be collected in randomized trials or by careful observation of "natural experiments" in a cohort of individuals who could be monitored continuously for an extended period of time; however, these studies have not been done.

There are, of course, uses of risk assessment that do not demand the standard of accuracy implied by Equation 8.4. For example, even though there may be a considerable amount of random error in risk assessments, using them to set insurance premiums may result in a more equitable price *on the average* than pricing based on the actuarial estimates. The truly important question, though, is whether or not risk appraisals can be taken as accurate measures of *individual* risk. To answer this question, it is important to know the nature of the errors built in to the present risk assessment devices, and how those errors affect individual estimates of risk. At present, it is uncertain that either 8.3 or 8.4 are satisfied in practice. Thus, advice about life style derived from the HHA and similar instruments may sometimes be incorrect and, on occasion, even harmful.

POLICY IMPLICATIONS OF IMPROVED PREDICTIONS

In the above discussion, it has been shown that both government and private sources have access to information they can use to estimate (with increasing accuracy) the probability of death or significant functional health status loss in a given population. From the point of view of public policy, the questions then are: "Should government do anything?" and, if so, "What methods should it employ?"

The first question depends largely on three factors: (1) the extent to which externalities accrue to society from health status prediction activities; (2) the extent to which these externalities can be predicted in terms of both magnitude and timing; and (3) how much precision in research findings is required by government before action can be taken, i.e., what are the confidence limits that have been used to ensure that government action avoid both Type I and Type II errors (e.g., failing to accept the hypothesis when it is true, and failing to reject the hypothesis when it is false).

On the first point, if, as a consequence of improving health status prediction, society reaps benefits or bears costs that do not accrue directly to individuals (i.e., externalities exist) or if the knowledge base for engaging in such prediction takes on the characteristics of a public good, governmental intervention is warranted. Since research and knowledge generation activities have the characteristics of a public good in the sense that one person's acquisition of that information does not preclude others from potentially acquiring it at the same time, social support for health status prediction research is warranted. The positive externalities of such research findings that accrue to society take the form of insights that can be used

to alter the health behavior of a younger generation, based on the knowledge of an older one, and thus avoid the costs linked to early mortality
and morbidity.

On the second point, as the methodologies described earlier become
more precise in their ability to predict the magnitudes and timing of health
status changes, society can reap the benefits of this knowledge more
quickly. In such instances, the returns resulting from social investments
become more obvious and tangible, thus implying more vigorous governmental support.

With respect to the third factor, research precision, a social welfare
calculation is always implicit in determining the accuracy and confidence
requirements for any findings before governmental action is warranted.
Zeckhauser (1975) and Acton (1977) point to instances where governmental
decisions have, ex post to the decision, valued life that varied from a low
of $20,000 to the $1 to $2 million range. In situations where there are no
clear losers from governmental action, or when the economic implications
are modest, research findings often can precipitate prompt action. On the
other hand, where there are large numbers of winners and losers and
where the economic stakes are great, e.g., where they involve the profit-
ability of large corporations, then government action is exceedingly slow.

Turning to the second question, "What methods should government
use?", there are several options. The government can develop the internal
capacity to produce information and resulting health status predictions.
The annual National Health Interview Survey conducted by the National
Center for Health Statistics is a representative example of this option
(National Center for Health Statistics, 1964). The Canadian government
decided to develop the same internal capability for appraising health risks
facing its population (*Morbidity and Mortality,* 1981). Another option is
for the government to subcontract with a private organization to process
and disseminate such information. The Research Triangle Institute (Raleigh-
Durham-Chapel Hill, North Carolina) represents one of many examples
of an organization that collects, processes, and disseminates information
related to health and nutrition.

The government can also implement a variety of taxes, regulations, or
subsidies to provide private organizations with incentives to pursue activities it would like established. Favorable tax treatment of research and
development costs represents another available option.

In a pluralistic society like the United States, there are additional issues
to be resolved from an implementation point of view. First, which level
of government should initiate action and have jurisdiction over the intervention process? It is common in the history of legislation in this country
that a state has acted prior to the federal government. (Schlesinger, 1974,

notes that interventions by states to provide Maternal and Child Health Services comprise one example where states acted prior to the federal government.) This is particularly true where the positive or negative externalities reveal themselves to a particular subset of the population that resides in one locale, e.g., the enactment of child labor laws in Massachusetts prior to their adoption in other parts of the country.

Second, jurisdictional issues often arise between governmental entities engaged in (1) monitoring data collection, (2) calculating risks, and (3) implementing various governmental interventions (alterations in health insurance premiums can change a potentially desirable intervention into one that cannot be implemented). While it often is easier to forget about such issues, debates regarding policy options increasingly require that they be addressed systematically. They represent part of the cost of obtaining the positive externalities envisioned from the intervention option under consideration.

Health Insurance

Perhaps the single most important set of policy implications regarding improved prediction of health risks and the factors associated with them is related to the area of health insurance. If it is known, for example, that smokers have a much higher probability of death and of contracting certain illnesses based on their previous and present smoking behavior, is it equitable for the rest of society to subsidize smokers by paying the same health insurance premiums? The most comprehensive review of the epidemiological evidence on smoking is the 1979 Report by the Surgeon General on Smoking. (See also Manheim, 1974.)

Virtually all health insurance pricing is based on an average cost principle, with everyone in the group paying the same premium and bearing an equal portion of the risk. It is commonly presumed that at some time in the future, all the individuals in the group will get their share. However, it is increasingly clear from empirical research findings that individuals have considerable influence over their own health status at any given point and throughout their life cycle. As a consequence, one policy option for consideration by both government (for Medicare and Medicaid) and private insurance carriers envisages individualized health insurance premiums based on key behavioral factors such as smoking, alcohol consumption, exercise and eating patterns (Belloc and Breslow, 1972; Belloc, 1973) and other microsocial and macrosocial and environmental factors associated with health status changes.

By altering premium structures in this manner, society would be achieving a different equity goal than has previously existed. The new goal would be to equate the individual marginal benefits and costs of health care across the population. The issue of adverse selection and how to deal with it amid improving competition and the related fallout is being increasingly addressed (Luft, 1981; Wennberg, 1979; Wennberg and Gittelsohn, 1980). These authors present data showing large cost differences between small areas in the same locale. Wennberg questions the equity of such occurrences.

Premium changes also would provide individual incentives to alter behaviors that clearly are adverse to health. Given that the demand for health insurance is not totally insensitive to price changes (Phelps, 1973), and that individuals are informed that the price of their policy is contingent on their own behavior, incentive structures can be established to elicit appropriate responses from the covered population.

Further, premiums for virtually every other line of insurance are not based on average cost but are individualized on certain specific characteristics related to differential risks. In automobile insurance, for example, a person's past driving record, driver education training, characteristics of the automobile, residence, age, and sex are considered in determining the individual's premium.

Similarly, age, occupation, health history, and other factors are reviewed by life insurance companies before completing a policy. Finally, for home owner fire insurance, the distance from a fire hydrant and the type of construction materials used in the house help determine the level of premiums. An individual makes marginal choices and if a person prefers to live at the top of the hill with no water, then the fire insurance premiums will reflect the increased risk that a blaze could destroy the property. If research findings, as indicated, are establishing significant differences in the risk of contracting health problems over time, why shouldn't premiums for health insurance reflect those differentials in risk, as they do for other forms of insurance?

Tax and Subsidization Policies

To the extent that society bears the costs of poor health among certain groups in the population, and to the extent that poor health status is related to the consumption of certain products, it is reasonable to suggest that consumption taxes be imposed to cover those costs. In the case of highways, a tax on gasoline is imposed on individuals who use them to finance the initial and recurrent costs of the road system. Similarly, for individuals wishing to continue to consume cigarettes and other products identified with adverse health risks, it is reasonable to impose taxes to pay the costs that society bears for maintaining those individuals who suffer premature functional health status loss or who require medical care earlier than would otherwise be expected. Given the increasing evidence of large health losses attributable to smoking cigarettes, taxes may well be increased to develop the funds necessary to pay for the premature health costs that society incurs.

It is important to point out that "health" taxes on such commodities as cigarettes and alcoholic beverages do not restrict individuals' freedom of choice to consume what they want, subject to their budget constraints, nor do these levies restrict producers from engaging in efforts to maintain or increase consumption. The imposition of these taxes merely provides society with the resources necessary to pay for the negative health externalities it must bear.

Similarly, to the extent that society benefits by increased levels of exercise so that health losses occur farther in the future, it may be useful to consider mechanisms by which goods used in the exercise process could be subsidized. Of course, the size of the health subsidy would take into consideration the possible adverse health costs that might accrue because of the increased use. For example, the jogging craze has increased the incidence of foot and other musculoskeletal problems requiring medical care. If these additional sports injury costs were borne privately, however, the social gross subsidy would not have to be reduced (Thomas, Lee, Franks, & Paffenberger, 1981).

For example, those who run regularly have a reduced risk of contracting certain major ailments such as coronary heart disease. An income tax deduction is a common way to subsidize the purchase of items deemed socially desirable, e.g., health insurance and houses. Why not extend the analogy to the purchase of items complementary to running or other forms of beneficial exercise? Further, if on-the-job stress were demonstrated to be related to mental health and the occurrence of significant life events—and an increasing body of research suggests such relationships (Syme & Reeder, 1967)—tax relief might be indicated for those who engaged in more stress-dissipating exercise and related activities. To minimize the adverse employment effects of subsidizing imported commodities, a tax distinction could be made between items manufactured in the United States and those produced elsewhere.

State and local governments also can use their own tax and subsidy options independent of the federal government. They provide health care services, finance other health costs for their population, and reap benefits from a healthier population. The incidence of positive and negative externalities of course may differ from one governmental jurisdiction to another, thus implying a different set of tax and subsidization practices.

To the extent that state and local governments jointly fund Medicaid, it is in their self-interest to know how the health status of the poor is affected by individual behavior and other environmental factors that may be amendable to one or more intervention options. The findings of Dunlop, Revo, and Tychsen (1980) and Grossman (1975) show that while the poor have lower health levels than those who are more affluent, such status can be augmented by individual behavior.

For all income groups, improved health status is positively associated with years of schooling. It is unclear exactly how education operates vis-à-vis health status. Undoubtedly it is related to the ability to obtain and process useful information in the environment. Such behavior certainly is more efficient. (See Grossman, 1972.) It is important, however, to learn how specific education technology affects knowledge, attitudes, and practice of improved self-health behaviors. It is not a priori clear that more schooling is the cost-effective approach.

Occupational Safety and Health Policies

A significant portion of adverse health risks are found in the workplace environment (Archer, 1981). As a consequence, society bears many negative externalities and finances direct health and rehabilitation costs of those who are injured or suffer function loss because of occupationally related disease. To pay for these costs, society may want to impose certain taxes on the final goods and services produced. For example, technologies used in textile manufacturing are said to expose workers to a higher risk of contracting brown lung disease. Similarly, many other manufacturing processes, such as some involving the use of asbestos, regularly expose workers to a high risk of injury or disease from many substances and circumstances. These situations represent instances where the final consumer must bear the cost through additional taxes imposed on consumption.

In the specific instances where there is a reasonable freedom of choice of occupation, however, the costs of occupational safety and health and/or of workers' compensation should be borne by individuals who make the choice to participate in that occupation. Examples include professional football players, airline pilots, and film stunt performers. These individuals should bear the full costs of the freedom of job choice they have decided to exercise.

To the extent that regulatory costs are incurred in monitoring occupational safety and health standards, these should be borne by society as a whole on public good or externality grounds. Exactly which type of regulatory strategy yields the greatest set of health and other benefits relative to the costs is unclear. However, since there have been regulatory changes by the Occupational Safety and Health Administration since its inception in 1970, it can be presumed that a "learning-by-doing" approach may be feasible.

Unresolved Issues

This chapter has not resolved the issue of imperfect knowledge. As in the section on methodology, the health risk of any particular individual at any moment in that person's life is not precisely defined. Presumably more research can be done to subclassify individuals according to health risks. However, many risks, such as those arising from environmental, pollution, and other contextual variables, are unavoidable at present. Thus, risk sharing via pooling will remain an integral part of health insurance pricing.

It is clear, however, that improvements can be made in the pricing of health insurance irrespective of the carrier, i.e., the government or private entities, given the improvements made over the last decade in predicting health status changes. These price changes also can set in motion many decisions by individuals about how to improve their own status by alternating health-related behaviors. The embodied incentive structure is consistent with other desirable social objectives as well, including the reduction in health care costs.

Another issue requiring resolution from a public policy point of view is jurisdictional in nature. Given that information regarding health risk is available, who or what governmental entity should be responsible for public communication? The following related questions also must be addressed:

- How can the public be informed?
- What perceptual distortions can be anticipated?
- How do these distortions vary across the population?
- Should the message or communications approach be changed if the size of the risks varies?
- If legal action is to be taken, who will be responsible for mounting the effort?

Clearly these policy implementation issues are of importance. Is the political process ready to address them forthrightly?

Finally, a related but distinct issue is how to address the social equity trade-offs. For example, what steps are taken, and by whom, if health risks are defined and causal linkages are supported? Will society or some subset thereof or individuals bear the cost? Specifically, in what proportions will they bear those costs?

Over the last decade many advances have been made in the assessment of health risks. Theoretical linkages of causality have been advanced; methodological breakthroughs have occurred involving health status index development and measurement technique. Improved data sets have emerged. More precise risk estimates are available, disaggregated by population characteristics. Many of these developments have been discussed.

The policy implications have not yet been analyzed or debated in full. This chapter has raised some of the important implications of these developments, particularly related to health insurance premium pricing and tax or subsidization strategies. There are many thorny implementation issues to be resolved as well as more basic measurement work to be accomplished. Policy makers, always facing an uncertain world, must decide when to act. It is clear that some policy areas, as discussed here, warrant action.

REFERENCES

Acton, J.P. Valuing lifesaving alternatives and some measurements. *Journal of Law and Contemporary Problems,* 1977.

Archer, V. Health concerns in uranium mining and milling. *Journal of Occupational Medicine,* July 1981, *237,* 502–506.

Belloc, N. Relationship of health practices and mortality. *Preventive Medicine,* March 1973, *2,* 67–81.

Belloc, N., & Breslow, L. Relationship of health status and health practices. *Preventive Medicine,* August 1972, *1,* 409–421.

Crocker, T., et al. *Methods development for assessing air pollution control benefits.* Environmental Protection Agency, Publication No. EPA-600/5-79-00). Washington, D.C.: February 1979.

Dunlop, D.W., Revo, L., & Tyschen, S. *Impact of employment and inflation on the health status of the poor.* (Final report to the National Center of Health Services Research and Development.) Hyattsville, Md.: U.S. Department of Health and Human Services, 1980.

Feldstein, M.S. *The rising cost of hospital care.* Washington, D.C.: Information Resources Press, 1971.

Gordon, T., Kannel, W., & Halperin, M. Predictability of coronary heart disease. *Journal of Chronic Disease,* 1979, *32*(6), pp. 427–440.

Grossman, M. The correlation between health and education. In N.E. Terleckji (Ed.), *Household production and consumption.* New York: Columbia University Press, 1975.

Grossman, M. *The demand for health: A theoretical and empirical investigation.* New York: Columbia University Press, 1972.

Hall, J., and Zwemer, J. *Prospective Medicine.* Indianapolis: Methodist Hospital of Indiana, 1979.

Kneese, A., & Schulze, W. Environmental health and economics—The case of cancer. *The American Economic Review,* February 1977, *67*(1), 325–332.

Kramer, D., Wiley, J.A., & Camacho, T. *A study of the predictive validity of the health hazard appraisal.* Berkeley, Calif.: California Department of Health Services, Human Population Laboratory, October 1980. (Working paper)

Luft, H. *Adverse selection: or, How to avoid helping to pay your neighbor's health care bills.* (Technical Briefing Memo). Washington, D.C.: National Health Policy Forum, October 30, 1981.

Manheim, L. *Health, health practices, and socioeconomic status: The role of education.* Unpublished doctoral dissertation, University of California, Berkeley, 1974.

McFadden, D. Conditional logic analysis of qualitative choice behavior. In P. Zarembka (Ed.), *Frontiers of Econometrics.* New York: Academic Press, 1973, pp. 105–143.

National Center for Health Statistics, U.S. Department of Health Education and Welfare, "Health Survey Procedure: Concepts, Questionnaire Development and Definitions in the Health Interview Survey," Series 1, No. 2, *Vital & Health Statistics,* May 1964.

Phelps, Charles E. *The Demand for Health Insurance: A Theoretical and Empirical Investigation,* Report No. R-1054-OEO, (Santa Monica, Calif.: RAND Corp., July, 1973)

Public Health Service. *Smoking and health: A report of the Surgeon General.* (Department of Health, Education, and Welfare, Publication No. (PHS) 79-50066). Washington, D.C.: U.S. Government Printing Office, 1979.

Robbins, L., & Hall, J. *How to practice prospective medicine.* Indianapolis: Methodist Hospital of Indiana, 1970.

Sacks, J., Krushat, W., & Newman, J. Reliability of the health hazard appraisal. *American Journal of Public Health,* July 1980, *70*(7), 730–732.

Schlesinger, E. The impact of federal legislation on maternal and child health services in the United States. *Milbank Memorial Fund Quarterly/Health and Society,* Winter 1974, *52*(1), 1–14.

Schulze, W., Ben-David, S., Crocker, T.D., and Kneese A. Economics and epidemiology: Application to cancer. In S. Mushkin & D.W. Dunlop (Eds.), *Health: What is it worth?* Elmsford, N.Y.: Pergamon Press, 1979.

Schwartz, M., Naierman, M., & Birnbaum, H. Catastrophic illness expense: Implications for national health policy in the U.S. *Social Science and Medicine,* June 1978, *12*(½), 13–23.

Spasoff, R.A., McDowell, I.W., Wright, P.A., & Dunkley, G.C. *Proposals for a revised Evalu* Life: Final Report of a Contract,* submitted to Department of National Health and Welfare, Ottawa, Ontario, Feb. 1981.

Syme, L., & Reeder, L. (Eds.). Social stress and cardiovascular disease. *Milbank Memorial Fund Quarterly/Health and Society,* April 1967, *45*(1). (Special issue)

Thaler, R., & Rosen, S. Estimating the value of a life: Evidence from the labor market. In N.E. Terleckji (Ed.), *Household production and consumption.* New York: Columbia University Press, 1976.

Thomas, G., Lee, P., Franks, P., & Paffenberger, R., Jr. *Exercise and health: The evidence and the implications.* Cambridge, Mass.: Oelgeschlager, Gunn and Hamm, Inc., 1981.

U.S. Centers for Disease Control, U.S. Department of Health and Human Services. *Morbidity and Mortality Weekly Report,* October 2, 1981, *30*(38), 487.

Wennberg, J. Factors governing utilization of hospital service. *Hospital Practice,* September 1979, *14,* No. 9, pp. 115–127.

Wennberg, J., & Gittelsohn, A. *A small area approach to the analysis of health system performance.* (Department of Health and Human Services, Health Resources Administration, Publication No. (HRA) 80–14012). Washington, D.C.: U.S. Government Printing Office, August 1980.

Wiley, J.A. Predictive risk factors do predict life events. Pp. 75–79 in *Proceedings of the 16th Annual Meeting of the Society of Prospective Medicine,* Tucson, Arizona, October, 1980.

Zeckhauser, R. Procedures for valuing lives. *Public Policy,* Fall 1975, *23*(4), 420–463.

Chapter 9

Structuring Information for Policy Development and Evaluation

Barnett R. Parker

The delivery of more effective personal health services (PHS), i.e., those that would offer a greater health "benefit" to a patient population, is a complex, multidimensional problem. In particular, the outcome of any effort to improve the PHS delivery mechanism, and/or the services themselves, is dependent upon policy issues emanating from several sectors of society (Milio, 1981). Thus, both health and nonhealth (energy, environmental, socioeconomic) sectors involve issues and considerations that directly or indirectly affect service delivery.

The multisectoral implications of the PHS problem are clarified by the oval diagram (Delp, Thesen, Motiwalla, & Seshadri, 1977) in Figure 9-1. The circles represent sectors and the arrows their interrelationships. The diagram is overly simplified since the purpose here is merely to emphasize the multidimensional nature of a complete or full-spectrum PHS intervention strategy. Such a strategy consists of a series of interventions (boxes), ranging from the normal activities of a PHS effort, e.g., disease treatment, to more developmental and environmental aspects.

The crucial consideration is that only by viewing these efforts as part of a synergistic whole, i.e., a system, can overall health status ultimately be enhanced (lower cycle) or, at least, degradation avoided (upper cycle). (A system may be defined as a set of objects and the relationships between the objects and their attributes (Hall & Fagen, 1968). The most basic of all systems consists of three essential components: one or more inputs, a conversion process, and one or more outputs.)

The full-spectrum PHS intervention strategy outlined in Figure 9-1 is inherently complicated, involving an interaction of technologies and communications across many sectors of society. Not surprisingly, programs and projects designed to encompass such intersectoral considerations must be based on efficient management capable of making effective, responsible decisions (Parker, 1981). A critical prerequisite for this is "a reasonable

Figure 9-1 Intersectoral Dimensions Crucial to a Full-Spectrum Personal Health Services Intervention Strategy: An Oval Diagram Representation

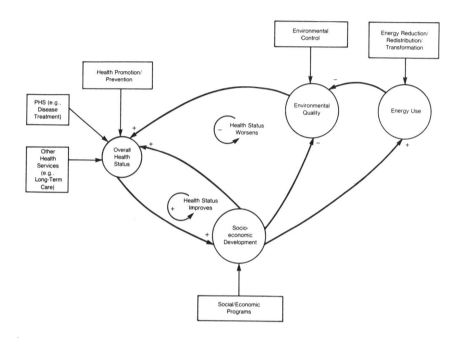

Explanation: The purpose of an oval diagram is to hypothesize the basic structure of interrelationships/interactions causing and perpetuating the problems or phenomena under study. An arrow with a positive (+) sign at its head indicates that the two factors connected by the arrow change in the same direction. A negative sign (−) indicates they change in opposite directions. A loop with an even number of negative signs is referred to as a positive feedback loop and reinforces factor changes in the same direction as the change. A negative feedback loop (odd number of negative signs) acts to resist factor changes, moving in a direction opposite to the change.

amount of information concerning problems, resources, and the possibility of intervention in an 'environment' in which specific actions are encouraged'' (Härö, 1980). That is to say, effective PHS policy making and decision making must be supported by appropriate, situation-responsive information.

This chapter analyzes several key aspects of information as they relate to PHS policy development and evaluation including:

- What information must be made available in providing an effective PHS policy support function, i.e., what constitutes "appropriate" or "good" information?

- What characteristics should this support information possess?
- Does such information exist on an a priori basis, e.g., in the form of Center for Health Statistics data bases?
- How really useful are existing data bases in PHS policy development?
- What requirements do the policy maker (as an individual) and the program/organization place on the needed information?
- How is the information acquired, developed, stored, and delivered to the appropriate policy maker or relevant organizational location?

OBJECTIVES AND EVALUATION: THE RELEVANCE TREE

In preparing to identify and describe the information required for support of a full-spectrum PHS strategy, it is necessary first to specify the relevant program/organizational goals and objectives and the corresponding measures of performance, i.e., evaluation criteria. A useful tool for this purpose is the relevance tree (Delp, Thesen, Motiwalla, & Seshadri, 1977). Relevance tree diagramming takes a hierarchical approach to analysis of a problem, commencing with identification of the overall mission. Given the mission, major goals relevant to it are established. Appropriate objectives, targets, and measures (criteria) are then developed for each goal, thus allowing a complex problem (system) to be disaggregated into more fundamental and manageable dimensions. This process is applied to the PHS problem in Figure 9-2. Full development is left to individual users; however, the example presented here involving PHS patient visit distribution is carried through in some detail.

Of particular importance to the question of information for policy development and evaluation is the quality of the performance measures specified in the diagram. Thus each instrument must be directly measurable and/or predictable from other measurable factors. Further, it must possess critical levels of reliability and validity. The latter is a particularly troublesome issue since outcomes in health care policy making often are difficult to quantify (Stimson, 1969). What normally must suffice, therefore, are proxy or surrogate measures of the original phenomena that are highly reflective of the often intangible concepts they purport to represent.

For example, many studies use time of travel or distance as a surrogate for "accessibility" of health services (ReVelle, Marks, & Liebman, 1970; Rojeski & ReVelle, 1970). While such instruments are easily measurable, they are valid only in certain situations such as emergency medical services where time of travel is, in fact, a critical aspect of accessibility (Volz, 1971). As for basic primary care services, however, accessibility is a more complicated concept involving such issues as out-of-pocket cost, hours of facility operation, and waiting time at the facility (Parker & Srinivasan, 1976).

Figure 9-2 A Relevance Tree Portrayal of the Full-Spectrum PHS Issue

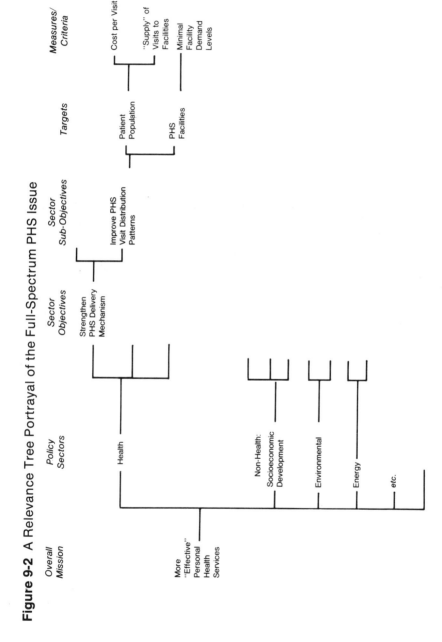

INFORMATION FOR PHS POLICY DEVELOPMENT

From Figure 9-2 it is evident that development of effective policy for any aspect of the PHS issue requires well-defined criteria for each objective/sub-objective. In general, these criteria (e.g., minimal facility demand levels) are, themselves, dependent upon a series of factors or variables. These factors constitute the information set or information base upon which formulation of policy for the appropriate objective(s) is based. Thus, if policy development requires determination of minimal facility demand levels, information on such factors as facility size, operating costs, and service mix are needed to measure (i.e., estimate) the demand levels. If such information is not available or easily measurable, or if it does not possess characteristics defined as appropriate for the situation, the policy development process may be hindered severely or interrupted entirely.

The key implication is that in order to effect meaningful PHS policy, information, as distinguished from data—raw facts and figures with no specified role—is required. Furthermore, the information must be "good" in the sense that it responds not only to the policy under development but also to whatever impinges on the policy development process: (1) the type of policy decision(s) being made, and the models/methodologies used in the process, (2) the perceived needs and requirements of the policy makers, and (3) the organizational context within which the policies are developed (Parker & Kaluzny, 1982).

These considerations are outlined in Figure 9-3, which depicts the generation of good, i.e., appropriate, information as a simple system. The process begins with some real-world situation, characterized in terms of classes or groups of objects, events, concepts, and people. Data are the symbolic surrogates or descriptors of these entities (Burch, Strater, & Grudnitski, 1979). For example, a series of infection rates resulting from a new strain of influenza across regions describes (i.e., is a surrogate for) the set of actual events—influenza illnesses summarized at the regional level. Such data may be stored subsequently or converted through either or both of two types of health information system: informal and formal. (The concept of a health information system is discussed in more detail later.)

The informal system consists of telephone calls, personal conversations, newspaper articles circulated among program/organizational personnel, etc. The formal system can embody processing operations ranging in complexity from hand calculations and manual filing to sophisticated computer methods. Both system types, however, are involved in the conversion, i.e., organization, transformation, retention, and retrieval of the data into forms useful to its recipient(s).

Figure 9-3 Generating Information for PHS Policy Support: A Simple Systems View

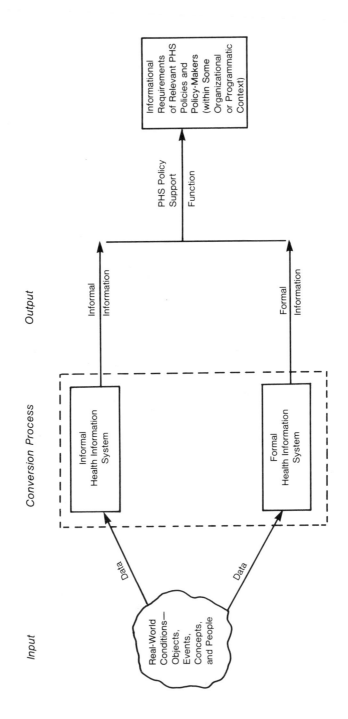

Source: Adapted from "A Manager-Based Assessment Module for Health Information Systems in Developing Countries," by Barnett R. Parker, in *Proceedings, Congreso Internacional de Sistemas,* Caracas, Venezuela, 1981.

At this point, the processed data become information. The information may be in terms of hunches, judgments, or opinions (informal information), or more structured forms, e.g., program performance reports, budget summaries, predicted future resource levels, etc. The principle purpose of this information, regardless of its form, is to support key policy-making decision-making efforts, thus allowing for improved PHS program performance. For the example given earlier, the influenza data may have little meaning to, say, the program budget officer. However, if cross-tabulated to help the epidemiologist predict future disease patterns by age and location, the data could become formal information capable of supporting more effective policy for the delivery of influenza services.

The requirements on information to be used in support of PHS policy development, noted here and in Figure 9-3, are substantial. However, establishing these requirements emphasizes the importance of avoiding poor or ineffective policy resulting from ill-designed input, commonly referred to as "garbage in–garbage out." The same policy may require different information (or information structured differently) as a function of variations across policy makers and/or organizational contexts.

For example, determination of cost per visit (Figure 9-2) may be defined differently (and thus may depend on different factors) when viewed by a consumer action group as opposed to a legislative committee or an academic researcher. Similarly, two legislators may use the same basic cost information but attach varying importances to different attributes (characteristics) of the information, e.g., accuracy vs. timeliness.

Given the basic requirements of information needed for support of PHS policy development, it is important to determine how such information can be identified in any given policy/decision situation. A methodology is offered next that fulfills this need. It is important to bear in mind, however, that while this procedure identifies the content and structure of appropriate (i.e., "good") information, it does not guarantee its availability or accessibility. These factors represent key constraints that need to be overcome if viability of the policy process is to be maintained. As explained, such conditions normally can be dealt with directly by the proposed methodology, particularly when interfaced with a suitable health information system (Figure 9-9, infra).

METHODOLOGY FOR STRUCTURING PHS INFORMATION

The methodology proposed here for structuring information appropriate for support of PHS policy making presupposes some analysis of the situation that would yield a relevance tree (or similar portrayal) of problem objectives and performance measures (as in Figure 9-2, supra). The methodology consists of three phases:

Phase 1: Determination of Informational Sets

For each performance or policy measure/criterion y_i, $i = 1, \ldots, m$ (listed in the far right-hand column of the relevance tree), identify the individual(s) who are organizationally "close" or "appropriate" to the corresponding objectives, i.e., those who are in the best or most feasible position to evaluate performance on the objectives. A form of Delphi or nominal group technique (Delbecq, Van de Ven, & Gustafson, 1975) is used at this point. A typical nominal group process involves the following routine: A question or problem is posed to the group. Each member writes as many responses to the question as possible. The group leader asks members to state ideas from their lists and records them on a chart visible to all. No discussion is permitted until all ideas have been listed. Then each item is discussed in an interacting group format. Based on this discussion, the participants rank-order the items according to their relative importance. The process may be repeated with intervening discussion and argument. The outcome is an overall ranking of the group's responses to the original question/problem.

This technique is used to determine from appropriate individuals what informational items or factors (i.e., independent variables) would be required to predict or otherwise measure y_i; that is, to identify the factors z_{ij}, $i = 1, \ldots, m$ and $j = 1, \ldots, n$ in Equation 9.1:

$$y_i = f_i (z_{i1}, z_{i2}, \ldots, z_{ij}, \ldots, z_{in}) \text{ for all} \qquad \textbf{(9.1)}$$
$$i = 1, \ldots, m$$

where: y_i = performance measure i;

z_{ij} = predictor/informational item j relevant to prediction/measurement of criterion i;

f_i = some (to-be-determined) function of the predictor variables as they relate to criterion y_i;

m = number of performance measures/criteria; and

n = number of predictors/informational items (assumed constant across all m criteria).

The assumption on n may be relaxed easily. Thus, if the number of informational items is assumed to be dependent upon, i.e., a function of, the criteria y_i, $i = 1, \ldots, m$, then we define n_i = number of items used/required to measure criterion y_i, where any n_i may differ from the original (constant) n. That is, previously, $n_i = n$ for all $i = 1, \ldots, m$; now n_i may be $\leq$, $=$, or $\geq n$.

Note that the Delphi determination of predictors for y_i may be supplemented by an analysis of the relevant literature since criteria used in health policy problems often are themselves the subject of study. Such work may provide support to and additional insights into the results of the Delphi effort. For example, a great deal of work has been done relating measures of health facility utilization to various socioeconomic, demographic, and geographic variables (e.g., "Utilization of Health Services," 1972; Hershey, Luft, & Gianaris, 1975), "enabling" factors (Andersen, 1968), and measures of patient satisfaction (Ashcraft, Penchansky, Berki, Fortus, & Gray, 1978). A typical output of these studies is the expression obtained by Galvin and Fan (1975) for number of physician visits:

$$NPV = 0.082DD + 0.015A + 0.633S - 0.244R - 0.015MS + \qquad \textbf{(9.2)}$$
$$0.056C - 0.030E + 1.027I - 0.042ST + 0.119NC$$

where:
NPV	= number of physician visits;	C	= occupation;
DD	= number of disabled days;	E	= education;
A	= age;	I	= (public) insurance;
S	= sex;	ST	= satisfaction; and
R	= race;	NC	= number of health
MS	= marital status;		conditions.

The factors $DD, A, \ldots, ST, NC$ in Equation 9.2 represent the z_{ij} terms of Equation 9.1, i.e., the relevant information base, while NPV corresponds to y_i, the criterion of interest.

In some cases, determination of the set of predictors, $\{z_{ij}\}$, i.e., z_{ij} for all $i = 1, \ldots, m$ and $j = 1, \ldots, n$, is even more straightforward than when based on an analysis of the literature. (A set is any well-defined collection of objects. It normally is denoted by a pair of brackets, { }, around the objects that constitute the set. In the example here, $\{z_{ij}\}$ represents all n informational factors ($j = 1, \ldots, n$) associated with all m criteria y_i, $i = 1, \ldots, m$.) Thus, if y_i is a measure determinable from a well-known mathematical expression or model, the factors may be directly identified. (A variation of this method of determining $\{z_{ij}\}$ is used later in an application of the proposed methodology.) A simple example of this type of situation involves the model for economic order quantity (EOQ) (Hillier & Lieberman, 1980). EOQ is the optimal quantity of some given product to be ordered for inventory under the most basic of conditions:

- constant and known demand, costs, and order quantities
- zero lead time (between placing and receiving an order)
- no stockouts (shortages)
- infinite replenishment rate

The relevant expression is:

$$Q^* = \sqrt{\frac{2DC_o}{C_h}} \qquad (9.3)$$

where: Q^* = economic order quantity;
   D = annual demand (units of product);
   C_o = cost per order (dollars); and
   C_h = annual holding cost per unit of product (dollars/ unit of product).

Thus, if it is known that D = 1,200 units annually, C_o = \$5.00, and C_h = \$1.20, the recommended policy is to order

$$Q^* = \sqrt{\frac{2(5.00)(1200)}{1.20}} = 100.0 \text{ units (per month).}$$

From this model, it is seen that measurement or prediction of Q^* is based on determination of D, C_o, and C_h. These three items thus represent the information set underlying or supporting any policy making concerning Q^*. It may be necessary in some cases to extend this informational analysis to members of a more basic information set. Thus, in this example, measurement of any of the three items D, C_o, and C_h may require determination of their own underlying factors, e.g., market conditions as they relate to demand, D.

An important implication of this last point is that during the implementation of Phase 1, some emphasis should be placed on keeping the number of predictors for each criterion small, preferably not more than six or seven. This is designed to maintain both costs and overall informational requirements at manageable levels as well as to generally control the complexity of the methodology and the interpretation of results.

Phase 1a: Specification of the Predictor-Criterion Relationships

In many cases, ad hoc or intuitive estimates of y_i can be made based on the z_{ij} factors. That is to say, the policy maker may possess a good mental or cognitive representation of the f_i functions of Equation 9.1, thus avoiding the need to specify them explicitly, e.g., statistically (King & Cleland, 1975). However, increasingly, there is a need in health care policy making to quantify issues, particularly if they are crucial to larger analyses (Warner & Holloway, 1978).

In the example begun earlier, facility demand levels may very well impinge on larger issues such as economic development and energy usage.

Given such considerations, explicit representation of the f_i functions becomes desirable. Without detailing the rationale here, the functions of Equation 9.1 may be assumed to be linear in form with little threat to their explanatory/predictive capabilities (Bettman, 1971; Dawes & Corrigan, 1974). Linear models offer powerful predictive validities in a variety of contexts because of a series of structural characteristics present in most decision situations (Dawes & Corrigan, 1974). These characteristics are outlined in the Appendix to this chapter. The model of Equation 9.1 thus may be expressed as:

$$y_i = b_{i1}z_{i1} + \ldots + b_{ij}z_{ij} + \ldots + b_{in}z_{in} = \sum_{j=1}^{n} b_{ij}z_{ij} \qquad \textbf{(9.4)}$$

$$\text{for all } i = 1, \ldots, m$$

where: y_i, z_{ij} are as previously defined; and
$\quad\quad b_{ij}$ = relative importance/contribution of factor j with
$\quad\quad\quad$ respect to criterion y_i.

Typically, a statistical procedure such as multivariable regression, i.e., regression involving more than a single independent variable, (Kleinbaum & Kupper, 1978) would be utilized to derive Equation 9.4. Thus, values of the criteria, y_i, $i = 1, \ldots, m$ would be regressed onto values for the factors $\{z_{ij}\}$ yielding the importance weights $\{b_{ij}\}$.

If instead the form of f_i was to be extracted from the literature, or based on some a priori management science or economic model, then Equation 9.4 would simply be replaced by the appropriately chosen function(s). For example, if an inventory policy problem was to involve determination of an EOQ, Equation 9.3 would be substituted for Equation 9.4 in the analysis.

With Equation 9.4, or some other functional form for f_i specified, the value of y_i may be determined for any values of the z_{ij}, $j = 1, \ldots, n$ considered within "normal" ranges, i.e., ranges for which the model is considered valid. Thus, y_i becomes directly estimable from the Phase 1 information base. This capability, tempered by the Phase 3 (infra) structural requirements on the information, helps define the overall support function (Figure 9-3) of information in PHS policy development. (See also Figure 9-9, infra.)

Phase 2: Determination of Informational Characteristics

Let $S_i = z_{ij}$, for some given i and all $j = 1, \ldots, n$, i.e., S_i = set of informational factors required to predict/measure criterion y_i alone. Now, define $\{x_k\}$ (i.e., x_k for all $k = 1, \ldots, q$) to be the set of q attributes or characteristics associated with generating, retrieving, transforming, sorting, and utilizing the information in any of the informational sets, S_i, $i = 1, \ldots, m$.

A simplifying assumption, similar to that in the discussion of Equation 9.1, is made here—namely, that the number of informational characteristics, q, is constant across information sets S_i. Thus, we assume $q_i = q$ for all $i = 1, \ldots, m$. As in the previous case, this assumption can be relaxed easily. However, research indicates that the set of attributes used to characterize a given product—here, information—remains relatively stable across related applications, e.g., across the sets S_i (Parker, 1977).

In general, these informational attributes are well known. They include such considerations as cost, validity/accuracy, origin, time horizon, form (Senn, 1978), accessibility, flexibility, and verifiability (Burch et al., 1979). Emphasis in this phase should be on identification of a cogent set of factors recognized in the literature as important to the policy use of information. Measurement of the factors' relative importances is left for Phase 3; here, the concern is simply with the fact that they have some reasonable influence on individuals' satisfaction with, and utilization of, information in PHS policy-making situations, i.e., that they are relevant.

As in Phase 1, but for different reasons, the number of attributes must be kept small. In Phase 3, individuals will be judging the informational sets S_i characterized in terms of these factors. The range of five to seven attributes generally is recognized as maximal since individuals have difficulty mentally processing more than this number of items simultaneously (Miller, 1956). Again, for the sake of simplicity, the final set of attributes, $\{x_k\}$, is considered appropriate for all informational sets, S_i, $i = 1, \ldots, m$.

Phase 3: Structuring the Phase 1 Informational Sets

Given an informational set for each policy criterion y_i, and structural (design) attributes of those sets, it becomes necessary to determine the relative importances of the attributes. As discussed later, this knowledge allows formulation of information sets and systems responsive to the needs and preferences of policy makers as well as to the organizational contexts within which they operate.

In this regard, consider the global measure: overall value of, or satisfaction with, the information in set S_i for supporting a policy decision/evaluation on criterion y_i. This perceptual valuation is to be made in terms of the Phase 2 informational attributes $\{x_k\}$ by policy makers organizationally close to objective(s) relevant to criterion y_i. The purpose of this exercise is to determine the relative importance of each attribute x_k, $k = 1, \ldots, q$, to these policy makers in utilizing S_i to support criterion y_i-based efforts. These importances might best be expressed through a series of weights or saliences, $\{w_{ik}\}$, across criteria $i = 1, \ldots, m$ and attributes $k = 1, \ldots, q$ (Srinivasan, Shocker, & Weinstein, 1973).

Conjoint analysis—a powerful methodology that has its roots in the psychological and marketing sciences (Green & Srinivasan, 1978)—may be utilized to delineate $\{w_{ik}\}$. These weights are as perceived by policy makers. More precisely, they are quantitative representations of the cognitive processes underlying the policy-makers' perceptions. An overview of the conjoint process as it applies to the information structure problem is given next. Some of the more technical details are offered in the Appendix.

Conjoint Analysis

Conjoint analysis is a quantification process that implicitly estimates the structure of an individual's or group's overall preferences/judgments for some "product" of interest (in the current case—information) in terms of the factors or attributes used to characterize the product. This normally is accomplished by a regression or mathematical programming model of the individual's stated preferences or judgments regarding a set of real or hypothetical products, i.e., product profiles, with respect to the attribute values constituting these profiles. Generally, the attributes (independent variables) are interval scaled, while the preferences/judgments (dependent variable) may be either interval or ordinal scaled (Green & Srinivasan, 1978). This choice of scale is of practical importance in cases where only a rank-ordering of products, rather than a direct interval rating, is possible or desirable. The procedure has been shown to yield significant levels of reliability and validity in a variety of decision contexts (Montgomery, Wittink, & Glaze, 1977; Parker & Srinivasan, 1976).

The conjoint procedure consists of the following steps:

Step 0: Preference/Judgment Model

Assume that t informational designs (profiles) exist, $r = 1, \ldots, t$, each characterized in terms of $\{x_k\}$. Let V_{ir} represent the value of any informational set S_i, with design/structure r, in terms of its ability to support policy development on criterion y_i. (This value is as perceived by the appropriate policy maker(s).) V_{ir} is hypothesized to be calculable from the following linear expression:

$$V_{ij} = \sum_{k=1}^{q} w_{ik}x_{kr} \quad i = 1, \ldots, m; \, r = 1, \ldots, t \qquad \textbf{(9.5)}$$

where: V_{ir} = perceived value of informational design/structure r with respect to its ability to support policy development through S_i on criterion y_i;

w_{ik} = perceived relative importance/contribution of design variable k to policy development on criterion y_i;

x_{kr} = level (number of units) of variable k present in informational structure r; and

m, q, t = number of criteria, design factors (attributes), and informational designs, respectively.

Step 1: Stimuli Construction

A series of $t \simeq 30$ (hypothetical) information design profiles is constructed, with each profile characterized in terms of the q design factors $\{x_k\}$. In general, the optimal number of profiles will depend upon the number of parameters, i.e., importance weights, to be estimated. For most cases, however, a sample of approximately 30 profiles (stimuli) is recommended. This number offers the best compromise between difficulty of task for the respondent and stability of the resulting importance weights (Green & Srinivasan, 1978). The levels of the factors $\{x_{kr}\}$ in Equation 9.5, and their interattribute correlations, are based on values considered historically realistic for the current problem context (Parker & Srinivasan, 1976).

A recommended procedure for construction of the profiles involves random sampling of factor values from a multivariate normal distribution, followed by trial-and-error checks to ensure that no single profile dominates any of the others. The objective is to force the respondent to make real trade-offs among the factors when any two profiles are compared on the overall utility measure developed in Step 3, infra.

Step 2: Stimuli Format

Each design profile is listed on a $3'' \times 5''$ stimulus card, the typical structure being:

Policy Decision Criterion: _____ (y_i) _____
accessibility: (number of "units" of accessibility, x_{1r}) _____
validity/accuracy: (number of "units" of validity/accuracy, x_{2r}) _____
flexibility: etc. _____
form: _____   _____   _____
et al.: _____

The same $t \simeq 30$ profiles of Step 1 are used for each of the $i = 1, \ldots,$ m criteria. That is, m sets of stimulus cards are constructed, each set differing only in the content of the first line—"Policy Decision Criterion: (y_i) ." (This is not exactly true. The order of the informational characteristics should be randomized across the sets of stimuli cards.)

Step 3: Respondents' Judgments

The criterion y_i set of design profiles is randomly ordered and presented to individual(s) considered organizationally close to the relevant objectives. "Close" here means that the person(s) are in a position to meaningfully rate or rank-order the profiles on the measure: "ability of the information design (profile) to support, through S_i, the policy development process on criterion y_i."

The choice of measurement scale for the respondents' judgments—direct rating (on an interval scale such as Likert) or an ordinal rank-ordering—should be based on such considerations as availability of time, total number of respondents, and complexity of the profiles, i.e., number and type of attributes. In general, ranking will yield more reliable data since it is easier for a respondent to express a measure of relative preference for one profile versus another, as opposed to a magnitude of preference/value for each single profile (Green & Srinivasan, 1978).

It is at this point that the methodology addresses the problem of data availability or accessibility that was raised earlier. Because of their central role in policy development, one or both of these constructs is almost always incorporated into the design profiles as an informational attribute. Now, when the respondent(s) express preferences among the profiles, they are, in essence, trading off among two or more attributes. If availability/accessibility is a major, possibly debilitating, issue (i.e., it has the potential for compromising the policy process), respondents, by design, will be likely to assign it a proportionately high importance.

This implies that relatively more of other attributes would willingly be "spent" to ensure information availability and/or accessibility, thus removing, or at least lessening, the threat of serious process constraints because of these factors. It is in this way that the conjoint procedure deals directly with the problem of information availability. (As discussed later in the chapter, final responsibility for such issues lies with the health information system, which is charged with actually providing the policy support information. See Figure 9-9, infra.)

Step 4: Estimation Process

The ratings/rankings of Step 3 together with the design factor values from the Step 1 profiles (stimuli) are entered into one of several coefficient estimation procedures such as LINMAP (Srinivasan & Shocker, 1973), PREFMAP (Carroll, 1972), or MONANOVA (Kruskal, 1965). Shocker and Srinivasan (1979) present a detailed discussion of the advantages, disadvantages, requirements, etc., of each of these procedures. Using a variety of methods, these procedures determine a set of optimal importance weights, $\{w^*_{ik}\}$, that, through Equation 9.5, yield V_{ir} values "as congruent as possible" in sequence with the respondents' actual preferences/judgments. This set of weights represents the respondents' underlying value or priority structure concerning the relative contribution of each design factor k to the policy development process on criterion y_i-based objectives.

OUTPUT OF THE METHODOLOGY

The methodology developed in the previous section generates a series of outputs that helps define the informational needs of a PHS policy development and evaluation process independent of the level of analysis. That is, the procedure operates equally as effectively on macroissues as it does on more microlevel policies.

To review, the methodology outputs are as follows:

1. A series of m informational sets S_i, $i = 1, \ldots, m$ that specify the information items or variables $\{z_{ij}\}$ seen as necessary to predict or otherwise measure each of m criteria identified as fundamental to the original policy problem (e.g., as in Figure 9-2).
2. Some form of model relating the items of S_i to each criterion, thus allowing a prediction of y_i for any given set of values $\{z_{i1}, z_{i2}, \ldots, z_{in}\}$.
3. The set of informational design/structural characteristics, $\{x_k\}$, considered most crucial to the use of all S_i sets in support of PHS policy development on the performance criteria y_i, $i = 1, \ldots, m$.
4. The relative importances, $\{w^*_{ik}\}$, of each design characteristic as it applies to the use of S_i in support of criterion y_i policy making.

Implications of the Methodology Output

What is now available to the PHS policy maker may be considered in less technical terms:

- information technically required for support (i.e., for measurement or prediction) of policy development relevant to PHS program objectives; and
- user-based/organization-based specifications for the structure or design of this information.

These provisions translate into a series of information bases constructed and designed in response to: (1) policies considered capable of effecting an improved PHS condition, (2) perceived needs and preferences of relevant PHS policy makers, and (3) the organizational context within which these policy makers operate.

The principles underlying the proposed methodology reflect the findings of a large number of research efforts. Thus, it is widely recognized that the effectiveness of managerial policy decisions can be substantially enhanced if the decisions are supported by appropriate information (Keen & Morton, 1978; Mason & Mitroff, 1973). In particular, organizational objectives will be better met if the information for decision support accounts for the type of decision, e.g., control, strategic, adaptive (Dickson, Senn, & Chervany, 1977; Mason & Mitroff, 1973; Parker & Kaluzny, 1982; Schonberger, 1980); its organizational location or context (Ein-Dor & Segev, 1978; Parker & Kaluzny, 1982); and decision maker needs, preferences, and requirements (Dickson et al., 1977; King & Cleland, 1975; Mason & Mitroff, 1973; Parker & Kaluzny, 1982). However, such information does not guarantee effective policy (Ackoff, 1967); rather, it suggests that an implicit upper limit on policy development and evaluation is created by the absence of information responsive to critical dimensions of the policy problem.

AN EXAMPLE OF IMPROVED POLICY MAKING

To further clarify the concepts developed thus far, a detailed example is presented. The objective is to show how and why appropriate information, as defined earlier, allows for more effective PHS policy making. As will be seen, identification of the required information (the factors $\{z_{ij}\}$ in Equation 9.1) is based here on a model that technically falls somewhere between the user-derived type expression of Equation 9.4 and the formal type policy model of Equation 9.3.

The problem, outlined in the relevance tree of Figure 9-2 (supra), considers how to best allocate patient visits in a given region to a series of PHS facilities. Assume that patients reside in three principal locations or supply points, L_1, L_2, and L_3, while there are four PHS facilities or demand points, F_1, F_2, F_3, and F_4. The policy to be developed involves deciding how many patient visits/year from each residential location should be directed to each facility so that some measure of societal cost is minimized.

Assume the following required information, as called for in Figure 9-2, is available:

Utilization cost, c_{ij} (in dollars) of a single patient from location L_i ($i = 1$, 2, 3) traveling to, and utilizing, facility F_j ($j = 1, 2, 3, 4$):

From Residential Location	To PHS Facility			
	F_1	F_2	F_3	F_4
L_1	12	15	3	20
L_2	20	22	7	5
L_3	9	11	20	19

Maximum number of patient visits/year, P_i, emanating from each residential (supply) location, L_i:

	Residential Location		
	L_1	L_2	L_3
Maximum Number Annual Visits, P_i	500	1,500	1,250

Minimum number of visits/year, D_j, at each facility, F_j, to maintain viability (i.e., minimum demand):

	PHS Facility			
	F_1	F_2	F_3	F_4
Minimum Annual Demand, D_j	850	1,000	900	500

This problem is diagramed in Figure 9-4.

Let x_{ij} = number of annual patient visits from location L_i to facility F_j. The values for all x_{ij} ($i = 1, 2, 3$; $j = 1, 2, 3, 4$) are what must be determined to solve the problem. Thus they are termed the control or policy variables. Given the problem's structure, a representation in terms of a formal policy model known as the transportation model (Hillier & Lieberman, 1980) appears reasonable.

Figure 9-4 Flow Diagram of Patient Visit Problem

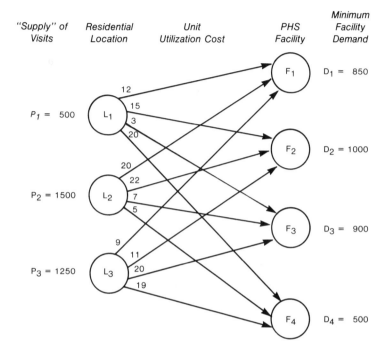

As noted earlier, a policy problem (or some part of one) often possesses a structure that allows it to be represented in terms of a specific off-the-shelf model. Such a representation generally strengthens the policy development process because of the more systematic analysis required by a formal model. However, effective use of such a model depends heavily on the quality of the input information—a point representing the main thrust of this chapter. Excellent discussions of the utility and application of formal mathematical models to the policy process are given by Greenberger, Crenson, and Crissey (1976) and Stokey and Zeckhauser (1978).

From the standpoint of informational requirements and solution, the transportation model is a cross between the types of Equations 9.3 and 9.4. Thus, like the former but unlike the latter, the information set is known a priori. However, like both models, the value of the criterion is obtained through application of a formal solution procedure. Further, the transportation model possesses a basic prespecified structure (like Equation 9.3), but requires some construction, and estimation of a specific set of parameters, i.e., c_{ij}, P_i, and D_j (as in Equation 9.4).

A verbal representation of the transportation model, as it applies to the current problem, is as follows:

minimize: total annual cost of all patient visits from locations L_i ($i = 1, 2,$ 3) to facilities F_j ($j = 1, 2, 3, 4$)

subject to: total number of annual patient visits from each location $\leq$ "supply" of possible annual patient visits from corresponding location

and:

total number of annual patient visits to each facility $\geq$ annual number of patient visits required for viability of corresponding facility

$\left.\begin{array}{c} \\ \\ \\ \\ \\ \\ \\ \\ \\ \\ \\ \end{array}\right\}$ Verbal Model (VM)

Thus it is possible to minimize annual visit (utilization) costs subject to a series of supply-and-demand constraints.

The problem now is formally structured by quantifying the verbal model (VM) with the information given earlier:

objective function:
$$\text{minimize } z = 12x_{11} + 15x_{12} + 3x_{13} + 20x_{14} + 20x_{21} + 22x_{22} \quad \textbf{(9.6)}$$
$$+ 7x_{23} + 5x_{24} + 9x_{31} + 11x_{32} + 20x_{33} + 19x_{34}$$

constraints:

As an example of the supply constraints, the total number of visits emanating from location L_1 cannot exceed the available level of 500. This is illustrated in Figure 9-5 and expressed quantitatively in Equation 9.7.

$$x_{11} + x_{12} + x_{13} + x_{14} \leq 500 \quad \textbf{(9.7)}$$

As an example of the demand constraints, the total number of visits to facility F_1 from all three residential locations cannot be less than the required level of 850. (See Figure 9-6 and Equation 9.8.)

$$x_{11} + x_{21} + x_{31} \geq 850 \quad \textbf{(9.8)}$$

Figure 9-5 The Supply Constraint for Location L_1

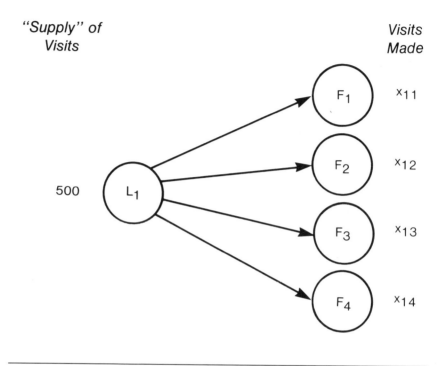

Figure 9-6 The Demand Constraint for Facility F_1

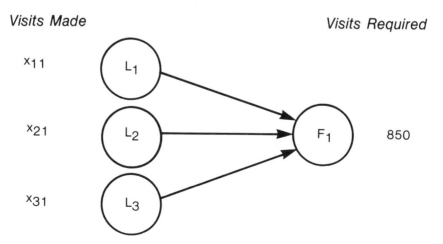

The complete model representing this problem is given by Equation 9.9:

$$\text{minimize } z = 12x_{11} + 15x_{12} + 3x_{13} + 20x_{14} + 20x_{21} + 22x_{22}$$
$$+ 7x_{23} + 5x_{24} + 9x_{31} + 11x_{32} + 20x_{33} + 19x_{34}$$

$$
\begin{aligned}
\text{subject to: } & x_{11} + x_{12} + x_{13} + x_{14} \leqslant 500 && \text{(9.9)}\\
& x_{21} + x_{22} + x_{23} + x_{24} \leqslant 1500\\
& x_{31} + x_{32} + x_{33} + x_{34} \leqslant 1250\\
& x_{11} + x_{21} + x_{31} \geqslant 850\\
& x_{12} + x_{22} + x_{32} \geqslant 1000\\
& x_{13} + x_{23} + x_{33} \geqslant 900\\
& x_{14} + x_{24} + x_{34} \geqslant 500\\
& x_{ij} \geqslant 0 \quad i=1, 2, 3; \quad j=1, 2, 3, 4
\end{aligned}
$$

Results of the Example

Solution of Equation 9.9 leads to a policy that recommends either of the following distributions of annual patient visits:

$$x_{11} = 500, \ x_{22} = 100, \ x_{23} = 900, \ x_{24} = 500,$$
$$x_{31} = 350, \ x_{32} = 900, \text{ all other } x_{ij} = 0. \quad \text{(9.10)}$$

$$x_{11} = 500, \ x_{21} = 100, \ x_{23} = 900, \ x_{24} = 500,$$
$$x_{31} = 250, \ x_{32} = 1000, \text{ all other } x_{ij} = 0. \quad \text{(9.11)}$$

Solution of this transportation model is simple and straightforward. This example is small enough, in fact, to be solved by hand using a procedure known as the "stepping-stone" method (Hillier & Lieberman, 1980). The distributions in Equations 9.10 and 9.11 are diagramed in Figures 9-7 and

---

Figure 9-7 First Alternative Distribution of Patients

From Residential Location	To PHS Facility F_1	F_2	F_3	F_4	Total
L_1	500	0	0	0	500
L_2	0	100	900	500	1500
L_3	350	900	0	0	1250
Total	850	1000	900	500	

9-8, respectively. The corresponding cost of either policy option is $30,050. Because of the properties of the transportation model, the solutions of Equations 9.10 and 9.11 represent the minimum cost (or optimal) patient distribution for the given information sets. That is, for the parameter values provided, there can be no patient visit distribution less costly than $30,050. What this implies is central to the purposes here: by providing information sets designed for a model able to realistically represent part or all of a PHS policy problem, the corresponding policy development process can be strengthened significantly, often leading to optimal or near optimal recommendations.

If a policy problem does not seem to correspond neatly to any well-known model or methodology, a slight restructuring, relaxation of assumptions, etc., might allow for such a representation. While the problem then may be changed somewhat from its original form, the benefits resulting from use of an existing model or framework with prespecified informational requirements is likely to be substantial (Morris, 1967). Such models lend a formality and systemization to the policy process, thereby helping to avoid ad hoc or intuitive type approaches. These latter modes of analysis may work sometimes but generally they cannot guarantee best, or even good, policy. Further, a replicability of policy cannot be ensured.

The key question for the policy maker then is: By relaxing assumptions, or otherwise adjusting the problem structure, how much validity of representation is traded off for a fundamentally stronger policy development process, and is the trade-off worthwhile? Such a question must be posed each time a model or methodology is contemplated for use in the policy process. The answer, as might be expected, depends upon circumstances.

Figure 9-8 Second Alternative Distribution of Patients

From Residential Location	F$_1$	F$_2$	F$_3$	F$_4$	Total
L$_1$	500	0	0	0	500
L$_2$	100	0	900	500	1500
L$_3$	250	1000	0	0	1250
Total	850	1000	900	500	

To PHS Facility

However, the policy maker invariably will generate a deeper understanding of the problem itself as a result of the analysis required to determine that answer.

Results of the Example: Further Discussion and Implications

The process outlined in the previous section generated a policy for a least-cost pattern of patient visits from some given set of locational sources to some given group of PHS facility sites. Not surprisingly, delineation of this policy was dependent on provision of appropriate information. From the relevance tree of Figure 9-2, and related discussions, the appropriate information was shown to involve three item classes:

1. the cost, c_{ij}, of a single patient from residential location L_i traveling to, and utilizing, facility F_j;
2. the "supply," P_i, of annual patient visits at residential location L_i; and
3. the minimum number of annual patient visits, D_j, required for viability of facility F_j.

These item classes, together, represent the basic information set required to generate a patient distribution policy using the transportation model. As such, they are analogous to the set of factors $\{z_{ij}\}$ in Equation 9.4 and the items D, C_o, and C_h in Equation 9.3. However, like the factors in Equation 9.3, they represent parameters of a model, as well as measures in and of themselves. As noted earlier, this implies that they may be easily measurable, i.e., directly determinable, or one or more may require estimation/prediction based on their own set(s) of predictors. Given the nature of these factors, the latter would seem to hold here. For example, the facility demand levels, D_j, would need to be determined from a function similar to Equation 9.12:

$$\text{facility demand level, } D_j = f_j \text{ (facility size, operating} \qquad \textbf{(9.12)}$$
$$\text{costs, service mix, etc.)}$$

where f_j is some (linear) function of the predictors. Equation 9.12 is identical to Equation 9.4 in the sense that the criterion—facility demand level—is specified in terms of factors considered relevant and directly obtainable/measurable. The true information set for this policy problem thus consists of the factors to be included in Equation 9.12 as well as those predictors relevant to the estimation of the P_i and c_{ij} parameters.

Thus far, discussion of the example and its results has concentrated on Phases 1 and 1a of the proposed methodology. As the methodology emphasizes, however, an information set in support of PHS policy making, no matter how complete its content, must be structured properly. For example, patient distribution policy requires determination of facility demand levels, which in turn are dependent upon, inter alia, facility size, operating costs, and service mix. But unless measurements of these factors are forthcoming in accordance with the Phase 2 structural characteristics, as weighted in Phase 3, the policy process is likely to become disrupted.

Why? Because, as the title suggests, it is the PHS policy maker who actually makes the policy. The information sets, constructed to support the policy process, must contain information structured/characterized in response to the needs and preferences of the user of that information (Mason & Mitroff, 1973). In the example here, it may be that the region of interest incorporates the metropolitan areas of two states, one in a growth period and one in a stage of decline. Given the likelihood of large movements of population within the region, information in support of the development of visit distribution policy should be accessible, timely, available quarterly, and numeric and/or graphic in form. Possibly less important would be aspects such as origin, completeness, and even cost. If this were the case, Phase 3 importance weights would necessarily be higher for the first set of characteristics than for the latter set.

The implications of this argument should be considered in relation to the PHS policy development process. A PHS policy problem has been formulated in terms of a powerful and widely available decision model. Given the information set required by this model (values for all c_{ij}, P_i, and D_j factors), an optimal or least-cost solution to the problem was made available. However, for this solution to be useful to the policy maker on a continuing basis, the information set must possess characteristics beyond its sheer relevance to the model. Thus, only when the information set is both sufficient in content and structurally responsive to existing conditions can it be considered truly complete and capable of being functionally supportive of the policy development process.

DATA BASES AND INFORMATION SUPPORT

An important question concerning support of the PHS policy development process is whether some or all of the required information sets exist a priori and, if so, whether they are structured properly. Usable existing data bases would be most advantageous in allowing at least a partial bypassing of the methodology proposed earlier. The actual process of generating the information also could be avoided. Under such conditions, a minimum application of the methodology still would be required, however, if only to identify guidelines on what information was needed and what basic characteristics the information should possess.

In seeking existing information for support of PHS policy making, it is necessary to address the fundamental question of data vs. information. As discussed earlier, information is properly processed data, not unlike a piece of fine furniture; the furniture represents the processed version of input raw timber, designed to suit the tastes of potential users. Satisfying such tastes (i.e., needs) in designing information involves meeting the requirements (listed earlier) of good information. As has been noted, this is a substantial task.

Thus, while many PHS and PHS-related data bases exist (e.g., *Public Health Reports,* 1981; "Computer Tapes," 1981), it is rare that such sources possess information sets that would be identified independently through the proposed methodology for a given policy problem. This is not to say, however, that such data sets are of no value. Often existing data can be used as information if the policy problem is restated or restructured in some definable way.

For example, the state of North Carolina has, since 1979, collected data on all services provided by every county health department during the month of March of each year. Data exist for a large number of service categories as well as for several classes of health employees. Typology of patients is by age, race, and sex. The resulting data base allows for a substantial evaluation of health services delivery in the state (Parker & Freund, 1982).

However, if it became necessary to develop policy based on the distribution of services by, say, socioeconomic status or education of the patient, the data would be of considerably less value. On the other hand, if a reasonable correlation between one of these factors and age or race were to be assumed or otherwise substantiated, the data then could be used under the stated assumption.

What should be emphasized is that existing PHS data bases normally exist as a result of some well-defined project, program, contract, etc. Their contents, formats, and other characteristics undoubtedly conform to the original purposes and objectives of the project. To seek utilization of such data as information in support of some other PHS policy problem normally will require a restating of the problem to conform with the properties of the data. Such an effort is similar in spirit to one discussed earlier in the chapter—restructuring the policy problem to conform with the assumptions and requirements of a given mathematical policy model.

In both of these situations, the decision called for is the same: evaluation of the trade-off between increased process efficiency/reduced cost, and loss of representativeness of the original policy problem. The PHS policy maker faces this dilemma every time an issue requiring further development and/or evaluation arises. As noted earlier, no patent rules exist for its solution.

INFORMATION SYSTEMS FOR POLICY DEVELOPMENT

The previous section centered on the utilization of existing, unprocessed data in support of PHS policy development. It was shown that use of raw data for such purposes normally is not fruitful, because requirements for appropriate information generally are not met by data generated for other than current purposes. In this regard, it should be recalled that the proposed methodology identifies the content and structure of appropriate support information. According to Figure 9-3 (supra), however, it is the information system that actually develops and delivers information considered suitable for policy support.

Effective PHS policy development therefore depends upon an interface between a health information system (HIS) and the informational requirements identified by the methodology. The associated process is outlined in Figure 9-9 in the form of a simple system with feedback. Such a system involves the feedback of one or more items of output information for the sole purpose of influencing future inputs in some specified manner. It should be noted in the chart that the flow from "data" to "support function" is identical with that of Figure 9-3 but now an output from the PHS policies and policy makers is generated and fed back as input to the HIS. This feedback is the critical stabilizing loop in the process. It represents the methodology's findings and recommendations for informational content (via $\{z_{ij}\}$) and structure (via $\{x_k\}$ and $\{w^*_{ik}\}$), for use by the HIS to selectively acquire, organize, transform, and, ultimately, deliver the requested information.

In order to complete this analysis of the role information plays in support of PHS policy development and evaluation, it is important to understand: (1) the basic structure of a health information system and (2) the formal role such a system plays in developing and delivering good information. As suggested by Figure 9-9, results from the proposed methodology should be considered "instructions" to the HIS, designed to properly guide its processing of data into PHS support information.

While a number of information system models exist in the literature (e.g., Davis, 1974; Senn, 1978), few have been developed that respond to the issues of Figure 9-3, i.e., the policy type, policy maker preferences, and organizational context. Fewer still have been applied within a health or health-related context. A conceptualization designed to overcome these

Figure 9-9 Simple Information System with Feedback for PHS Policy Support

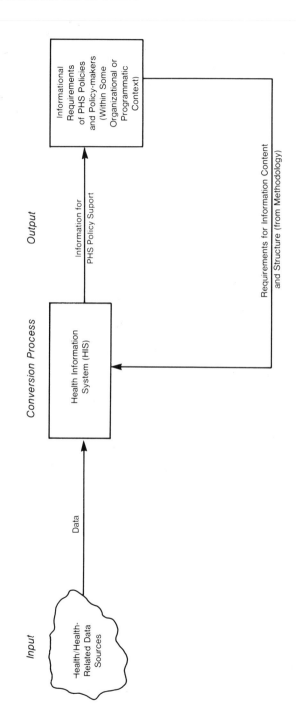

problems is presented in Figure 9-10. This framework applies the important insights of Mason and Mitroff (1973), who state that:

> an information system consists of at least one PERSON of a certain PSYCHOLOGICAL TYPE who faces a PROBLEM within some ORGANIZATIONAL CONTEXT for which he needs EVIDENCE to arrive at a solution (i.e., to select some course of action) and that the evidence is made available to him through some MODE OF PRESENTATION.

The lower portion of Figure 9-10 represents the generator of EVIDENCE, or information system, while the upper portion characterizes the ORGANIZATIONAL CONTEXT within which the information system exists. The interface of the two (dotted line) consists of all policy makers/decision makers (PSYCHOLOGICAL TYPES) who are users of the system.

The organization is viewed in terms of three critical design variables: (1) resource flows—patients/clients, funds, equipment, and personnel; (2) organizational subsystems—management, adaptive, maintenance, and production; and (3) policy/decision type—control, strategic, and adaptive (Parker & Kaluzny, 1982). All of the design variables are defined in Parker and Kaluzny. They are not repeated here since the variables are used only to offer a conceptual view of the organization useful to a discussion of an HIS.

With four levels on each of the first two variables, and three on the last (designated C, S, and A), the matrix representation has $4 \times 4 \times 3 = 48$ cells. Depending upon the organization type being represented, the number of relevant cells can range from 3 or 6 to 48.

For example, a simple organizational structure (Kaluzny, Warner, Warren, & Zelman, 1982) possessing all flows and policy types would be represented by $12 \times 2 = 24$ cells in the "management" and "production" rows. Each cell actually is a point or location in organizational "space" and, as such, has specific informational requirements. These may vary significantly, depending upon the composition of the factor levels. The information delivered to the organization from the HIS (Figure 9-9, supra) is shown here as a flow from the right.

The HIS (EVIDENCE Generator) consists of features that are common to all resource flows as well as those that are unique to specific flows. The proper levels and mix of these features are identified as information system design, a topic of enormous current interest (e.g., King & Cleland, 1975; Parker, 1982; Parker & Kaluzny, 1982). The input and feedback to the HIS shown in Figure 9-9 ("data" and "requirements for information con-

Figure 9-10 Structure of a Health Information System (EVIDENCE Generator)

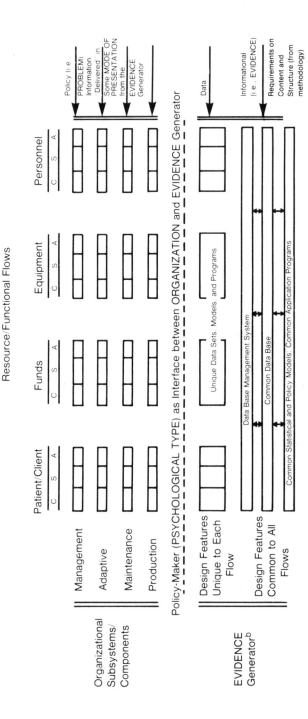

[a]Policy/Decision type abbreviations are: C = control; S = strategic; A = adaptive.

[b]Representation adapted from *Management Information Systems: Conceptual Foundations, Structure, and Development*, 2nd ed., by Gordon B. Davis, McGraw-Hill Book Company, © 1974.

Source: Reprinted with permission from "Structuring Information Systems for More Effective Disease Control Programs" by Barnett R. Parker and Arnold D. Kaluzny, *Journal of Medical Systems*, © 1982.

tent and structure," respectively) are depicted here as flows from the right.

Overall, Figure 9-10 offers a detailed look at the interface of HIS and information requirements and the support role this plays in PHS policy development. The support process begins with the introduction of raw data and relevant specifications for information to the HIS (southeast corner of the diagram). The HIS then processes the data according to these (proposed) specifications. The specifications have been developed in response to: the policy (PROBLEM), policy maker (PERSON of a certain PSYCHOLOGICAL TYPE), and ORGANIZATIONAL CONTEXT. The resulting "tuned" information or EVIDENCE is then delivered in a specified form/format (MODE OF PRESENTATION) for use in the PHS policy development process occurring at various points in the organizational "space."

It is in this manner, then, that the proposed methodology instructs the HIS to develop and deliver information capable of supporting key PHS policy-related activities. The author's position is that without this process and the information (EVIDENCE) it generates, the effectiveness of any PHS policy development effort will necessarily be limited. However, as noted earlier, the process does not guarantee effective policy; it only allows for such policy, since, for example, the information may not be utilized appropriately or, in the worst of cases, not used at all (Ackoff, 1967).

CONCLUSION

This chapter began with a brief description of the complexities inherent in the delivery of effective personal health services (PHS). The problem was shown to be multisectoral in nature, thus requiring significant movements of technology and communications across a series of societal subsystems. The argument was made that successful policy development and evaluation within such a context was incumbent upon the identification and provision of good or appropriate information. In particular, effective PHS policy was seen to be critically dependent upon:

1. Information (i.e., properly processed data) that was responsive, in both content and structure, to the (a) policy class or type and any models and methodologies to be used in formulating the policy; (b) needs, preferences, and beliefs of the relevant policy maker(s); and (c) requirements of the organizational/programmatic structure within which the policy development process occurs; and
2. A health information system (HIS) that implemented the requirements of (1) by first converting input data into the needed information and then delivering it to the appropriate organizational "locations."

Thus, a well-designed information base and interfacing HIS are considered strategic elements in the effort to generate and evaluate effective PHS policy. It is important to note that the support role of these elements is made independent of both the level of analysis and the nature or position of the policy maker. The proposed methodology for structuring information, and the HIS framework (Figure 9-10), therefore may be applied with equal confidence to PHS problems at the macrolevel or microlevel. The policy makers may be professional analysts, consumer groups, regional and state officials, or higher authorities. Thus, it makes little difference, for example, whether the patient visit distribution issue (Figure 9-2) is dealt with at the county or state level, or whether the policy makers are consumers, HSA officials, or state legislators.

The principal objective of this chapter has been to characterize, and provide a means for structuring, an information-based support system for PHS policy development. However, a series of cautions must be noted in conjunction with this effort. Originally identified in the now-classic paper by Ackoff (1967), these considerations make clear the fact (noted earlier) that merely designing "good" information does not necessarily lead to more effective PHS policy. Four potential problems apply here; each is listed briefly, together with suggestions for its control:

1. *Overabundance of irrelevant information is not helpful:* The lack of relevant information in support of policy development is no less serious than the problem of overabundance of irrelevant information. *Control:* Evaluate output of both the methodology and the HIS for their emphasis on supplying relevant information as well as avoiding or eliminating irrelevant information. In so doing, consider the weightings assigned to such informational attributes as uniqueness and clarity.
2. *Requested information is not necessarily required information:* In a general sense, the proposed methodology assumes that policy makers know what information they need. Information they request, however, may not represent what actually is required. *Control:* Emphasize the use of validated empirical models and/or formal decision models (as exemplified by Equations 9.2 and 9.3) in the policy development process. Characterizing the required information then becomes a much less subjective process.
3. *Availability of needed information does not necessarily improve policy making:* A methodology-HIS interface (Figure 9-9) that provides the policy maker with appropriately structured information requires that the individual use that information effectively in order to enhance the resulting policy. This may not always occur. *Control:* Emphasize,

as in the preceding point, the use of objective decision rules and models. In addition, implement a feedback mechanism for the purpose of identifying and describing to policy makers any shortfalls in their use of information previously provided them.

4. *Policy makers may not understand how the HIS functions:* Although not discussed in this chapter, an important aspect of the policy development process involves the evaluation and, if necessary, adjustment of the HIS design/structure (Parker, 1982). This normally is a difficult task because policy makers generally do not understand the operating characteristics of an HIS. *Control:* Train the HIS user or policy maker, who may also be the individual queried in the proposed methodology, to evaluate and hence control the information system. Simplified modules, such as that given by Parker (1981), are useful in this effort.

In conclusion, the authors believe that application of the methodology for structuring information and implementation of the HIS framework, adjusted where necessary by the control measures of these four points, will lead to significantly more effective PHS policy decisions. This, in turn, should allow for the delivery of personal health services offering a greater health benefit to specified patient populations.

Appendix 9-A

Estimating the Structure of Individuals' Preferences/Judgments through Conjoint Analysis

A great deal of support exists for the representation of an individual's preferences or judgments concerning some product or service as a multidimensional function of the product's attributes (Wilkie & Pessemier, 1973). Earlier work in this area was based heavily on the Fishbein-Rosenberg class of expectancy-value models (Fishbein, 1967; Rosenberg, 1956) represented in Equation 9.13:

$$A_{kj} = \sum_{r=1}^{t} I_{kr}B_{kjr} \tag{9.13}$$

where: A_{kj} = attitude of individual k toward object/product j;
$\quad I_{kr}$ = importance (salience, etc.) assigned attribute r by individual k;
$\quad B_{kjr}$ = belief (expectancy, etc.) of individual k as to the extent to which attribute r is offered by product j; and
$\quad t$ = number of attributes.

Equation 9.13 involves a compositional or build-up approach in that the product's attribute levels and corresponding attribute importances are separately and explicitly estimated by the respondent (Green & Srinivasan, 1978). Because of the following conditions, however, such an approach presents serious difficulties in the design of PHS policy support information:

- while the number of design factors is small (five to seven), the number of criteria may be large, thus leading to an unmanageably large number of weights to be estimated;
- given a continuum of criteria, it may be difficult for some individuals to explicate the precise contribution of each and every design factor to a variety of performance criteria; and, more generally,

- because of the nature of the measurements, a number of classic biases may arise, including halo effects and central tendency errors (Beckwith & Lehmann, 1975; Parker, 1977).

In an effort to avoid the problems of Equation 9.13 while maintaining a multiattribute view of individuals' preferences, the method of conjoint analysis is employed here. Broadly speaking, conjoint analysis refers to any decompositional procedure that estimates the structure of an individual's preferences or judgments, e.g., via importance weights, given the person's overall evaluations of a set of product alternatives that are characterized in terms of levels of relevant attributes (Green & Srinivasan, 1978). This concept can be considered as it applies to the current informational design problem:

Assume that there are t different (real or hypothetical) informational designs (stimuli) that are described in terms of q attributes or characteristics. Let x_{kr} represent the known value of attribute $k = 1, \ldots, q$ in information design $r = 1, \ldots, t$. Given that the PHS system must respond to a series of goals, y_i, $i = 1, \ldots, m$, and that only certain individuals/ policy makers are organizationally appropriate or close to each goal, let w_{ik} represent the relative importance of attribute k to goal y_i (as perceived by the appropriate individual(s)). These weights are to be estimated.

Now, the (unknown) value of informational design r with respect to support of policy development on measure y_i, represented by V_{ir}, is hypothesized to be some function of the w_{ik} and x_{kr} values (Green & Srinivasan, 1978). It has been shown that in most decision contexts, a simple linear function of the form in Equation 9.5 (supra) represents well individuals' judgment or preference processes (Dawes & Corrigan, 1974). Factors contributing to this situation include the following:

- conditionally monotone relationships between predictors and the criterion, i.e., more extreme values of the former lead to correspondingly more extreme values for the latter;
- deviations from optimal weights do not make much practical difference; and
- measurement error exists in the predictor (independent) variables.

The implication is that Equation 9.5 acts as a good analog or paramorphic representation of the judgment process, i.e., it simulates the process rather than identifying the true cognitive structure underlying the process (Hoffman, 1960).

A simulation is all that is necessary when process prediction is of interest. Thus, there is less concern here about model structure than the overall ability to predict individuals' judgments or preferences for some given set of informational designs using the model. In some instances the linear model actually is more complex than the underlying process, while in other situations the reverse is true (Einhorn, 1971). It is the case, in fact, that two or more process models might be (1) structurally different yet equally valid (predictively), or (2) structurally equivalent yet represent entirely different underlying processes, e.g., $y_i = x_{i1} + x_{i2}$ and

$$y_i' = \sqrt{x_{i1}^2 + 2x_{i1}\,x_{i2} + x_{i2}^2} \tag{9.14}$$

(Parker, 1977).

To be sure, significant evidence exists showing that such estimates of human judgment may actually be more valid, predictively, of the overall (global) criterion of interest than the original ratings upon which the model, i.e., importance weights, actually was based (Dawes & Corrigan, 1974).

Given these arguments, it is fair to assume a confidence in the use of Equation 9.5 as a valid model of individuals' judgments with respect to informational design. A conjoint analysis is then employed to identify those importance weights ($\{w_{ik}^*\}$) that satisfy individuals' ratings of informational designs $r = 1, \ldots, t$ "as closely as possible." In particular, if an individual prefers design r to r' with respect to policy development on goal y_i, the weights $\{w_{ik}^*\}$ yielding $V_{ir} \geq V_{ir'}$ would be sought.

If the opposite occurs, i.e., $V_{ir} < V_{ir'}$, then the weights are not reflecting the true design judgments of the individual. Thus, the optimal weights should necessarily minimize the number of discrepancies between the calculated V_{ir} levels and the actual design ratings. Such weights are said to represent the individual's internal (cognitive) policy or value structure with respect to the product attributes $k = 1, \ldots, q$ (Parker & Skinner, in press).

REFERENCES

Ackoff, R.L. Management misinformation systems. *Management Science,* December 1967, *14,* B147–B156.

Andersen, R. *A behavioral model of families' use of health services* (Research Series 25). Chicago: University of Chicago, Graduate School of Business, 1968.

Ashcraft, M., Penchansky, R., Berki, S., Fortus, R., & Gray, J. Expectations and experience of HMO enrollees after one year: An analysis of satisfaction, utilization and costs. *Medical Care,* January 1978, *16*(1), 14–32.

Beckwith, N.E., & Lehmann, D.R. The importance of halo effects in multiattribute attitude models. *Journal of Marketing Research,* August 1975, *12,* 265–275.

Bettman, J.R. The structure of consumer choice processes. *Journal of Marketing Research,* November 1971, *8,* 465–471.

Burch, J.G., Strater, F.R., & Grudnitski, G. *Information systems: Theory and practice* (2nd ed.). New York: John Wiley & Sons, Inc., 1979.

Carroll, J.D. Individual differences and multidimensional scaling. In R.N. Shepard, A.K. Romney & S.B. Nerlove (Eds.), *Multidimensional scaling: Theory and applications in behavioral sciences* (Vol. 1). New York: Seminar Press, 1972, pp. 105–155.

Davis, G.B. *Management information systems: Conceptual foundations, structure, and development*. 2nd ed. New York: McGraw-Hill Book Company, 1982.

Dawes, R., & Corrigan, B. Linear models in decision making. *Psychological Bulletin,* February 1974, *81,* 95–106.

Delbecq, A.L., Van de Ven, A.H., & Gustafson, D.H. *Group techniques for program planning: A guide to nominal group and Delphi processes*. Glenview, Ill.: Scott, Foresman and Company, 1975.

Delp, P., Thesen, A., Motiwalla, J., & Seshadri, N. *Systems tools for project planning.* Bloomington, Ind.: International Development Institute, 1977.

Dickson, G.W., Senn, J.A., & Chervany, N.L. Research in management information systems: The Minnesota experiments. *Management Science,* May 1977, *23,* 913–923.

Ein-Dor, P., & Segev, E. Organizational context and the success of management information systems. *Management Science,* June 1978, *24,* 1064–1077.

Einhorn, H. Use of nonlinear, noncompensatory models as a function of task and amount of information. *Organizational Behavior and Human Performance,* January 1971, *6,* 1–26.

Fishbein, M. A behavior theory approach to the relations between beliefs about an object and the attitude towards the object. In M. Fishbein (Ed.), *Readings in attitude theory and measurement.* New York: John Wiley & Sons, Inc., 1967, pp. 389–399.

Galvin, M.E., & Fan, M. The utilization of physicians' services in Los Angeles County, 1973. *Journal of Health and Social Behavior,* March 1975, *16*(1), 74–94.

Green, P.E., & Srinivasan, V. Conjoint analysis in consumer research: Issues and outlook. *Journal of Consumer Research,* September 1978, *5,* 103–123.

Greenberger, M., Crenson, M., & Crissey, B. *Models in the policy process: Public decision making in the computer era.* New York: Russell Sage Foundation, 1976.

Hall, A.D., & Fagen, R.E. Definition of system. In W. Buckley (Ed.), *Modern systems research for the behavioral scientist.* Chicago: Aldine Publishing Company, 1968, pp. 81–92.

Härö, A.S. Information systems for health services at the national level. In G. McLachlan (Ed.), *Information systems for health services.* Copenhagen: World Health Organization, 1980.

Hershey, J.C., Luft, H.S., & Gianaris, J.M. Making sense out of utilization data. *Medical Care,* October 1975, *13*(10), 838–854.

Hillier, F., & Lieberman, G. *Introduction to operations research* (3rd rev. ed.). San Francisco: Holden-Day, 1980.

Hoffman, P.J. The paramorphic representation of clinical judgment. *Psychological Bulletin,* February 1960, *57,* 116–131.

Kaluzny, A., Warner, M., Warren, D., & Zelman, W. *The management of health services.* Englewood Cliffs, N.J.: Prentice-Hall, Inc., 1982.

Keen, P.G., & Morton, M.S. *Decision support systems: An organizational perspective.* Reading, Mass.: Addison-Wesley Publishing Company, 1978.

King, W., & Cleland, D. The design of management information systems: An information analysis approach. *Management Science,* November 1975, *22,* 286–297.

Kleinbaum, D.G., & Kupper, L.L. *Applied regression analysis and other multivariable methods.* North Scituate, Mass.: Duxbury Press, 1978.

Kruskal, J.B. Analysis of factorial experiments by estimating monotone transformation of the data. *Journal of the Royal Statistical Society,* 1965, Series B27, 251–263.

Major data systems of the National Center for Health Statistics, 25th anniversary of the National Health Survey. *Public Health Reports,* May-June 1981, *96*(3), 200–201.

Mason, R.O., & Mitroff, I.I. A Program for research on management information systems. *Management Science,* January 1973, *19,* 475–487.

Milio, N. *Promoting health through public policy.* Philadelphia: F.A. Davis Company, 1981.

Miller, G. The magical number seven, plus or minus two: Some limits on our capacity for processing information. *Psychological Review,* March 1956, *63,* 81–97.

Montgomery, D.B., Wittink, D.R., & Glaze, T. A predictive test of individual level concept evaluation and trade-off analysis (Research Paper No. 415). Stanford, Calif: Stanford University, Graduate School of Business, 1977.

Morris, W.T. On the art of modeling. *Management Science,* August 1967, *13,* B-707–B-717.

National Center for Health Services Research and Development; Health Services and Mental Health Administration. *Computer tapes available from 20 health services research projects.* Washington, D.C.: U.S. Department of Health and Human Services, National Center for Health Services Research, 1981.

Parker, B.R. *On the relevance of consumer behavior theory to health care delivery planning: Development of a patient health benefit function.* Paper presented at the Operations Research Society of America Conference, San Francisco, 1977.

Parker, B.R. A manager-based assessment module for health information systems in developing countries. *Proceedings, Congreso Internacional de Sistemas,* Caracas, Venezuela, 1981.

Parker, B.R. A user-based, multiple goal methodology for evaluation and design correction of a health information system. *Management Science,* submitted 1982.

Parker, B.R., & Freund, D. Cost per service in local health departments: Concepts and illustrations. *Journal of Community Health,* submitted 1982.

Parker, B.R., & Kaluzny, A.D. Structuring information systems for more effective disease control programs. *Journal of Medical Systems,* 1982.

Parker B.R., & Skinner, B.D. Improving the selection of family medicine residents through development of multidimensional policy models. *Health Policy and Education,* in press.

Parker, B.R., & Srinivasan, V. A consumer preference approach to the planning of rural primary health-care facilities. *Operations Research,* September-October 1976, *24,* 991–1025.

ReVelle, C., Marks, C., & Liebman, J. An analysis of private and public sector location models. *Management Science,* June 1970, *16,* 692–707.

Rojeski, R., & ReVelle, C. Central facilities location under an investment constraint. *Geographical Analysis,* October 1970, *2,* 343–360.

Rosenberg, M.J. Cognitive structure and attitudinal affect. *Journal of Abnormal and Social Psychology,* November 1956, *53,* 367–372.

Schonberger, R. MIS design: A contingency approach. *MIS Quarterly,* March 1980, *4,* 13–20.

Senn, J.A. *Information systems in management.* Belmont, Calif.: Wadsworth Publishing Co., Inc., 1978.

Shocker, A.D., & Srinivasan, V. Multiattribute approaches for product concept evaluation and generation: A critical review. *Journal of Marketing Research,* May 1979, *16,* 159–180.

Srinivasan, V., & Shocker, A.D. Estimating the weights for multiple attributes in a composite criterion using pairwise judgments. *Psychometrika,* December 1973, *38,* 473–493.

Srinivasan, V., Shocker, A.D., & Weinstein, A.G. Measurement of a composite criterion of managerial success. *Organizational Behavior and Human Performance,* February 1973, *9,* 147–167.

Stimson, D.H. Utility measurement in public health decision making. *Management Science,* October 1969, *16,* B17–B30.

Stokey, E., & Zeckhauser, R. *A primer for policy analysis.* New York: W.W. Norton & Company, Inc., 1978.

The utilization of health services: Indices and correlates—A research bibliography. Washington, D.C.: U.S. Department of Health, Education, and Welfare, 1972.

Volz, R. Optimum ambulance location in semirural areas. *Transportation Science,* May 1971, *5,* 193–203.

Warner, D.M., & Holloway, D.C. *Decision making and control for health administration: The management of quantitative analysis.* Ann Arbor, Mich.: Health Administration Press, 1978.

Wilkie, W.L., & Pessemier, E.A. Issues in marketing's use of multiattribute attitude models. *Journal of Marketing Research,* November 1973, *10,* 428–441.

Chapter 10

Policy Issues in the Delivery of Personal Health Services in Public-General Hospitals

Laurel A. Files

Public-general hospitals play a distinct role in the delivery of health care in the United States. While they perform the same functions as other short-term, acute care hospitals, public-general hospitals have a mission that sets them apart. They usually are the medical care provider of last resort, taking responsibility for the care of the medically indigent and those otherwise unserved or underserved by the broader health system.

Changing social expectations and economic forces have generated pressures upon and within the health system that threaten its composition and configuration. One effect of this turbulence is that the very existence of public-general hospitals as a class may be in jeopardy, in that they appear to be particularly vulnerable to such pressures (Friedman, 1980). If these hospitals are unable to meet the challenges they face, there could be a significant void in the health care delivery system and there no longer would be a medical or health care "safety net" for the poor and near-poor who have come to depend upon it.

This chapter examines the traditional and current role of public-general hospitals, the viability of possible alternatives to this role, and the policy questions regarding adequate care for those who are unable to provide for themselves.

It also explores the strategic planning process as it might relate to public-general hospitals' strengthening themselves from within and identifies some of the policy issues involved in the implementation of this process in a public institution. This includes consideration of expanding their community health role.

Finally, because of the significant role in medical education and research that the public teaching hospitals have played, issues specific to this group of institutions are addressed.

HISTORICAL ROLE OF PUBLIC-GENERAL HOSPITALS

Approximately 25 percent of the hospitals in this country are public-general. These city, county, district, and state institutions constitute almost a third of the subset of nonfederal, short-term, acute care hospitals, which make up more than 80 percent of the total facilities in the nation. Two other groupings in this subset are the not-for-profit, or voluntary hospitals (47 percent of all facilities), owned and run by community associations or religious organizations; and the proprietary hospitals (10 percent), which are investor-owned and operated for profit (AHA, 1981).

In the late 1700s and early 1800s, voluntary hospitals began to evolve as the physician's "workshop" and as a setting for the training of medical students. These hospitals admitted both indigent and paying patients and were supported financially by both private philanthropy and local government. In contrast, the genesis of today's public-general hospitals was in the 18th-century almshouses, whose basic mission was custodial—to feed and shelter the poor; they were providers of medical care only as absolutely necessary. It was not until the late 1800s that the hospital departments of the almshouses developed as independent public medical care institutions. By then, the hospital was more generally accepted for the care of acute illness and injury and had become "a curative institution in which communities concentrated their health care resources in support of the practicing physician for the benefit of all" (Dowling & Armstrong, 1980, p. 128).

In keeping with their origins, the public-general hospitals have developed into the primary providers of inpatient, short-term, acute medical care for the medically indigent, and those in areas unserved or underserved by private providers.

Most other unmet health needs of the public have been addressed through the broader public health system, including health departments, programs for communicable diseases and maternal and child health, community mental health centers (CMHCs), and public assistance for specific groups such as crippled children, the aged, the blind, the disabled, and poor families with dependent children. The public delivery of health care thus has been two-track: one, primarily curative general hospitals; the other, public health agencies and programs, primarily preventive in focus and providing only limited nonacute medical care.

In describing the role of the public-general hospital in the delivery of personal health services, it is helpful to compare the roles of the different types of institutions in each of the three spheres of health care: primary, secondary, and tertiary.

These areas of care are defined as follows (*Discursive Dictionary,* 1976):

> *Primary Care:* Basic or general health care . . . and the care of the simpler and more common illnesses. . . . Primary care is comprehensive in the sense that it takes responsibility for the overall coordination of the patient's health problems, be they biological, behavioral, or social.
>
> *Secondary Care:* Services provided by medical specialists who generally do not have first contact with patients. . . . In the United States, however, there has been a trend toward self-referral . . . rather than referral by primary care providers.
>
> *Tertiary Care:* Services provided by highly specialized providers . . . [which] frequently require highly sophisticated technological and support facilities. The development of these services has largely been a function of . . . basic and clinical biomedical research.

Historically, the three types of short-term hospitals have focused on different spheres of care. All have been providers of inpatient secondary care. But while the proprietary hospitals generally have offered no significant amount of primary or tertiary care, the voluntary and public-general institutions have been active in these spheres. In particular, the public-general hospitals have been significant providers of primary care in urban areas and in rural areas with limited access to private physicians, and of tertiary care in the urban teaching hospitals, especially those that are the major affiliate of a medical school, state-owned or university-owned.

ENVIRONMENTAL TURBULENCE AND HEALTH CARE DELIVERY

By the early 1980s, the health care system was facing an increasingly turbulent environment, with the potential of altering the structure of the system as well as the historical roles of its institutions. The growing national budget deficit has contributed to increasing discomfort on the part of policy makers pressed by continually rising expenditures of public funds on health care, especially hospital costs. The Department of Health and Human Services' Health Care Financing Administration has estimated inpatient and outpatient care, financed by government and private hospitals, to be $112 billion for fiscal year 1981, a 17 percent increase over the previous year (Brazda, 1982).

This concern has been translated into a desire to cap medical care expenditures through both supply-side and demand-side mechanisms. Thus, the levels of government support of hospitals and other health facilities (i.e., departments of public health, neighborhood health centers, CHMCs) are no longer secure; the level and source of reimbursement for medical care to the indigent, the disabled, and the elderly (Medicaid and Medicare) are being questioned; the nature and extent of other third party reimbursements is in transition; and new forms of competitive service delivery structures are being encouraged and supported in the hope that a "freer" market will drive prices down. Tougher regulations are also in the offing if other means of cost control prove unsuccessful.

Increasingly, policy questions are being framed in terms of cost-benefit ratios and short-term efficiency, and often are grounded in the unquestioned and unproved assumption that all constituencies have an equitable role in forming policy and the resultant structure of the system thus, at minimum, would be satisfying to all concerned.

The issues of who is the appropriate bearer of the burden (namely, financial risks and losses) involved in delivering certain kinds of services and care, and how these can be delivered most effectively, are not often dealt with explicitly. To turn this around and make it explicit, the question to be asked is:

> What is perceived to be the government's (federal, state, local) responsibility and role with regard to health care for the medically indigent and those with otherwise unmet health needs?

In response, the nation could decide that the government has all, some, or no, responsibility for these activities. If the government accepts any responsibility, its role can be direct (through public institutions, i.e., run by government employees) and/or indirect (through financial mechanisms).

If it is determined that there is a role for public institutions, then it is critical that the development of health-related policies should include formal or informal consideration of their impact on these institutions to ensure internal consistency, i.e., so that the intentions of one policy are not undermined by the implementation of other policies. Thus, if the role of public-general hospitals as the medical care providers of last resort is confirmed, it is critical that policy makers be cognizant of the impacts of various other policies on these institutions and on those who consume their care.

Public-general hospitals should not be allowed to continue to exist by default. This could have undesirable financial and human costs. If they are to continue to perform desired societal functions—historical and/or new ones—they should be able to do so with the support of public policies and regulations rather than in spite of them.

HEALTH POLICIES AND BIASED EXTERNALITIES

Policy decisions with regard both to the dynamics of the health care system and to the role of public hospitals within that system will have a tremendous influence on shaping the roles of public and private hospitals for the rest of the 1980s and beyond. Because of those institutions' traditionally different service delivery patterns, however, the nature and extent of change will continue to vary, depending on the type of hospital, and the different types of patient populations and other constituencies they serve.

Policy intentions can be stated explicitly or can evolve from ad hoc decisions. In either case, they affect the nature and quality of related service delivery. Furthermore, this effect may radiate throughout an entire service delivery system, with positive and/or negative implications for its organizational structure. Some of these system impacts may be known, or suspected, and deliberately planned. Others may be externalities, or unplanned effects, that also may be positive and/or negative. Although the concept of externalities by definition acknowledges that policy makers and planners are not omniscient, it certainly is desirable that any negative effects be minimized to the extent possible.

When health policies (and subsequent regulations) lead to undesirable externalities, they ultimately can be a matter of life and death. Policies motivated predominantly by economic criteria, such as minimum cost and maximum efficiency, with little regard for social factors such as individual needs and benefits, may increase the level of undesirable externalities unnecessarily. It may be expected and acceptable that some policies may threaten the viability of some institutions. If the result is a weeding out of the poorest performing institutions, whose clientele then is absorbed by other, better-operating ones, the system and the public may benefit. However, if the policies have an unpredicted, negative effect on only certain types of institutions and, consequently, on only certain classes of clients, reconsideration or adaptation of these courses of action could be critical.

Monitoring and feedback on undesirable externalities therefore is important if emerging policies are to be consistent with the expected and desired social roles of public institutions.

SHOULD THERE BE PUBLIC-GENERAL HOSPITALS?

The historical role of public-general hospitals is well established. Whether they need to continue to exist, whether they should continue to perform the same roles as in the past, and whether their existence should be governmentally protected are not questions that have clear-cut answers.

An important factor in determining the current and future need for public-general hospitals, and underlying the elaboration of their role, is whether the initial assumption is that there is a one-class or two-class system of health care in this country. If a one-class system is assumed, that approach leads to a different set of policy alternatives than does assuming a two-class system. If the nation behaves as if it has a one-class system but in fact does not, this may encourage policy makers to ignore problems and to limit options for improvement. If the country behaves as if it has a two-class system, it may perpetuate stereotypes and squelch potential social and economic development.

A One-Class System of Care?

If a one-class system of health care is determined to be both desirable and possible, at minimum a policy framework should be generated to address directly the task of (1) effectively mainstreaming the indigent into the private sector, (2) developing options for geographic or service areas in which there is no private sector alternative, and (3) determining which, if any, existing public providers represent investments that should continue to exist, then upgrading those facilities as needed and developing them into mainstream self-supporting purveyors of care, i.e., attractive to a market beyond the indigent.

Mainstreaming the Indigent

A one-class system should mean that the indigent always receive their care from the same providers and in the same institutions as do all other clients. Medicare and Medicaid are a step in this direction, with certain drawbacks. Medicare and Medicaid patients are identifiable to the provider and so—in particular for Medicaid—those individuals may be treated differently from others. Thus there might be a one-class system structurally but a two-class system in practice. Vouchers for purchasing health care from the consumer's choice of provider might facilitate entry of the poor into the private sector even further but still would identify them as poor and so would not guarantee them first-class care.

Income maintenance solutions, negative income tax, and other schemes to put more money into the hands of the poor, with which they then could buy health care from any provider they chose, might avoid the stigma but would not necessarily result in any better service. Any restrictions to earmark the use of this money would raise other administrative control issues.

National health insurance is another type of mechanism that could facilitate financial access to services for the poor without singling them out. The pros and cons of national health insurance and the likelihood of its becoming a reality have been discussed at great length in many other forums and are not pursued here.

From the consumer's perspective, making any of these mechanisms work properly would involve educating the indigent to new utilization patterns and to making prudent and appropriate health care purchases.

Another solution might be to emulate the automobile insurance industry and identify a pool of high-risk patients who then are assigned to mainstream providers (fee-for-service physicians, private hospitals, etc.). This again raises the question of stigma as well as freedom of choice (of both consumers and providers) and still does not guarantee high-quality care.

Availability of Services

Unless there were incentives to assure the availability of services in areas of need (geographic/physical location, and specific service needs) as well as incentives to providers in general, vouchers or money in hand might be useless to the poor. The possible development of "Medicaid mills" (and second-class care) raises the issue of incentives vs. overregulation.

Limited provider resources is not an unsolvable problem but does have to be addressed systematically. The Rural Health Initiative was a public response; was it sufficient and did it mainstream? The Robert Wood Johnson Foundation-funded Rural Health Program was a private initiative but was limited in application. Funding seems to be necessary and should be relatively long term in order to redistribute providers and services and keep them in place long enough to guarantee their existence beyond the period of external funding.

The availability of certain types of sophisticated and specialized tertiary care also tends to be highly dependent on developmental funding and may not be accessible to poor patients unless they are subsidized publicly.

Public Provider's Role in a One-Class System

Mainstreaming public health would not necessarily mean the demise of public-general hospitals as institutions. However, it could involve a redefinition of their roles, goals, and functions.

Most of these hospitals represent a significant commitment of services to the poor, who could not immediately—and perhaps not ever completely—be absorbed by the private sector. As a partial illustration of the size of this commitment, estimates of bad debts have been as high as 10 percent of total patient charges in nonprofit and public hospitals in certain locations (Dowling & Armstrong, 1980, p. 127), and charity/collection losses have been estimated at the level of $2.0 billion annually at the 270 nonfederal teaching hospitals with major college of medicine affiliations (Colloton, 1981, p. 25).

Even if a transition to a totally private system of care were possible, and even if this were carried out gradually, any risk of failure would be borne by the current users of public hospitals. These are not only the poor but also—disproportionately—certain subclasses of the poor. For instance, a 1981 study indicated that more than three times as many minority elderly (22 percent) received their health care through institutions such as hospital outpatient departments than did the white elderly (Bernstein & Berk, 1981).

Many of those dependent upon public hospitals might be ineligible for entry to private facilities, e.g., illegal aliens might not qualify for vouchers but do receive treatment in public hospitals. It can be assumed that the failure of alternate (private) care might disproportionately affect racial, ethnic, and other minorities. Thus, the public hospitals would need to continue to be available as a fail-safe mechanism against private system failure.

Finally, many of the public hospitals also represent a considerable capital investment by taxpayers and deserve a close evaluation in terms of institutional mainstreaming.

Separate but Equal (Adequate)?

Speaking to the other side of this question, Elliot Roberts, director of the Cook County Hospital in Chicago, asserted that the nation had yet to address realistically the problem of providing health care for the poor, which he felt should begin with accepting the fact that a two-class system of medical care was in operation. What must be done, he declared, is to decide how best to perform, given that setting (Punch, 1981b).

What Is a Two-Class System?

The common stereotype of a two-class system refers to quality of care, i.e., better and worse. In health care, this might mean anything the patient can afford vs. some absolute minimum necessary for the survival of those who cannot pay their own way. Although two-class often is expressed in institutional terms—private vs. public hospitals—it probably is described more accurately in patient terms: private vs. public (medically indigent) patients. It is not uncommon in public hospitals for private patient clinics to be physically separate from the public clinics, or for the admissions department to practice "creative scheduling" so that private patients are not in outpatient waiting rooms at the same time as the indigent, or for private clients to be treated by medical faculty and perhaps by house staff, and public patients primarily by medical students, supervised by house staff and medical faculty.

A more sensitive and caring two-class system could be developed, however. If Roberts's suggestion that it be determined how best to perform in such a system were pursued, the analysis might begin by defining two-class as the equivalent of two tracks, running parallel but providing a different array of services to two different groups of passengers. In other words, the second track should be "no frills" rather than "no good." Determining what are frills and what are necessities is, of course, in the eye of the beholder—or, more appropriately, of the recipient of services—and would be no simple policy task.

Public Role of the Private Provider

A two-track health care system does not dictate a public sector vs. private sector dichotomy or any other specific structural division. Nevertheless, there is no reason to believe that the current public-private structure will not survive, with the public system continuing as the provider of last resort for the medically indigent and the private sector being more exclusive.

There also is reason to expect that the private provider will continue to offer some services to public clients. The extent and nature of any public role for the private sector is a policy question, however, especially if that sector is to be subsidized in this role and the public sector simultaneously is to be upgraded. Furthermore, if the private sector is to continue to be used for public purposes, it will have to be determined to what extent indigent patient mainstreaming should be encouraged in the two-track model, and how. For which patients? For what services? Paid for through what mechanisms and from what sources? The role of provider incentives, public-private competition, most appropriate use of services, and consumer needs and preferences all need to be considered carefully.

Defining the Future of Public-General Hospitals

> Only the purest romantic would assert that public hospitals have done no wrong. . . . But the decision to close, convert, or reduce [their] size . . . should be based on each hospital's relationship with its community, its stated mission . . . and how well it is accomplishing that mission . . . [not on] cost . . . or . . . ownership alone . . . (Friedman, 1980).

Whether the health care system is one class or two, substantial human and capital investment already is involved in the subsystem of public-general hospitals that would seem to assure many of them a necessary and continuing role in providing services. What the future configuration of these institutions will be, both as individual facilities and as components of the larger medical-health care system, will depend not only on the management expertise of individual hospital chief executive officers and their institutional policy decisions but on such determinations at all levels of government.

The central public policy question is that of the financial infrastructure of the entire system. The key question for public hospitals involves financial responsibility for the medically indigent—whether there is a means for equitable distribution of this responsibility or whether it will fall more heavily on one segment of society than on another.

Who Should Be Responsible for the Medically Indigent?

Hospital-based care for the indigent is supported by the funding of institutions, i.e., public hospitals, and of individual patient care. Institutional support comes from local, state, and federal government general tax revenues in many forms, including access to the capital market through tax-exempt bonds. Primary federal funds for subsidizing care of individual patients—Medicaid and Medicare—are derived from special trust accounts, while similar programs at local levels (state and community) usually are supported by general tax revenues. Some inner-city hospitals are dependent upon the state and federal government for as much as 80 percent of patient care revenue (Altman, 1981).

In addition, hospitals attempt to redistribute their costs through the controversial "hidden tax," namely, cost shifting (Friedman, 1982). Cost shifting is the process by which hospitals charge one group of patients a higher price for care in order to compensate, at least in part, for the fact that another group (those supported by government assistance programs as well as other charity or bad debt patients) is not paying its share. The effect of this practice is that Blue Cross and the commercial health insurers—and their policy holders, if the costs are passed on—as well as self-paying patients bear a disproportionate share of the cost of care for the medically indigent. In a sense, the better-off sick are being financially penalized for being sick.

It has been predicted that 1,000 hospitals will be forced to close by 1990 because of federal reimbursement reductions and the "resultant increase in cost shifting" (*Hospital Week,* 1982). The implication of this is that self-paying patients and third party payers are quickly reaching the limit in their willingness to absorb additional costs of indigent and charity care. But if this care is to be provided, someone has to pay. So far, no one has been willing to focus directly on the human side of cost cutting, i.e., withholding or reducing basic health services.

The policy and operational issues that surface under the umbrella of cost shifting are, in fact, the generic factors involved in determining who pays. These issues include the following:

Who Bears the Cost?	*Issue*
The hospital attempts to absorb the loss.	1. There is no issue except for the hospital's bottom line, if costs elsewhere cannot be reduced.
	2. Nonpublic hospitals may refuse to accept medically indigent patients, "dumping" them on the public institutions and thus compounding this problem for the latter.
	3. Public hospitals that have no financial slack could be put out of business by dumping unless their sponsoring body (local or state government) picks up the costs, in which case the actual bearer of the expenses is the local or state taxpayer. David Rosenbloom, Boston's commissioner of health, predicted that public hospitals would close rather than be trapped by the private hospitals' freezing out of undesirable patients (Punch, 1981a).

Local or state taxpayers bear the cost.

1. There may be no issue except for the ironic twist that in the poorer cities, counties, and states, where the level of indigent care is higher, patients' and the taxpayers' ability to pay for care may be lower.

The hospital shifts costs to private patients by adjusting prices upward.

1. At some point, hospitals with greater indigent patient loads will become less competitive. They may suffer a drop in patients by losing self-referrals and physician referrals. They may lose HMO contracts. The recent experience of a county hospital in one of the southern states probably is a sign of the times:

Announcing a 23 percent increase in private room rates to compensate for a $2 million-a-year cut in Medicaid and Medicare payments, the hospital was faced with the wrath of one local industry—concerned with escalating insurance costs—that protested the rate hike by advising its employees to use local private hospitals instead. That was an "innovative" response, said a spokesman for another local firm.

2. Hospitals with large indigent patient populations and small numbers of private patients, such as inner-city public facilities, may have few options for shifting costs.

3. Economist Uwe Reinhardt raises the issue as to whether it is ethical to charge the sickest

patient the most (Friedman, 1982).

4. Hospitals may feel forced to discount prices for some groups (a particular health maintenance organization, Blue Cross), thus raising even higher the costs to commercially insured patients.

Costs are shifted to commercial insurers.

1. When costs are shifted to commercial insurers, but Blue Cross contracts are more favorable, the former may be made noncompetitive (HIAA, 1982).

The federal government pays for Medicare and Medicaid but seeks cost cutting.

1. The issue appears to be that of the federal government's "fair share" for those to whom coverage has been promised vs. its perception that costs can be held down more than hospitals have been doing.

In the short run, how these issues are resolved is intimately related to the policy statement evolving as the new federalism of the early 1980s. Basically, this is a question of how dominant a role the national government should play in health and welfare, an area many still feel should be totally a prerogative of the state. However, the rising expectations of consumers and the increasing tendency of states to tighten, rather than loosen, their purse strings, could lead to an irreconcilable gap. Furthermore, the balance between freedom for private entrepreneurship and public oversight through regulation and direct provision of services must be worked out within this broader framework.

STRATEGIC PLANNING FOR SURVIVAL

There is no question that whatever the role of public-general hospitals is to be, they certainly are going to be expected to be more efficient, more effective, and more accountable than many of them have been perceived to be. This will involve internal policy making and decision making by the individual hospitals to reconcile their basic public mission with what it takes for them to stay alive as organizations.

One means of surviving economic pressures is for public-general hospitals to branch out into a broader range of revenue-producing activities. In this way, they might be better able to support their public mission as well as to become mainstream providers. A critical step in their preparation for such an expanded role is strategic planning, and this, too, raises public policy issues.

An organization's strategy is its blueprint (either formalized, informally understood, or implicit in its combined activities) for reconciling its internal capabilities and the personal values of its key personnel with its environment, i.e., external opportunities and constraints (Hofer & Schendel, 1978; Shirley, Peters, & El-Ansary, 1976). One of the most important aspects of strategic planning is that it is not unidimensional but rather involves developing a hierarchy of organizational strategies: (1) corporate, (2) strategic business unit (SBU), and (3) functional area.

At the corporate level, the strategic question is: What business(es) should the corporation be in? For a public-general hospital, the responses might include, for example, developing a home care program, merging with a public health department, developing a chronic long-term care capability (e.g., purchasing a long-term care facility, building a new facility, developing swing beds—beds regularly maintained for both short- and long-term use, depending on need).

At the SBU level, the strategic focus is on how to compete effectively. For the public-general hospital, this would include decisions as to whether and how to increase market share (proportion of the home care, public health, or long-term care market, for example), to maintain its growth, or to maximize its profits.

At the level of the functional areas, the focus is on maximizing productivity. Functional area decisions include those that pertain to geographic coverage (e.g., regional public health center vs. local public health services), to markets (e.g., market development—increase share of home care market or stimulate greater demand for such services), to product line (skilled nursing facilities vs. intermediate care facilities, rehabilitation vs. psychiatric beds).

Policy Issues in Strategic Planning

A primary constraint in hospital strategic planning involves its historically perceived mission and the nature of its "product."

While industry typically is an "economic enterprise with social overtones," the hospital is a "social enterprise with deepening economic overtones" (Johnson, 1979). Whereas a hospital trustee holds a public trust, a corporate director is responsible to shareholders. The mission and product of the not-for-profit hospital are primarily social in nature and theoretically have been driven by perceptions of social good (derived from the accumulation of individual patient benefits). In contrast, while the for-profit corporation has a mission and product similar to the not-for-profits, the former are shaped further by the profit-and-loss statement.

Strategic planning, as conceptualized and practiced in the business world, facilitates economic-reactive rather than socially proactive planning. Thus proprietary hospitals, to the extent that their economic goals actually dominate their social goals, already are in a posture appropriate to implementing strategic planning. To deal with the more technical questions of implementing a strategic planning process, the not-for-profit hospitals and those who support them financially first must come to terms with the more fundamental question: What is the proper role of economics in the decision-making equation of this social institution?

A second issue is whether it is legitimate for government-supported facilities to become involved in strategies that may involve competing with nongovernment facilities. Many feel that the public hospital already has an unfair competitive edge in the form of public funds, tax advantages, protective legislation, and other preferential factors. Public hospitals, on the other hand, see many of these "advantages" as constraints, feeling that their burdens outweigh their supports, that their potential for good business management often is hampered by their governmental status, that they are subjected to a higher level of restrictive regulation than are the proprietaries and community not-for-profits, and that they are captive to a system that makes them accountable to an almost infinite array of often-conflicting constituencies.

The truth as to the ability of public hospitals to compete effectively may lie somewhere in between these two extreme views and, because of the high level of environmental uncertainty, probably is in flux. The issue as to whether it is legitimate for them to compete is related to these questions but ultimately is a policy question—judgmental in nature.

Finally, is survival of the public hospital under conditions of competition compatible with the expectation that it be the provider of last resort? A proprietary hospital's strategic plan might include divesting itself of losing businesses such as services that cost more than it can recover through patient revenues or those with low profit margins. Depending upon the service—emergency care for the urban poor, for example—the public hospital may not have the moral or social flexibility to eliminate losers short of closing down entirely. A proprietary hospital can diversify into nonhealth and/or profit-making enterprises so as to build and strengthen the corporation. Would it be acceptable for the public hospital to plan for such developmental growth? Would such diversification be acceptable, on the other hand, in order to support a hospital's public service activities, i.e., to offset the losses produced by fulfilling its public trust?

Some of these issues are touched on in Loebs, Johnson, and Summers's adaptation (1982) of the Hofer and Schendel (1978) strategic planning model for application by rural primary care centers.

Community Health Care Strategies

The strategic planning process, implemented systematically, should enable hospitals to develop strategies that are in their own best interest. As a policy issue, however, there is potential conflict between this process of strategic planning, or constructing an organizational survival map, and the public interest. Consciously assessing choices with a "business" mindset may crystallize these conflicts between hospital survival and community needs (Cunningham, 1981). "Perhaps the toughest aspect of strategy is selecting the appropriate balance between social responsibility and economic performance" (Webber, 1982, pp. 69–70).

A brief scenario can illustrate this. Let it be assumed that University General Hospital uses the Boston Consulting Group's (BCG) Business Portfolio Matrix to help it identify the best business(es) it should be in (Hedley, 1977; Hofer & Schendel, 1978). Let it also be assumed that this analysis leads University General to the conclusion that Obstetrics (OB) is, in BCG's jargon, a "dog"; the hospital's relative competitive position is low for OB and the growth of the industry is low. In other words, University General's current share of the OB market is small as compared to South Memorial (a private hospital that has the highest number of deliveries in the area), and the area's birth rate—and thus the future need for OB services—is stable or declining.

In cold business terms, the corporate-level decision should be to discontinue OB at University General and focus primarily on its "stars," the services where its market share and the industry growth rate are high. This would be in University General's best interest. But what if University General is providing OB care for most of the indigent women in the area and is the only hospital within a reasonable driving distance that has been willing and able to take on high-risk maternity patients? It may not be in the community's best interest for University General to discontinue its OB services.

As resources continue to decline and economic performance becomes more critical to survival, this is the kind of strategic dilemma that increasingly faces public-general hospitals and their communities. Such dilemmas are not caused by strategic planning but the process may surface them more systematically and explicitly. Therefore, it would be constructive for hospitals to use this process to formulate public policy issues and to increase their leverage in the development of public policy frameworks that link individual hospital strategies and broader community health care needs. In the example above, the community might develop a framework for identifying, prioritizing, and subsidizing specific services for indigents at University General.

This leads to the suggestion that one arena for potential public policy focus relevant to personal health services might be in the development of hospital-based community health care networks. Since 1947, a variety of public commissions has encouraged an expanded community role for hospitals, especially the public-general hospitals:

- The Commission on Hospital Care (1947) recommended an integrated program between general hospitals and chronic long-term care institutions (e.g., mental hospitals, TB facilities), as well as with other community agencies.
- The National Commission on Community Health Services (1967) called for "comprehensive personal health care through a network of appropriate alternative settings" (p. 30).
- The 37th American Assembly (of nationally recognized authorities in health care and related fields) recommended restructuring the role of the hospital to enable it to play a more prominent part in developing a comprehensive health care system (*Health of Americans,* 1970).
- The Commission on Public-General Hospitals (1978) described a "major role" for such hospitals in "planning and arranging for neighborhood-based primary care services" as well as for ensuring coordination with other human services programs (pp. 23–25).

Many others writing in this area have visualized the public hospital as the hub of a community health care delivery system or network (Bryant, Ginsberg, Goldsmith, Olendzki, & Piore, 1976; Crosby, 1970; Herman & McKay, 1968; Kissick, 1978; Newman, 1982; Somers, 1971).

Until the middle and late 1970s, the availability of seemingly unlimited resources and a tolerable level of governmental regulation combined to produce a hospitable health care environment. The environment, while not placid, also was not turbulent; rather, it was relatively unchanging, with interorganizational encounters either infrequent, random, or mostly predictable (Emery & Trist, 1965). This allowed hospitals (and other health care providers) to equate organizational self-interest with organizational autonomy. Communitywide health networks had little relevance for individual hospitals.

As the health and the broader socioeconomic environments have become increasingly turbulent, and sufficient resources for all has become less and less likely, a state of "resource dependence" (Pfeffer & Salancik, 1978) has developed among many health care providers. Hospitals, in need of patients, personnel, capital, and other resources, are frequently being forced to recognize their need for interorganizational interaction. Growth in the hospital industry is declining (Table 10-1). Stabilization through diversification and formation of coalitions emerges as the more appropriate organizational response to the environment (Longest, 1979).

Lehman (1975) suggests that "rising public expectations about what constitutes an adequate array of health services, along with a concern for the costs involved, have led to a broad agreement that comprehensive and economical medical care can flow only from pluralities of units coordinating their activities" (p. 212). Hospital mergers are one form of stabilization and possibly are even a prerequisite to the "outreach programs envisioned by those devoted to comprehensive, uniformly available care" (Starkweather, 1981, p. 4). Hospital-based or hospital-initiated networks of community health care could be a stabilization strategy with, as a byproduct, the dovetailing of public-general hospital interests and community public policy on economic needs and social responsibility.

As public-general hospitals begin to think, plan, and develop strategically, one set of alternatives may be to diversify within the health care field in terms of both services and clientele, providing a broader array of personal health services to a broader market, i.e., the mainstream consumer. Increasingly, there is a "creaming" of self-paying and insured patients by for-profit hospitals, free-standing surgicenters and emergicenters, HMOs, etc., for high-volume, low provider-cost services—e.g., simple elective surgery, ambulatory and other less acute care, preventive care, and health promotion. Many of these services traditionally have been offered by hospitals and public health agencies.

Hospitals need to give attention to redefining their relationships with other providers (Feldstein, 1981). With a pooling of talent and resources,

Table 10-1 Growth in Short-Term Nonfederal Hospitals and Beds

	1960–1970	1970–1980	Interdecade Growth Rate
Number of Hospitals	+ 8.5%	+ 0.8%	−91%
Number of Beds	+32.9%	+16.8%	−49%

Source: Adapted from Guide to the Health Care Field, American Hospital Association, © 1981.

these public institutions could redesign their delivery of these services so as to be attractive to a broader market. Simultaneously, this could increase the availability and accessibility of a more comprehensive range of services for indigent patients. Further, the reduction of conflict among public providers could strengthen the hand of the public organizations in developing relationships with the privates. Relationships with private sector health care providers such as HMOs and nursing homes should be explored, as these could lead to broader referral networks for both routine inpatient care and tertiary care (in the case of the teaching hospitals).

A bottom line policy consideration is that such developments probably depend on governmental interest and funding. Shonick's study (1980) of the motivations, outcomes, and implementation process of the merging of the local public health department and the local public-general hospital in several urban centers provides evidence of how essential it is that there be local governmental support, federal funding, and a perceived need of participating agencies if such system realignments are to be successful.

Shonick concludes that it is in the overall public policy interest to support publicly operated local networks of integrated, regionalized health systems, even though public hospitals are eroding and there is minimal general discussion of this issue. He feels this would tend to guarantee reasonably priced good health care for the poor while also providing a "*truly* pluralistic system wherein persons who preferred publicly operated services would have a viable public alternative available to them" (p. 30).

For heuristic purposes, this analysis has taken the perspective of the public-general hospital as the focal organization in providing an impetus for a community health care strategy because this could be congruent with its organizational health. However, it probably is unrealistic to expect such an initiative to originate in the hospitals without a preliminary push from governmental funding sources. The basic point is that hospital-based community health care strategies (1) are relevant for both public-general hospitals and their communities, (2) could be an appropriate arena for hospitals to develop a balance between social responsibility and economic performance, and (3) should be pursued aggressively in a public policy forum.

THE PUBLIC TEACHING HOSPITAL: A SPECIAL CASE

Distinguishing Characteristics

A teaching hospital is one that expresses some level of commitment to clinical medical education; public teaching hospitals are a subset of public-general hospitals. For many years, public teaching hospitals have been stereotyped as large, urban institutions and specialty care centers, providing a disproportionate amount of outpatient care, with substantial support from public and philanthropic sources.

In 1973, the Association of American Medical Colleges' (AAMC) Council of Teaching Hospitals identified 13 variables it felt described teaching hospitals more accurately:

1. size of intern and resident staff
2. number of fellowship positions
3. range of undergraduate clerkships
4. volume of research
5. medical faculty integration with hospital medical staff
6. nature of affiliation arrangements
7. existence of full-time salaried chiefs of service
8. number of other salaried physicians
9. number of special service programs
10. complexity of diagnostic mix of patients
11. staffing patterns and ratios
12. scope and intensity of laboratory services
13. financial arrangements and volume of service in outpatient clinics and emergency rooms (AAMC, 1981b, pp. 7–8).

Eight years later, AAMC's Department of Teaching Hospitals refined this checklist in an attempt to present a richer portrait of the operating environment of such institutions (AAMC, 1981b, pp. 8–20). Five broad areas (discussed next) were proposed to differentiate teaching hospitals from nonteaching hospitals; these factors also differentiate teaching institutions from each other in that the extent of the presence of each of these features varies from one facility to the next. The AAMC concluded that "it is difficult to define common needs, to generalize about priorities, and to take shared, mutually beneficial actions in the face of broad questions of public policy" (AAMC, 1981b, p. 21); however, these characteristics do define parameters that clarify some of the problems unique to teaching hospitals and that should facilitate consideration and development of future public policies.

The following discussion does not distinguish among types of teaching hospitals, but it should be assumed that the impact of any public policy will vary depending upon where the hospital is classified on a continuum from participation in a single residency program to being a university-owned teaching institution or the primary site of clinical education for a medical school.

The five characteristics identified by the AAMC in 1981 are as follows:

Multiple Objectives

Teaching hospitals are committed to providing and monitoring patient care, to health professionals' training, and to clinical research. The implementation of these missions involves values and activities that may be in conflict with each other and that can lead to the suboptimization of one mission at the expense of another. Frequently, activities that would enhance the competitiveness of patient care services have lower priority than other functions; for example, a marketable and revenue-producing ambulatory care department may be "sacrificed" to the interests of medical education and research.

Environmental and External Controls

In addition to the constraints and regulations under which all hospitals operate, the teaching institution may be particularly subject to values and demands of the medical school, various research foundations, medical school department chairmen, university policies, government appropriations regarding indigent health care, changes in medical school enrollment and curriculum, and controls over residency programs. The teaching hospital, therefore, is not always able singlemindedly to pursue activities that per se will advance the facility's efficiency and effectiveness.

Medical Staff Structure

The teaching hospital medical staff is distinguished by its size and complexity: formal departmentalization; full-time, salaried, appointed clinical service chiefs; full-time medical school compensated teaching physicians alongside nonteaching community physicians; medical school department chairmen; house staff. There is an organizational schizophrenia for department chairmen between the bureaucratic and interdepartmental demands related to effective hospital management and the relatively autonomous nature of the internal organization of the medical school. This dual role can create for the chairmen a "conflict with some of the hospital's greatest concerns: cost containment, effective resource allocation, efficient patient care scheduling, utilization review, and interdepartmental communication and cooperation" (AAMC, 1981b, p. 15).

Pursuit of Innovation

An ongoing and sophisticated biomedical research program results in frequent changes in medical education programs, demands for access to the most up-to-date techniques and technologies, and a continuous need to develop new services and recruit additional and new types of staff, all in the absence of proved cost efficiency or effectiveness but important to development.

Cost and Financing

"No matter how efficient or well managed a teaching hospital is, it is unlikely that [its] average costs will ever be lower than those of other hospitals" (AAMC, 1981b, p. 17) because, it is often claimed, of the added costs of medical education, the provision of more intense care to sicker patients, the high level of uncompensated care, and, typically, financial losses through outpatient departments. (It should be understood, however, that there is not always, or in all areas of the hospital, a direct relationship between teaching and costs.)

In short, the intraorganizational and interorganizational environment of teaching hospitals is considerably more complex than that of our public-general facilities so a greater range of public policies influences their functioning. Their role as providers of medical education and of tertiary care—often as regional referral centers—means they both have unique strengths and unique vulnerabilities in the turbulence of the health care environment.

Price Competition and Teaching Hospitals

Public hospitals, because of their historical mission (often accompanied by some degree of social stigma), suffer from a form of adverse utilization: they attract a significant proportion of patients who are a financial liability. This is exacerbated in the case of those hospitals that have a concentration of tertiary care since that level of care is complex and thus involves more expensive and longer hospitalizations and because many charity cases fall into that category. When this adverse utilization depresses the patient revenues flowing into teaching hospitals, they cannot always compete on a financially equitable basis with either the other public-general hospitals or in the total health care marketplace.

Furthermore, policies that on their face seem equitable among hospitals, in terms of there being no differential effects except with regard to survival of the fittest, sometimes have a biased impact on the teaching institutions. For example, it has been claimed that the National Health Planning and Resources Development Act of 1974 (P.L. 93-641), which created health system agencies (HSAs), did not acknowledge any unique role of teaching hospitals and "legitimized a disorganized, costly, time-consuming questioning of the pattern of activity that has long been a feature of teaching hospitals" (Sanders & Bander, 1980, p. 33). It has been similarly contended that the federal government's intention to restrain health care costs by controlling reimbursement of medical expenses, which is reflected in Medicare Section 223, was implemented through a methodology that was prejudiced against larger, older, urban teaching hospitals (Goldblatt, 1979, 1980).

If teaching hospitals have a significant role to play in the delivery of health care in this country, and if public policies such as these inadvertently have a negative effect upon these institutions as a class, it is then in the public interest to reassess such legislation, taking these impacts into account.

A potential threat to public teaching hospitals seems to be price competition stemming from the proliferation of providers of primary, secondary, and selected tertiary health care and the wider availability of medical specialists and subspecialists—whether or not this competition is stimulated, encouraged, and/or supported by federal, state, or local legislation. An increase in health care providers could lead to a wider dispersion of mainstream revenue-generating patients among those not burdened with heavy social responsibilities such as indigent care, medical education, and research. This could result in an erosion of an important and necessary segment of the teaching hospitals' existing and potential patient base.

Add to this threatened and actual cutbacks in direct support to hospitals and a trend away from cost-based reimbursement and it is conceivable that the public teaching hospitals, as a class, stand on very shaky ground.

Several papers in the early 1980s explored potential areas of difficulty for teaching hospitals as price competition became a more pervasive pressure in health services delivery. These areas, discussed next, include: undergraduate and graduate medical education, allied health sciences education, research, tertiary care and case mix, charity care, ambulatory care, and faculty practice plans (AAHC, n.d.; AAMC, 1981a; Colloton, 1981). While some of these issues may be more speculative than real, and while there may be some ax grinding among those views, developing a sensitivity to those areas of concern can encourage proactive rather than reactive policy making.

Undergraduate Medical Education

Undergraduate medical education is one factor in the higher institutional cost of care in teaching hospitals. There is the direct cost involved in the supervision of students and the indirect expense of lowered productivity because of the increased time absorbed by student-delivered services.

There also may be an opportunity cost in the loss of patients who do not want to be subjected to student learning needs and who thus avoid using teaching hospitals.

As competition increases, community hospitals and ambulatory care institutions that make settings available for student training may not be able to absorb these costs any longer and still remain competitive and so may begin to discontinue all, or the least cost-effective, medical school affiliations. The loss of these teaching sites could have a domino effect on the quality of medical education: students would be exposed to a more limited range of hospital and medical care delivery settings, there might be an insufficient number of patients available for high-quality student training, and there probably would be a less appropriate mix of patients in terms of the number and types of diagnoses to be observed.

Additional effects of such disaffiliations might include greater stress on university teaching hospitals to pick up the slack, thus exacerbating all of their other problems; pressure on students to provide more direct services, at the cost of time for more focused learning; reduced contributions by voluntary faculty in the university, who might not want to cover the loss of physician supervision in the community facilities; and greater pressure on full-time salaried university hospital and medical school faculty, some of whom subsequently might abandon teaching for private practice.

Graduate Medical Education

All of the direct and indirect costs outlined with regard to undergraduate medical education apply similarly to graduate medical education. By 1982, HMOs and other alternative delivery systems that sought sources of inpatient care for their clients were often reluctant to utilize teaching hospitals for anything but the most complex cases. These and other disruptions of patient referral patterns could well reduce the critical mass of patients necessary for high-quality advanced medical education; that, in turn, could result in the teaching hospitals' having to reconsider the number and types of specialized educational programs they could mount and maintain for postgraduate medical fellows.

Allied Health Sciences Education

Teaching hospitals provide an opportunity for the training and practice of innumerable allied health programs, many of which are dependent upon these institutions for their existence. The number and quality of training programs in such areas as dietetics, medical records, medical technology, nursing, occupational and physical therapy, physician's assistants, and so on, could be seriously jeopardized if price competition forced some of the teaching hospitals to close.

Clinical Research and Its Applications

Any activities that deplete the patient base reduce the potential for and/ or effectiveness of biomedical research. In addition, the initiation of new treatment modalities and other sophisticated medical research products usually is dependent upon large developmental expenditures, both those that are project-specific and those that are related to maintenance of a total environment supportive of and conducive to advanced research. Teaching hospitals and medical schools have relied only partially upon patient revenues for financial support for such research.

However, if federal policies on funding biomedical and other health-related research continue to tighten, patient revenues will become more crucial and probably will be insufficient to meet the need. The extent and quality of research could suffer. Moreover, if greater and greater portions of the cost of research were allowed to be shifted to routine patient charges, these hospitals would become less and less competitive in the open marketplace. (States with rate review regulations, however, are slow to allow such cost shifts.) Confounding these problems is the fact that initial applications of research often are neither cost-effective nor always productive in terms of improved patient outcomes.

Tertiary Care and Case Mix

The importance of an adequate base of tertiary care patients and an appropriate case mix for both teaching and research purposes has been described. The high cost of this care is not always reimbursed adequately and often may be subsidized by primary and secondary care fees and repayments. Changes in federal and state reimbursement policies could force some changes in institutional pricing and cost allocation policies. To the extent that tertiary care costs increase as a result, teaching hospitals, for the most part still would retain a competitive edge—when they were the sole provider of these services. However, it is not clear which, if any, services could become self-supporting in teaching hospitals. If cross-subsidization and other financial support were eliminated, it might not always be possible for these institutions to maintain an optimal case mix for educational purposes.

Furthermore, the AAMC has suggested that a hospital that is serving only a tertiary care population could produce a stressful and undesirable work environment, thus contributing to institutional personnel shortages and staff problems.

Charity Care

Cross-subsidization of unsponsored patients by fees from sponsored patients has been discussed. If competitive needs should force the discontinuation of cross-subsidization structures, and care for the indigent were reduced in the teaching hospitals, this could result in educational costs (i.e., depletion of patient base for teaching purposes), as well as social costs.

Ambulatory Care

Ambulatory care in hospitals and in other educational settings seems to have higher costs than it does in free-standing clinics and physicians' offices. Some of these expenses, however, are not necessarily "real" costs or deficits but are the result of hospital accounting procedures developed to cope with third party regulations. For example, cost reimbursement guidelines sometimes force higher than actual overhead costs onto the outpatient clinics; specifically, costs for hospital support services calculated on the basis of space, rather than on the actual expense of constructing and maintaining the space, often work to the financial disadvantage of the outpatient clinics.

The practice of separate billing for medical and hospital support fees reduces physician accountability for the cost of the total patient care package and may contribute to higher overall outpatient fees. At the same time, it is not unusual for outpatient-produced revenues, such as for ancillary services, to be integrated into general hospital revenues in a way that inhibits the institution's ability to assess ambulatory care financial performance.

Teaching hospitals also often load higher costs onto their outpatient services in other ways. Several factors contribute to this: More space is needed in educational settings, resulting in higher overhead costs. Educational costs allocated to clinics on the basis of number of trainees reflect the number of students who need training rather than the number of students required to provide the services. A broader spectrum of professional services usually is provided. There is a wider range of complex problems that are costly to treat in the teaching hospital outpatient setting.

In part, the problem of ambulatory care deficits (real or paper) has been absorbed by higher inpatient charges. New reimbursement regulations disallowing compensating cross-subsidization of outpatient clinic costs could create both accounting and management problems for these hospitals.

From an economic perspective, it is important to maintain the teaching hospital's capacity for good outpatient care because, as Colloton (1981) points out, there are longer-range economic benefits of training in ambulatory care settings, namely, that this may lead to the more frequent practice of methods of diagnosis and therapeutic care that can obviate expensive inpatient hospitalization.

Faculty Practice Plans

Teaching hospitals are under pressure to price hospital and medical services together, rather than separately (as often is the case). As this pressure intensifies, the higher teaching hospital cost component will need to be offset by reduced medical fees if this service package is to remain competitive. This could lead to the physicians' admitting more and more patients to other hospitals with which they are affiliated; obviously, that will decrease patient volume in the teaching hospitals and, in a vicious cycle, merely increase these institutions' overall problems. In addition, this could result in an increased incentive for medical faculty to leave teaching for private practice.

The Teaching Hospital: Final Thoughts

It is important that teaching hospitals recognize and focus on management inefficiencies that may be constraining their ability to be financially competitive. But they also need to separate problems stemming from internal management inefficiencies from those resulting from external sources related to the nature of the institution, so that the most appropriate responses can be made to each.

Friedman (1980) suggested that with "extensive manipulation of the voluntary sector," medical education could be provided in private institutions (p. 84). There is no evidence, however, that high-quality and/or cost-effective education could be better provided, or maintained at all, in that manner. And Friedman did qualify her statement by adding that this could be done only if the funding were available.

The key question, then, is whether funding for any and/or all forms of medical/health education should be made available as a matter of public policy. If the decision is affirmative, then the question of appropriate provider must be addressed. If it is determined that the public teaching hospitals should remain as the primary providers of this education, then it is important to develop means for separating hospital and medical provider expenses from educational costs to the extent possible (which may be quite limited), and then to subsidize hospitals directly for their educational funding needs. This would force the teaching hospitals to become competitive in their other components but would also facilitate their ability to do so.

CONCLUSION

In addition to the negative impact it is claimed that competition will have on public teaching hospitals, it has been seen that numerous federal and state funding regulations clearly have a significant influence on all hospitals. Friedman (1981) summarized several of these constraints, which are reviewed briefly next, in terms of some additional policy issues they could generate for teaching and/or all public-general hospitals:

- Medicaid program limits on inpatient days: For hospitals with a significant portion of indigent patients, who are sicker and/or have more complex problems and who therefore require longer lengths of stay than the average patient, how will the costs of nonreimbursable days be covered? Will these patients have to be denied appropriate care?
- Medicaid reimbursement cuts, abandonment of cost-based reimbursement, per diem caps: Will indigent patients be denied care or at least the full range of appropriate services? Will more expensive services be limited or withheld from them? If so, what will be the effect on quality of care? What will be the effect on teaching and research if the number and type of "observations" are reduced?
- Nonreimbursement by Medicaid for use of the emergency department for nonemergency care, and outpatient department limits: Will specific service cutbacks such as these limit the role of public hospitals in primary care? Will nonreimbursement constrain a source of referrals for inpatient secondary and tertiary care? Will it affect case mix? Will it result in an excess of inappropriate inpatient utilization?
- Reduced Medicaid eligibility: Will lowered eligibility increase the public hospital's burden with regard to uncompensated patients? Will transfers of ineligible patients from proprietary hospitals ("dumping") increase? Will some public hospitals be overtaxed to the point of closure? If so, will there be any provider of last resort?

As Friedman (1981) points out, such procedural changes have different impacts on states, on cities, and on types of hospitals. Thus, procedure implicitly shapes policy.

- Cost shifting: The teaching and other public-general hospitals that practice cost shifting to privately sponsored patients, in order to cut charity care losses and to support education-related expenses, will be at a considerable disadvantage as commercial carriers and HMOs refuse to tolerate higher costs and either limit reimbursement for services to their members or refuse to enter into unfavorable contracts with these institutions.

- Cuts in nursing home reimbursement: such reductions, plus restrictions on construction of new beds, plus an increase in the elderly population, will lead to placement problems for long-term/chronic patients. These pressures, coupled with length-of-stay restrictions and/or denied reimbursement for inappropriate hospitalization (i.e., a long-term patient in an acute care bed), will lead to significant financial losses for hospitals with long waiting lists for long-term placements— usually the public hospitals.
- Funding cuts in many specialty areas: These will increase the strain on public hospitals even further because they are often the primary providers for this type of care. This includes rural health services; deinstitutionalized mental health patients; the Indian Health Service; and care for refugee populations, undocumented aliens, migrants, etc.

The purpose of this recapitulation is to underline, one final time, the fact that there are many governmental activities that are initiated for one purpose (such as visible cost control, aimed at eliminating inefficient hospital practices and inefficient hospitals), but that can produce undesirable externalities (such as weakening needed hospitals that otherwise could survive).

What is advocated is a policy-making process that (1) determines what is socially desirable in the delivery of personal health services, (2) translates these social values into explicit policy decisions, (3) projects the impact of proposed legislation upon activities and institutions that implement these values, and (4) attempts to maximize the congruence between legislation and policy values.

Such a proactive program is not always feasible, or may not always be so in all aspects. At minimum, however, there should be continuous monitoring of the effect of legislation and administrative regulations on policy objectives so that timely adjustments can be made, as necessary and appropriate, to ensure that the health system comes as close as possible to producing what the nation desires.

REFERENCES

Altman, S.H. Decade ahead will challenge financial viability of hospitals. *Hospitals,* 1981, 55(2), 87–92.

American Hospital Association. *Guide to the health care field.* Chicago: Author, 1981.

Association of Academic Health Care Centers. Competition and academic health centers. Washington, D.C.: Author, n.d. (Mimeographed)

Association of American Medical Colleges. *Price competition in the health care marketplace: Issues for teaching hospitals.* Discussion paper approved by the AAMC Executive Council. Washington, D.C.: Author, March 1981. (a)

Association of American Medical Colleges. *Toward a more contemporary public understanding of the teaching hospital* (Rev. ed.). Washington, D.C.: AAMC Department of Teaching Hospitals, May 1981. (b)

Bernstein, A., & Berk, M. *Perceived health status and selected indicators of access to care among the minority aged.* Washington, D.C.: National Center for Health Services Research, Division of Intramural Research, 1981.

Brazda, J.F. Washington report. *The Nation's Health,* March 1982, p. 3.

Bryant, J.H., Ginsberg, A.S., Goldsmith, S.B., Olendzki, M.C., & Piore, N. *Community hospitals and primary care.* Cambridge, Mass.: Ballinger Publishing Co., 1976.

Colloton, J.W. *An analysis of proposed competitive health system plans and the implications for teaching hospitals.* Paper presented at the Sixth Private Sector Conference, Duke University Medical Center, Durham, N.C., March 1981.

Commission on Hospital Care. *Hospital care in the United States.* New York: Commonwealth Fund, 1947.

Commission on Public-General Hospitals. *The future of public-general hospitals: An agenda for transition.* Chicago: Hospital Research and Educational Trust, 1978.

Crosby, E.L. Hospitals as the center of the health care universe. *Hospitals,* 1970, *44*(1), 53–56.

Cunningham, R.M. *The healing mission and the business ethic.* Chicago: Pluribus Press, 1981.

A Discursive Dictionary of Health Care. Prepared by the staff for the Subcommittee on Health and the Environment of the Committee on Interstate and Foreign Commerce. U.S. House of Representatives, Washington, D.C.: U.S. Government Printing Office, 1976.

Dowling, W.L., & Armstrong, P.A. The hospital. In S.J. Williams & P.R. Torrens (Eds.), *Introduction to health services.* New York: John Wiley & Sons, Inc., 1980.

Emery, F.E., & Trist, E.L. The causal texture of organizational environments. *Human Relations,* 1965, *18*(1), 21–32.

Feldstein, P.J. Economic success for hospitals depends on their adaptability. *Hospitals,* 1981, *55*(2), 77–80.

Friedman, E. Public hospitals: Is "relevance" in the eye of the beholder? *Hospitals,* 1980, *54*(9), 83–93.

Friedman, E. Biting the bullet: The states begin funding cutbacks. *Hospitals,* 1981, *55*(1), 55–60.

Friedman, E. Shifting the cost—and the blame. *Hospitals,* 1982, *56*(6), 93–97.

Goldblatt, S.J. The teaching hospital under Medicare: A prejudiced position. *Health Care Management Review,* 1979, *4*(3), 67–79.

Goldblatt, S.J. The Medicare Section 223 schedule of limits: A continuing struggle. *Health Care Management Review,* 1980, *5*(2), 35–39.

Health Insurance Association of America. *Hospital cost shifting: The hidden tax.* Washington, D.C.: Author, 1982.

The health of Americans: Report of the 37th American Assembly. New York: Arden House, 1970.

Hedley, B. Strategy and the "business portfolio." *Long-Range Planning,* 1977, *10*(1), 9–15.

Herman, H., & McKay, M.E. *Community health services.* Washington, D.C.: International City Managers' Association, 1968.

Hofer, C.W., & Schendel, D. *Strategy formulation: Analytical concepts.* St. Paul, Minn.: West Publishing Company, 1978.

Hospital Week (newsletter), 1982, *18*(10).

Johnson, R.L. Revisiting "the wobbly three-legged stool." *Health Care Management Review,* 1979, *4*(3), 15–22.

Kissick, W.L. Community health and medical care: A perspective. In A.R. Kovner & S.P. Martin (Eds.), *Community health and medical care.* New York: Grune & Stratton, Inc., 1978.

Lehman, E.W. *Coordinating health care: Explorations in interorganizational relations.* Beverly Hills, Calif.: SAGE Publications, 1975.

Loebs, S.F., Johnson, J.L., & Summers, R.L. Managing the future through planned organizational change. In G.E. Bisbee, Jr. (Ed.), *Management of rural primary care: Concepts and cases.* Chicago: The Hospital Research and Educational Trust, 1982.

Longest, B.L., Jr. *A response theory of organizational strategy formulation: The case of community hospitals* (Working Paper #24). Evanston, Ill.: Northwestern University Center for Health Services and Policy Research, March 1979.

National Commission on Community Health Services. *Health is a community affair.* Cambridge, Mass.: Harvard University Press, 1967.

Newman, H. Medicaid's unanswered questions. *Hospitals,* 1982, *56*(1), 65–69.

Pfeffer, J., & Salancik, G.R. *The external control of organizations: A resource dependence perspective.* New York: Harper & Row Publishers, Inc., 1978.

Punch, L. Public hospitals straining to survive federal assault on healthcare costs. *Modern Healthcare,* 1981, *11*(12), 54, 55, 58. (a)

Punch, L. Winning finance control offers needed protection. *Modern Healthcare,* 1981, *11*(12), 55–56. (b)

Sanders, C.A., & Bander, K.W. Multi-institutional arrangements in a teaching hospital setting. *Health Care Management Review,* 1980, *5*(2), 25–33.

Shirley, R.C., Peters, M.H., & El-Ansary, A.I. *Strategy and policy formation: A multifunctional orientation.* Santa Barbara, Calif.: John Wiley & Sons, Inc., 1976.

Shonick, W. Mergers of public health departments with public hospitals in urban areas: Findings of 12 field studies. *Medical Care,* 1980, *18,* 30. (Supplement)

Somers, A.R. *Health care in transition: Directions for the future.* Chicago: The Hospital Research and Educational Trust, 1971.

Starkweather, D.B. *Hospital mergers in the making.* Ann Arbor, Mich.: Health Administration Press, 1981.

Webber, J.B. Ideas outpace reality of hospital strategic planning, but do they pinpoint the future? *Hospitals,* 1982, *56*(7), 68–71.

Chapter 11

The Health Professions: Policies and Issues

Thomas J. Bacon and
Suzanne J. Kotkin

Just as the health services industry has taken a greater and greater share of the total United States gross national product in recent years, so the personnel segment of that industry has become an increasingly important issue from a policy standpoint. Approximately two-thirds of the value of the health sector in this country is represented by the professional and nonprofessional component, with the remainder shared between physical capital such as plant and equipment and intermediate goods and services such as drugs, supplies, and so forth (Sorkin, 1977).

This chapter deals with professional staff involved in the health services sector and several important associated policy issues. Data are presented on levels of employment among major provider groups as well as on existing and future outputs of health professional schools. Federal health professions legislation in the past 30 years is reviewed, with particular attention to significant public policy shifts in those measures. Finally, several significant policy interventions in this arena are analyzed, with the focus on their long-term impact on the supply, distribution, and quality of health care providers.

EMPLOYMENT IN THE HEALTH SECTOR

The term health personnel includes a broad range of workers, from professionals, who traditionally are thought of when reference is made to health care providers (e.g., doctors, nurses, dentists), to large numbers of others with only minimal formal training such as aides and orderlies and those in related fields. The number of persons employed in health-related occupations has grown dramatically since 1970 (PHS, 1981a). From 1970 through 1979 the number of persons reporting themselves as holding health-related jobs grew from 3.1 million to nearly 5 million, an increase of 60 percent (Table 11-1), with gains in every occupational group within the field.

Although public attention focused on the growth in the supply of physicians during this period, and the gains in M.D.s exceeded 50 percent, even more dramatic increases occurred among the allied health fields. The numbers of persons employed as therapists, health technologists, and technicians more than doubled during the 1970s. The table also shows that

Table 11-1 Employment in Health-Related Jobs

Persons 16 and Older in Selected Health-Related Occupations: United States, Selected Years, 1970–79

(Data based on household interviews with a sample of the civilian noninstitutionalized population)

Occupation	1970[1]	1975	1976	1977	1978	1979
	(Number of Persons in Thousands)					
Totals	3,103	4,169	4,341	4,517	4,753	4,951
Physicians, medical and osteopathic	281	354	368	403	424	431
Dentists	91	110	107	105	117	131
Pharmacists	110	119	123	138	136	135
Registered nurses	830	935	999	1,063	1,112	1,223
Therapists	75	157	159	178	189	207
Health technologists and technicians	260	397	436	462	498	534
Health administrators	84	152	162	175	184	185
Dental assistants	88	126	122	123	130	134
Health aides, excluding nursing	119	211	229	234	270	281
Nursing aides, orderlies, and attendants	718	1,001	1,002	1,008	1,037	1,024
Practical nurses	237	370	381	371	402	376
Other health-related occupations[2]	210	237	253	257	254	290

1. Based on the 1970 decennial census; all other years are annual averages derived from the *Current Population Survey,* compiled by the U.S. Bureau of the Census. These data differ from those published by the National Center for Health Statistics in various editions of *Health Resource Statistics* because the latter are derived from a variety of sources.
2. Includes chiropractors, optometrists, podiatrists, veterinarians, dietitians, embalmers, funeral directors, opticians, lens grinders and polishers, dental laboratory technicians, lay midwives, and health trainees.

Sources: Census of Population, 1970, Detailed Characteristics, Final Report PC1-(D) by U.S. Bureau of the Census, Government Printing Office, February 1973. Also: *Employment and Earnings,* Vol. 25, No. 1, January 1978; Vol. 26, No. 1, January 1979; and Vol. 27, No. 1, January 1980, and unpublished data, by U.S. Bureau of Labor Statistics, Government Printing Office.

the field of health administration grew by almost 550 percent from 1970 through 1979, affirming that the increases were not limited to clinical fields.

Employment in the health services industry in general (including those not in health occupations) reached just under 7 million in 1979, up from 4.2 million in 1970 (Table 11-2). This represents a jump of some 61 percent in just nine years, with the largest absolute increases occurring in hospitals and the greatest percentage growth in convalescent institutions, offices of other health practitioners, and other health service sites. These increases in health sector employment far surpassed the rise in the nation's general labor force and accounted for health employment's growing share (nearly 5 percent in 1979) of the total work force.

Although this chapter deals in part with general employment in health-related fields and all their occupations regardless of location of job, its particular focus is on three major professional groups: physicians, dentists,

Table 11-2 Employment in the Health Services Industry by Place of Employment: United States, 1970–79

(Data based on household interviews with a sample of the civilian noninstitutionalized population)

	Year					
Place of Employment	1970[1]	1975	1976	1977	1978	1979
	(Number of Persons in Thousands)					
Totals	4,246	5,365	6,122	6,328	6,673	6,849
Offices of physicians	477	607	641	877	753	755
Offices of dentists	222	327	325	321	360	385
Offices of chiropractors	19	30	27	29	—	—
Hospitals	2,890	3,394	3,568	3,845	3,781	3,843
Convalescent institutions	509	884	945	949	1,009	1,035
Offices of other health practitioners	42	60	68	75	83	84
Other health service sites	288	563	548	632	687	747

1. April 1, derived from decennial census; all other data years are July 1 estimates. All totals exclude persons in health-related occupations working in nonhealth industries, as classified by the U.S. Bureau of the Census, such as pharmacists employed in drugstores, and nurses working in schools or in private households.

Sources: 1970 Census of Population, Occupation by Industry, Subject Reports, Final Report PC(2)-7C, by U.S. Bureau of the Census, Government Printing Office, October 1972. Also, *Employment and Earnings,* Vol. 24, No. 3, March 1977; Vol. 25, No. 1, January 1978; Vol. 26, No. 1, January 1979; and Vol. 27, No. 1, January 1980, and unpublished data, by U.S. Bureau of Labor Statistics Government Printing Office.

and nurses. These provide a major share of personal health services in this country and are the focus of much of the health professions policy decisions of the last two decades. The rest of this chapter addresses issues primarily concerning one or more of these three groups.

THE SUPPLY OF HEALTH PROFESSIONALS

The number of physicians, dentists, and registered nurses in the United States has grown dramatically since 1950. Table 11-3 shows that the gains for physicians occurred not only in absolute terms but also relative to population growth. Physicians per 100,000 population rose from 142 in 1950 to 197 in 1980. The supply of dentists, on the other hand, just kept up with the population growth and actually fell slightly during the 1950s and 1960s. The supply of nurses grew very rapidly in three decades despite the widespread shortages being reported by hospitals and other nurse-employment agencies.

From a national supply of 335,000 in 1950, the 1980 supply of 1,164,000 nurses represented a 347 percent increase during the 30-year period. In terms of R.N.s per 100,000 population, the increase was from 218 to 520 during the same period, or about 138 percent.

The significant overall increases in supply of health professionals resulted primarily from a rapid expansion of training programs and student positions for all major types of providers. As described in detail later, much of the increases in graduates occurred as a direct result of federal interventions in the training process, starting with the Health Professions Edu-

Table 11-3 Selected Health Professions and Active Professionals

Per 100,000 Population for 1950, 1960, 1970, 1975, and 1980

	1950	1960	1970	1975	1980
Total Physicians	219,900	259,500	323,200	378,600	444,000
Physicians per 100,000 Pop.	142	142	155	174	197
Total Dentists	79,190	90,120	102,220	112,020	126,240
Dentists per 100,000 Pop.	51.5	49.4	49.6	52.2	56.4
Total Registered Nurses	335,000	527,000	750,000	961,000	1,164,000
Nurses per 100,000 Pop.	218.1	289.1	363.9	448.1	519.9

Source: Supply and Characteristics of Selected Health Personnel by Department of Health and Human Services, U.S. Public Health Service, Health Resources Administration, Division of Health Professions, Publication No. (HRA) 81-20, U.S. Government Printing Office, 1981, pp. 22, 39, 48, 58.

cational Assistance Act of 1963, P.L. 88-129. Table 11-4 demonstrates the rapid growth in both graduates and schools training health professionals, with the most significant increases during the 1970s. The number of graduates from medical schools rose nearly 260 percent during the 28-year period, with those from dentistry schools more than doubling. Pharmacy schools' output was not listed in 1950, but in the years 1960–1978, this grew more than 220 percent. The number of schools did not increase so substantially, indicating that the rise in graduates was caused by increased enrollments in existing schools as well as a slower growth in construction of new schools. For example, while the number of schools of medicine increased by 57 percent (79 schools to 124 schools), graduates grew nearly threefold.

THE DEMAND FOR HEALTH PROFESSIONALS

There has been considerable interest in recent years at all levels of health professions policy development as to the adequacy of the existing and projected supply of major health providers relative to requirements. While the most visible policy debates have centered on physician supply in relation to demand, attention also has focused increasingly on shortages of nurses. Several major studies have been undertaken to better estimate the needs for health providers in order to guide policy decisions. Some of the major ones are described next.

The Graduate Medical Education National Advisory Committee (GMENAC) was created by the Secretary of Health and Human Services (then HEW) in 1976 to provide advice on the number of physicians required to meet the nation's health needs into the future in terms of total supply, specialty mix, and geographic distribution. The committee's charter stated specifically that a surplus (or a shortage) of physicians should be avoided and that a balance between supply and requirements should be achieved through modifications in the numbers of training positions in graduate medical education. The summary report of the committee (PHS, 1980c) generated considerable debate in the health policy arena.

The most significant finding of GMENAC, and the one that became most controversial, was that there would be a surplus of about 70,000 physicians by 1990 and 145,000 by the year 2000. The surpluses were projected to be particularly large in certain specialties, including virtually all surgical subspecialties and most medical subspecialties (Table 11-5). The only specialties for which no surpluses were expected were general and child psychiatry, emergency medicine, and preventive medicine. Major primary care specialties were projected to be at or near balance between supply and requirements.

Table 11-4 Graduates of Health Professions Schools and Number of Schools, by Profession

Selected 1950–78 Estimates and 1980 and 1990 Projections

(Data are based on reporting by health professions schools)

	Profession				
Year	Medicine	Osteopathy	Dentistry	Optometry	Pharmacy
Number of Graduates					
1950	5,553	373	2,565	961	—
1960	7,081	427	3,253	364	3,497
1970	8,367	432	3,749	445	4,758
1975	12,714	702	4,969	806	6,886
1978	14,393	963	5,324	1,011	7,785
Projections					
1980	15,346	1,029	5,380	1,046	6,900
1990	17,604	1,685	5,460	1,046	6,900
Number of Schools					
1950	79	6	42	10	—
1960	86	6	47	10	76
1970	103	7	53	11	74
1976	114	9	59	12	73
1978	124	14	60	13	72
Projections					
1980	124	14	60	13	72
1990	124	14	60	13	72

Sources: A Report to the President and Congress on the Status of Health Professions Personnel in the United States by Department of Health, Education, and Welfare, Health Resources Administration, Bureau of Health Manpower, DHEW Publication No. (HRA) 78-93, Hyattsville, Md., August 1978. Also, Supply of Manpower in Selected Health Occupations, 1950–1990 by Department of Health, Education, and Welfare, Health Resources Administration, Bureau of Health Professions, Division of Manpower Analysis, DHEW Publication No. (HRA) 80-35, Hyattsville, Md., January 1980, and selected data.

Table 11-5 Ratio Percent of Projected Supply of Physicians to Estimated Requirements, United States, 1990

	Ratio % of Requirements	Requirements	Surplus (shortage)
Shortages			
Child Psychiatry	45%	9,000	(4,900)
Emergency Medicine	70%	13,500	(4,250)
Preventive Medicine	75%	7,300	(1,750)
General Psychiatry	80%	38,500	(8,000)
Near Balance			
Hematology/Oncology—Internal Medicine	90%	9,000	(700)
Dermatology	105%	6,950	400
Gastroenterology—Internal Medicine	105%	6,500	400
Osteopathic General Practice	105%	22,000	1,150
Family Practice	105%	61,300	3,100
General Internal Medicine	105%	70,250	3,550
Otolaryngology	105%	8,000	500
General Pediatrics and Subspecialties	115%	36,400	4,950
Surpluses			
Urology	120%	7,700	1,650
Orthopedic Surgery	135%	15,100	5,000
Ophthalmology	140%	11,600	4,700
Thoracic Surgery	140%	2,050	850
Infectious Diseases—Internal Medicine	145%	2,250	1,000
Obstetrics/Gynecology	145%	24,000	10,450
Plastic Surgery	145%	2,700	1,200

TABLE 11-5 continued

	Ratio % of Requirements	Requirements	Surplus (shortage)
Allergy/Immunology—Internal Medicine	150%	2,050	1,000
General Surgery	150%	23,500	11,800
Nephrology—Internal Medicine	175%	2,750	2,100
Rheumatology—Internal Medicine	175%	1,700	1,300
Cardiology—Internal Medicine	190%	7,750	7,150
Endocrinology—Internal Medicine	190%	2,050	1,800
Neurosurgery	190%	2,650	2,450
Pulmonary—Internal Medicine	195%	3,600	3,350
*Physical Medicine and Rehabilitation	75%	3,200	(800)
*Anesthesiology	95%	21,000	(1550)
*Nuclear Medicine	N/A	4,000	N/A
*Pathology	125%	13,500	3,350
*Radiology	155%	18,000	9,800
*Neurology	160%	5,500	3,150

*The requirements in these six specialties were estimated crudely after a review of the literature. They should be considered as very rough approximations, and tentative. Supply numbers for nuclear medicine are not available.

Source: Summary Report of the Graduate Medical Education National Advisory Committee to the Secretary, Department of Health and Human Services, U.S. Public Health Service, Health Resources Administration, Publication No. (HRA) 80-651, 1980.

Despite overall surpluses, GMENAC found that geographic maldistribution of physicians would continue, with shortages most severe in very rural areas (e.g., counties with less than 10,000 population). Subsequent sections of this chapter deal with the distribution issue in more detail.

While the general consensus among both scholars and policy makers was that GMENAC represented a landmark study in the United States, it was subject to certain criticism. Although an entire volume of the GMENAC report (PHS, 1980c) deals with the issues of geographic distribution of physicians and the difficulty of even defining appropriate geographic units of measure to address the problem, much more public attention focused on the overall surplus issue. Some of those concerned with nagging distribution problems feared that any cuts in enrollments and training opportunities would affect most acutely the geographic areas already suffering the greatest shortages and the specialties that already were in balance or in short supply.

Others criticized GMENAC's use of expert panels to determine the service requirements for care by their respective specialty. If slight changes were made in estimating levels of productivity, substitutions by other specialties, and the proportion of physicians entering nonclinical positions in the health field, quite different results would be obtained that would not project such significant surpluses as the GMENAC report forecast. Nevertheless, the GMENAC study provides a systematic, vigorous analysis of physician supply and requirements by specialty and will likely serve as the standard for some years.

The question of demand for dentists is much more difficult to assess because of the economic characteristics of dental practice. Since health insurance covers dental care for only a small percentage of the population, demand for such services is clearly associated with income levels. Thus, while a number of studies have documented significant levels of dental disease and the consequent need for care among both child and adult populations, the lack of ability to pay for such services depresses the demand substantially.

As Sorkin (1977) and others have pointed out, increases in the demand for dental services are a function of three factors: (1) population growth, (2) rise in real per capita income, and (3) gains in the proportion of the population covered by dental insurance. Since about 1970, each of these factors has grown only slightly. With continuing increases in both total active dentists and, more importantly, in dentists per 100,000 population, the supply could be exceeding demand. Considerable anecdotal evidence indicates this indeed could be the case. Dental school graduates reported increasing difficulty in setting up private practices in many parts of the country. This is despite the fact that in terms of availability of dentists by size of place, rural areas and small towns are significantly less served than are urban areas.

The question of the adequacy of the supply of nurses has received as much attention since the late 1970s as any health provider issue. Despite the dramatic growth in both total supply and nurses per 100,000 population since 1950 (from 335,000 to 1.164 million in 1980), studies in the early 1980s consistently showed a significant shortage of registered nurses, particularly in hospital settings, in virtually all parts of the country. Estimates of up to 100,000 budgeted vacancies for R.N.s in hospitals alone focused attention on the nature and extent of the shortage and on efforts to reduce its size and impact on the health care system.

Part of the problem in determining the degree of overall shortage for nurses involves the method chosen for estimating current and future requirements. For example, one of the most detailed and comprehensive studies of nursing requirements was conducted by the Western Interstate Commission for Higher Education (WICHE, 1978). Using a needs-based approach to determine patient utilization rates as well as nurse staffing pattern changes as suggested by a panel of experts, the WICHE study projected very high requirements for nurses. Its estimate of requirements, even at the lower bound, substantially exceeded existing levels of R.N. utilization in hospitals, nursing homes, and other health care institutions in the United States. The panel thus projected a need for 1.4 to 1.9 million R.N.s in 1982, a figure far exceeding the 1978 supply of almost 1.2 million R.N.s (WICHE, 1978). These projections also exceeded others on the need of R.N.s based on utilization patterns, even when those patterns were modified to consider changes in educational levels, insurance patterns, and the organization of health care (Galambos, 1979).

Regardless of the level of shortage, there is considerable debate as to how to address the problem of bringing nurses back into the workplace once they have left. A publication by the U.S. Department of Health and Human Services (PHS, 1981b) summarized several nursing studies conducted in single states. A consistent pattern among all of those studies was that while the number of graduates of nursing schools and the number of active nurses had risen dramatically, shortages as measured by budgeted vacancies remained a serious problem. Nursing school enrollment actually declined slightly, starting in 1979, leading some to fear that gains in R.N.s in the work force would not keep pace with losses.

Salary levels clearly are an important factor in whether or not nurses choose to enter and remain in the work force. Nevertheless, many studies, including that of the National Commission on Nursing (1981) have shown that working conditions, style of management, staffing patterns, working relationships with physicians, and other factors often are as important as financial considerations in recruiting and retaining well-qualified nurses in hospitals and other health agencies. The institutions that have had the most success in turning their staffing situation around generally are those that have taken a multiple approach and have sought to improve the environment for nursing practice in as many ways as possible. More systematic research is clearly needed in this area if long-term progress is to be made.

GEOGRAPHIC DISTRIBUTION OF HEALTH PROFESSIONALS

While the debate continues over the adequacy of the overall supply of physicians and other health practitioners in the United States, there is general agreement that significant problems still exist in their geographic distribution. For several types of health providers, as the total supply has increased after 1950, the gap between underserved and well-served areas of the country has widened rather than lessened.

These differences are perhaps best demonstrated by trends in the supply of physicians in metropolitan and nonmetropolitan areas of the country during the years 1970 to 1978. While the nonmetropolitan counties showed increases in both the total supply of M.D.s and M.D.s per 100,000 population, the gains by metropolitan counties far exceeded them (Table 11-6). The ratio of physicians per 100,000 in nonmetropolitan areas increased only 17 percent (75.3 to 88.3) during this period, compared to 24 percent (166.0 to 206.0) for metropolitan areas, with the absolute differences widening dramatically.

There are substantial differences in physician resources by states and major geographic regions of the country as well (Table 11-7). Physician ratios ranged from a high of 524 per 100,000 population in the District of Columbia to just over 100 per 100,000 in Mississippi and South Dakota. As a region, the New England area is richest in physician supply, with parts of the South Central region having the fewest physicians in relation to population.

The number of active dentists rose steadily from a nationwide average of 47.4 per 100,000 population in 1970 to 54.9 in 1980. The regional differences in dentist ratios indicate that the South has gained the greatest number of dentists, with a ratio of 35.3 in 1970 to 44.4 in 1980—an increase of 9.1 per 100,000 population. However, the South still has the lowest dentist/population ratio of any region in the country. The largest increase in the ratio in any subregion occurred in New England, which increased its ratio by 13.2 dentists per 100,000 population (Table 11-8).

Table 11-6 Number and Percent Distribution of Active Nonfederal M.D.s and Physician-to-Population Ratios

By Metropolitan Areas and Nonmetropolitan Counties: December 31, 1970, and Adjusted Data for 1975 and 1978

Area Classification, By Population	1970			1975[1]			1978[1]		
	Active Nonfederal Physicians		Active Nonfederal Physicians per 100,000 Civilian Population	Active Nonfederal Physicians		Active Nonfederal Physicians per 100,000 Civilian Population	Active Nonfederal Physicians		Active Nonfederal Physicians per 100,000 Civilian Population
	Number	Percent Distribution		Number	Percent Distribution		Number	Percent Distribution	
All Areas[2]	278,855	100.0	137.3	332,224	100.0	156.5	380,151	100.0	174.7
Metropolitan areas	230,312	82.6	166.0	285,795	86.0	184.4	329,016	86.5	206.0
5,000,000 or more	55,189	19.8	214.2	57,068	17.2	237.0	60,517	15.9	259.9
1,000,000–4,999,999	95,228	34.2	179.2	124,734	37.5	196.8	148,785	39.1	221.1
500,000–999,999	39,898	14.3	147.1	46,009	13.8	165.1	52,377	13.8	191.1
50,000–499,999	39,997	14.3	122.3	57,984	17.5	146.1	67,337	17.7	160.3
Nonmetropolitan counties[3]	48,543	17.4	75.3	46,429	14.0	81.0	51,135	13.5	88.3
Potential metropolitan	11,777	4.2	113.3	6,298	1.9	129.0	5,422	1.4	155.8
50,000 or more	14,898	5.4	95.2	16,013	4.8	98.8	20,752	5.5	112.6

25,000–49,999	11,547	4.1	67.5	13,519	4.1	82.6	14,315	3.8	84.9
10,000–24,999	8,329	3.0	50.6	8,551	2.6	56.0	8,663	2.3	58.5
Less than 10,000	1,992	0.7	40.9	2,048	0.6	44.9	1,983	0.5	45.8

1. Numbers of active physicians for 1975 and 1978 are adjusted to include about 90 percent of those either with unknown address or not classified as to status or activity by the American Medical Association.
2. Excludes physicians in United States possessions.
3. Nonmetropolitan counties are classified by county population.

Sources: Data for 1970 (unadjusted) *Physician Distribution and Medical Licensure in the U.S., 1970* from American Medical Association, Center for Health Services Research and Development. Adjusted data for 1975 and 1978 from U.S. Department of Health, Education, and Welfare, Health Resources Administration, Bureau of Health Professions, Division of Health Professions Analysis.

Table 11-7 Ratio of Active Nonfederal M.D.s to Population in Metropolitan Areas and Nonmetropolitan Counties

By Region, Division, and State: December 31, 1979

Geographic Area	All Areas	Metropolitan Areas, by Population			Nonmetropolitan Counties, by Size of Central City		
		Total	1,000,000 or More	Under 1,000,000	Total	10,000 or More	Under 10,000
		Active Nonfederal Physicians per 100,000 Civilian Population					
UNITED STATES	176.9	213.0	242.6	177.9	89.5	115.9	63.2
NORTHEAST	221.9	240.1	274.9	184.8	119.9	117.5	125.7
New England	230.2	249.9	330.5	207.6	152.5	146.0	166.7
Connecticut	240.7	250.4	*	250.4	99.8	99.8	*
Maine	151.6	228.8	*	228.8	122.0	135.0	103.2
Massachusetts	253.7	257.8	330.5	150.5	146.8	122.0	156.6
New Hampshire	166.0	136.4	*	136.4	178.7	122.6	514.7
Rhode Island	211.4	229.2	*	229.2	132.4	132.4	*
Vermont	214.0	*	*	*	214.0	277.4	137.4
Middle Atlantic	219.1	237.2	266.2	170.2	104.0	104.2	103.4
New Jersey	182.9	190.8	209.4	165.8	95.2	91.6	102.9
New York	256.0	274.7	294.2	202.3	114.0	124.6	87.4
Pennsylvania	186.2	207.6	244.1	143.9	98.1	89.9	119.5

NORTH CENTRAL	157.7	191.1	209.5	164.4	81.7	112.8	55.4
East North Central	159.1	182.9	206.6	148.5	80.3	98.9	59.4
Illinois	180.2	203.0	212.5	156.3	80.3	104.9	58.2
Indiana	128.8	154.0	221.4	121.5	75.5	99.6	47.9
Michigan	152.7	168.6	168.2	169.2	82.9	112.1	63.2
Ohio	160.1	180.9	232.4	133.3	77.3	85.1	54.6
Wisconsin	153.6	197.7	199.6	195.8	87.2	108.6	69.1
West North Central	154.5	220.9	220.6	221.5	83.5	136.5	52.2
Iowa	124.5	133.7	*	133.7	119.1	244.5	54.7
Kansas	151.7	229.6	275.3	198.9	84.7	105.3	61.2
Minnesota	187.8	248.3	219.3	354.5	76.9	103.6	62.4
Missouri	158.8	218.7	209.9	279.6	54.2	89.9	37.9
Nebraska	148.1	237.9	*	237.9	75.8	116.3	54.4
North Dakota	127.5	239.2	*	239.2	94.2	150.2	57.1
South Dakota	102.5	228.8	*	228.8	80.2	144.0	45.4
SOUTH	158.0	200.6	233.7	181.5	80.9	114.1	56.1
South Atlantic	177.7	218.5	259.0	187.8	97.8	134.2	67.0
Delaware	166.7	194.9	*	194.9	106.4	106.4	*
District of Columbia	524.4	524.4	524.4	*	*	*	*
Florida	186.7	198.7	244.8	169.9	110.6	130.5	88.8

Table 11-7 continued

Active Nonfederal Physicians per 100,000 Civilian Population

Geographic Area	All Areas	Metropolitan Areas, by Population			Nonmetropolitan Counties, by Size of Central City		
		Total	1,000,000 or More	Under 1,000,000	Total	10,000 or More	Under 10,000
Georgia	143.8	190.7	193.9	185.7	81.4	131.7	43.5
Maryland	242.3	264.7	268.2	54.0	118.4	136.8	89.9
North Carolina	152.3	233.6	*	239.2	85.0	94.9	75.8
South Carolina	131.8	186.7	*	186.7	80.4	95.5	67.3
Virginia	168.0	188.7	190.2	188.0	128.7	229.9	68.6
West Virginia	139.0	176.1	*	176.1	118.1	221.2	65.2
East South Central	132.2	192.6	108.7	195.7	66.9	103.6	44.5
Alabama	123.6	163.6	*	163.6	58.5	85.7	37.7
Kentucky	133.3	207.5	108.7	226.8	72.2	129.5	50.2
Mississippi	107.4	193.4	*	193.4	76.0	111.3	44.2
Tennessee	152.3	207.3	*	207.3	59.7	90.8	43.2
West South Central	143.7	177.8	201.1	160.8	65.8	85.9	51.1
Arkansas	118.3	197.2	*	197.2	68.7	90.3	56.2
Louisiana	145.9	197.4	258.9	146.2	57.5	71.2	42.9
Oklahoma	128.9	172.5	*	172.5	73.7	103.3	46.6
Texas	150.3	171.9	186.9	156.0	66.1	86.2	54.4
WEST	199.4	222.7	247.3	178.9	106.0	123.7	76.3
Mountain	163.7	208.9	257.9	193.0	94.3	118.0	70.5
Arizona	181.4	218.7	*	218.7	72.1	82.7	56.0
Colorado	199.1	221.0	257.9	136.3	107.0	153.7	92.3

The Health Professions 305

Idaho	111.8	*	174.6	98.8	140.0	58.2
Montana	130.2	*	174.6	116.0	177.5	68.1
Nevada	131.2	*	142.9	80.2	171.1	51.6
New Mexico	145.8	*	253.2	91.6	96.5	76.7
Utah	166.8	*	193.2	70.5	96.5	59.7
Wyoming	104.5		*	104.5	120.0	87.5
Pacific	211.9	246.9	168.4	117.7	127.3	87.6
Alaska¹	120.1	—	—	—	—	—
California	224.4	247.0	177.2	120.2	127.2	96.8
Hawaii	202.4	*	214.9	152.1	152.1	*
Oregon	175.5	260.2	132.5	113.5	126.7	73.3
Washington	173.7	236.0	143.1	109.2	119.3	84.8

*There is no area in this state with the count of population indicated in the column heading.

1. Alaska is not divided into counties and therefore only the ratio for the entire state is computed.

Source: Estimated by U.S. Department of Health, Education, and Welfare, Health Resources Administration, Bureau of Health Professions, Division of Health Professions Analysis, based on data from the American Medical Association, Center for Health Services Research and Development.

Table 11-8 Number of Active Civilian Dentists and Dentist-to-Population Ratios

By Region, Division, and State: December 31, 1970, 1975, and 1980

Geographic Area	1970		1975		1980	
	Active Civilian Dentists	Active Civilian Dentists per 100,000 Civilian Population	Active Civilian Dentists	Active Civilian Dentists per 100,000 Civilian Population	Active Civilian Dentists	Active Civilian Dentists per 100,000 Civilian Population
UNITED STATES	95,680	47.4	106,740	50.5	121,240	54.9
NORTHEAST	28,601	58.9	31,983	64.8	32,536	65.2
New England	6,117	51.9	7,147	58.8	8,171	65.1
Connecticut	1,835	61.0	2,061	66.9	2,290	73.1
Maine	350	36.2	386	36.9	505	45.4
Massachusetts	3,024	52.9	3,683	63.5	4,079	68.2
New Hampshire	311	41.5	379	46.3	482	55.5
Rhode Island	425	46.9	442	47.5	522	54.4
Vermont	172	38.5	196	41.3	293	59.4
Middle Atlantic	22,484	61.1	24,836	66.8	24,365	65.3
New Jersey	4,056	57.3	4,308	58.8	4,860	64.9
New York	12,397	68.9	13,793	76.5	12,841	71.6
Pennsylvania	6,031	51.6	6,735	57.0	6,664	55.9

NORTH CENTRAL	26,129	46.3	28,146	48.9	31,036	53.1
East North Central	18,423	45.9	19,910	48.7	21,856	52.7
Illinois	5,503	50.0	5,870	52.9	6,214	55.2
Indiana	2,045	39.2	2,180	40.8	2,370	44.0
Michigan	4,285	48.1	4,520	49.6	5,085	54.7
Ohio	4,405	41.5	4,929	45.9	5,337	49.6
Wisconsin	2,185	49.6	2,411	52.5	2,850	59.8
West North Central	7,706	47.4	8,236	49.4	9,180	54.0
Iowa	1,306	46.7	1,364	47.7	1,497	51.6
Kansas	924	41.6	1,038	46.2	1,095	47.6
Minnesota	2,222	58.1	2,379	60.4	2,588	64.1
Missouri	1,983	42.3	2,079	43.6	2,404	49.6
Nebraska	809	55.0	876	56.8	985	61.9
North Dakota	232	38.0	249	39.6	302	48.9
South Dakota	230	34.8	251	36.9	309	45.0
SOUTH	22,025	35.3	25,255	37.5	32,095	44.4
South Atlantic	10,865	35.8	12,840	38.6	16,634	46.0
Delaware	213	38.6	239	41.8	261	43.7
District of Columbia	655	88.3	611	86.7	562	82.8
Florida	2,564	38.2	3,230	38.8	4,578	48.0
Georgia	1,351	29.4	1,670	34.1	2,142	40.7
Maryland	1,586	40.3	1,952	47.9	2,500	57.8

Table 11-8 continued

Geographic Area	1970		1975		1980	
	Active Civilian Dentists	Active Civilian Dentists per 100,000 Civilian Population	Active Civilian Dentists	Active Civilian Dentists per 100,000 Civilian Population	Active Civilian Dentists	Active Civilian Dentists per 100,000 Civilian Population
North Carolina	1,484	29.8	1,675	31.4	2,203	38.6
South Carolina	648	25.4	806	29.3	1,086	36.6
Virginia	1,770	39.4	2,027	42.1	2,549	49.0
West Virginia	594	34.0	630	35.1	753	40.7
East South Central	4,175	32.6	4,654	34.7	5,914	42.1
Alabama	1,009	29.4	1,096	30.6	1,380	36.7
Kentucky	1,129	35.2	1,263	37.7	1,584	44.9
Mississippi	608	27.9	613	26.4	786	32.6
Tennessee	1,429	36.0	1,682	40.5	2,164	49.7
West South Central	6,985	36.2	7,761	37.6	9,547	43.3
Arkansas	597	31.4	656	31.5	793	35.7
Louisiana	1,256	34.8	1,470	39.1	1,669	42.7
Oklahoma	932	36.6	1,031	38.0	1,237	43.7
Texas	4,200	37.4	4,604	38.1	5,848	44.7
WEST	18,925	54.9	21,356	57.3	25,573	63.7
Mountain	3,780	45.5	4,273	44.6	5,952	56.0
Arizona	699	38.1	826	37.2	1,212	47.5
Colorado	1,136	51.9	1,270	50.4	1,743	62.5

Idaho	325	44.9	352	43.2	476	53.5
Montana	311	44.3	349	47.3	467	59.3
Nevada	209	41.4	256	43.8	353	54.0
New Mexico	364	36.4	364	32.2	558	45.1
Utah	582	54.8	683	57.0	917	69.5
Wyoming	154	46.2	173	47.8	226	55.8
Pacific	15,145	57.9	17,083	61.6	19,621	66.5
Alaska	87	28.1	125	38.9	214	54.9
California	11,310	57.4	12,783	61.4	14,346	64.7
Hawaii	458	63.8	485	60.0	599	67.6
Oregon	1,376	65.2	1,463	63.4	1,779	72.9
Washington	1,914	57.0	2,227	64.6	2,683	74.2

Source: Estimated by U.S. Department of Health, Health Resources Administration, Bureau of Health Professions, Division of Health Professions Analysis, based on data from the American Dental Association, Bureau of Economic and Behavioral Research.

Data as of December 31, 1979, estimated the number of dentists per 100,000 population for metropolitan and nonmetropolitan counties. As expected, the ratios ranged from a high of 65.7 in the largest metropolitan areas to 30.9 in the least populated rural counties.

SPECIALTY DISTRIBUTION OF PHYSICIANS

The specialty distribution of health care providers, particularly physicians, has been an issue of long-standing concern to policy makers. Since World War II, the proportion of the total physician supply in general practice and related primary care specialties has declined steadily until the mid-1970s. Two-thirds of all physicians in 1950 were considered generalists but by 1970 the situation was reversed, with nearly two-thirds practicing in a specialty field. Table 11-9 documents this shift for the period 1965–1978, showing the continued decline in general and family practice in both absolute numbers and as a ratio of physicians to population. Although these declines were observed in general and family practice, other primary care physicians increased their numbers substantially. Since 1965, the number of both general internists and pediatricians more than doubled, with comparable increases in the ratio of these specialties to population (Table 11-10).

A number of national studies called for decreasing the number of residency positions available in the surgical specialties and the oversupplied medical subspecialties. However, little progress ensued, although the growth in primary care residency positions increased such opportunities as a proportion of the total. Specialty findings of GMENAC could lead to further serious policy considerations in this area.

REGULATION OF HEALTH PROFESSIONS

This section discusses the ways the regulatory process acts as a constraint on the options that policy makers, health educators, and the professions themselves develop to meet the nation's needs most effectively. The health care industry suffers no less than others from a wide array of regulations (some self-imposed), and new ones are issued frequently. This chapter does not examine the effects of all regulation affecting the industry other than to state that compliance adds to the costs that ultimately are borne by the consumer. The most important regulations affecting the education and utilization of health care personnel are the professional licensure laws. The rest of this section addresses the issues involving occupational licensure.

Milton Friedman (1962) was an early critic of licensure as a means of assuring quality of services. He identified licensure as an inflationary factor in the delivery of health services as well as a process used to restrict entry into a profession and limit the availability of care. Since then, a number of medical sociologists and economists have accused the medical profession of using the licensure laws as a means of safeguarding its position from competition rather than protecting the public from poor care (Friedson, 1970).

During the 1960s and early 1970s, a large number of practitioner groups, following the lead of the medical profession, attempted to secure for themselves the protection of occupational licensure. Since then, doubts have been expressed about occupational licensure in general and in the health field in particular. Professional leadership, state governments, and the American Hospital Association all have come forth at one time or another with criticisms of licensing, citing such regulation as restricting experimentation in the medical care industry and thereby adding to the expense of health care.

According to those opposed to licensure, it limits the number of practitioners available to perform health care functions and serves as a mechanism to help keep prices high because it keeps supply low. Licensing also impacts on geographic distribution of health professionals. If a large number of professionals is available, there should be some tendency for them to move into other, perhaps underserved, terrain. The licensing laws also limit patients' freedom of choice, according to this line of reasoning. Some patients would like to have the choice of an alternative technology to the therapeutic modalities espoused by high technology medicine. Yet licensure, and accompanying reimbursement regulations, restrict the types of health professionals who can bill for their services directly to the patient rather than through third party payers.

The licensure laws also specify the educational requirements for each profession. These, as they function in actual practice, affect consumers in several ways. Consumers absorb the expense of lengthy professional education by subsidizing cost directly through state and federal taxes. Patient fees in health care are closely related to level of education. The high education costs also limit entry into the profession and depress the supply of personnel.

Regulation, according to its detractors, also constrains the expanded functions that midlevel practitioners could perform. Nurse practitioners, physician's assistants, and nurse-midwives are required to be under the supervision of physicians, although the nature and extent of that oversight varies from state to state. Independent practice does not exist for these practitioners. Much more is at stake here than control over the quality of

Table 11-9 Number of Active M.D.s and Physician-to-Population Ratios

By General and Specialty Practice
Selected Years, December 31, 1965–1978[1,2]

Type of Practice	1965[3] Number	1965 Physicians per 100,000 Population	1970 Number	1970 Physicians per 100,000 Population	1975 Number	1975 Physicians per 100,000 Population	1978 Number	1978 Physicians per 100,000 Population
All Active	277,575	139.9	310,845	148.7	340,280	156.1	375,811	168.3
General and family practice[4]	64,943	32.6	57,948	27.7	54,557	25.0	56,197	25.1
Medical Specialities	61,435	31.0	77,214	36.9	95,087	43.6	109,743	49.2
Allergy	1,541	0.8	1,719	0.8	1,716	0.8	1,537	0.7
Card ovascular Diseases	4,311	2.2	6,476	3.1	6,933	3.2	8,506	3.8
Dermatology	3,407	1.7	4,003	1.9	4,661	2.1	5,105	2.3
Gastroenterology	1,344	0.7	2,010	1.0	2,381	1.1	3,314	1.5
Internal Medicine	33,892	17.0	41,872	20.0	54,331	24.9	62,641	28.0
Pediatric Allergy	270	0.1	391	0.2	446	0.2	437	0.2
Pediatric Cardiology	311	0.2	487	0.2	538	0.2	588	0.3
Pediatrics	14,255	7.2	17,941	8.6	21,746	10.0	24,545	11.0
Pulmonary Diseases	2,104	1.1	2,315	1.1	2,335	1.1	3,070	1.4
Surgical Specialities	73,185	36.7	86,042	41.1	96,015	44.1	102,414	45.9
General Surgery	25,643	12.9	29,761	14.2	31,562	14.5	32,059	14.4
Neurological Surgery	2,041	1.0	2,578	1.2	2,926	1.3	3,098	1.4
Obstetrics and Gynecology	16,379	8.2	18,876	9.0	21,731	10.0	23,963	10.7
Ophthalmology	8,380	4.2	9,927	4.7	11,129	5.1	11,933	5.3
Orthopedic Surgery	7,557	3.8	9,620	4.6	11,379	5.2	12,657	5.7

Otolaryngology	4,851	2.4	5,409	2.6	5,745	2.6	6,117	2.7
Plastic Surgery	1,167	0.6	1,600	0.8	2,236	1.0	2,624	1.2
Colon and Rectal Surgery	715	0.4	667	0.3	661	0.3	679	0.3
Thoracic Surgery	1,473	0.7	1,809	0.9	1,979	0.9	2,042	1.0
Urology	4,979	2.5	5,795	2.8	6,667	3.1	7,242	3.2
Other Specialities	78,012	39.1	89,641	42.8	94,621	43.4	107,457	48.1
Aerospace Medicine	1,603	0.8	1,188	0.6	684	0.3	584	0.3
Anesthesiology	8,592	4.3	10,860	5.2	12,861	5.9	14,246	6.4
Child Psychiatry	1,154	0.6	2,090	1.0	2,581	1.2	2,926	1.3
Neurology	2,198	1.1	3,074	1.5	4,131	1.9	4,923	2.2
Occupational Medicine	2,801	1.4	2,713	1.3	2,355	1.1	2,351	1.0
Pathology[5]	8,233	4.1	10,483	5.0	11,910	5.5	12,854	5.8
Physical Medicine and Rehabilitation	1,162	0.6	1,479	0.7	1,664	0.8	1,900	0.8
Psychiatry	17,333	8.7	21,146	10.1	23,922	11.0	25,596	11.5
Public Health[6]	3,988	2.0	3,833	1.8	3,454	1.6	3,096	1.4
Radiology[7]	9,686	4.9	13,360	6.4	16,240	7.5	18,407	8.2
Other and Unspecified	21,262	10.7	19,415	9.3	14,819	6.8	20,574	9.2

1. Includes physicians in federal service and those in United States possessions.
2. Ratios are based on total population plus civilian population in United States possessions.
3. Because of a change in the AMA classification procedure, 1965 data have been adjusted to be comparable to figures for the later years.
4. Family practice is included beginning in 1970.
5. Includes forensic pathology.
6. Includes general preventive medicine.
7. Includes both diagnostic and therapeutic radiology.

Source: American Medical Association, Center for Health Services Research and Development, *Physician Distribution and Medical Licensure in the U.S., 1978*; also for annual issues for 1970 and 1975 data. The 1965 adjusted data are from the AMA report *Reclassification of Physicians*, 1968.

Table 11-10 Number of M.D.s Active in Primary Care, and Primary Care Physician-to-Population Ratios

By Type of Practice: December 31, Selected Years 1965–1978, and Adjusted Data for 1978–1980

Year	Primary Care Physicians[1]	Total Population (Thousands)[2]	Primary Care: Physicians per 100,000 Population	Type of Primary Care Practice					
				General and Family Practice[3]		Internal Medicine		Pediatrics	
				Number	Physicians per 100,000 Population	Number	Physicians per 100,000 Population	Number	Physicians per 100,000 Population
1965	113,090	198,357	56.8	64,943	32.6	33,892	17.0	14,255	7.2
1970	117,761	209,096	56.3	57,948	27.7	41,872	20.0	17,941	8.6
1975	130,634	217,966	59.9	54,557	25.0	54,331	24.9	21,746	10.0
1976	135,881	219,648	61.9	55,479	25.3	57,911	26.4	22,491	10.2
1977	140,948	221,419	63.6	55,159	24.9	61,830	27.9	23,959	10.8
1978	143,383	223,274	64.2	56,197	25.2	62,641	28.0	24,545	11.0
1978[4]	154,370	223,274	69.1	58,740	26.3	66,910	30.0	28,720	12.8
1979[4,5]	157,480	225,099	70.0	58,980	26.2	68,780	30.6	29,720	13.2
1980[4,5]	166,640	227,911	73.1	61,620	27.0	73,220	32.1	31,800	14.0

1. Includes physicians in federal service and those in United States possessions.
2. Total population includes civilians in United States possessions.
3. Family practice is included beginning in 1970.
4. These numbers are adjusted to include most physicians whose address or activity status are unknown.
5. Adjusted numbers for 1979 and 1980 are based on estimates.

Sources: Data for 1965 through 1978 (unadjusted) compiled by U.S. Department of Health, Education, and Welfare, Health Resources Administration, Bureau of Health Professions, Division of Health Professions Analysis, based on data from the American Medical Association, Center for Health Services Research and Development, *Physician Distribution and Medical Licensure in the U.S., 1978*; also prior annual issues. All adjusted data for 1978 through 1980 also by HRA. Other data from U.S. Bureau of the Census, *Current Population Report* P-25, Nos. 542, 603, 704, and 812.

care provided by the midlevel practitioners. The right of supervision gives physicians control over the number of their competitors and the tenor of their practice, according to critics.

The licensure laws also are accused of impeding the development of cost-effective prevention programs. It has been demonstrated that less intensively trained personnel can safely do much of the work necessary in prevention work. It has been estimated that as high as 80 percent of the routine well-baby care normally provided by pediatricians can safely be delegated to nurse practitioners or other than non-M.D. providers. Routine foot care by podiatrists and eye care by optometrists also have been shown to be safe and cost-effective alternatives to physician treatment yet these remain controversial in many states because of efforts by organized medicine to restrict expansion of the functions of these types of providers.

A list of seven criteria (Dolan, 1980) to be considered in deciding whether to experiment with alternative personnel configurations for delivering services offers these choices:

1. between alternative therapeutic ideologies, both of which can make reasonable claims to a scientific base (say, obstetricians vs. midwives)
2. between practitioners offering to provide services where mistakes usually are not serious and make themselves known over time (dentists vs. dental hygienists)
3. between less-trained practitioners' services and no services (underserved rural and urban areas) when such practitioners have a reasonable amount of training
4. between permitting people to prepare for the performance of services in nontraditional routes such as apprenticeship programs and on-the-job training programs (institutional licensure) or rejecting that approach.
5. between a delivery environment in which de facto review of services is easy and nearly certain (institutional licensure) and a tight control
6. between a modest decrement or increase in formal training or certification (podiatrists vs. M.D.s or certified M.D.s vs. noncertified M.D.s or R.N.s vs. N.P.s)
7. between a traditional approach and an alternative one that claims to be safe, a stance that is supported circumstantially by reasonably reliable studies in other countries or other locations in the United States.

Those who favor continued strong licensure laws point to the importance of protecting the public from lower quality health care. They note that in the case of highly technical, complex services such as many medical procedures, the average patient has no means of evaluating alternative choices for treatment as to their efficacy. Their argument therefore is that the professions themselves are the only ones who can validly make the decisions about who are qualified to practice and to set the standards for licensure.

During the 1970s a number of states created licensure review commissions, often known as "sunset commissions," to review the necessity of state regulatory practices and licensure boards. Without exception, these commissions, while praised at the outset for their intention to streamline the licensure process and to abolish unnecessary laws, found implementation of such ideas difficult. Consumers as well as providers have risen up in virtually every state to oppose any moves that might be viewed as a weakening of the process. In several states, consumers have been added to licensure boards. Other states have adopted legislation tightening the process so that standards of quality are enforced more strictly and violators of regulations can be disciplined more readily by their peers. Nevertheless, licensure of individual practitioners continues as the major mechanism by which the practice of health care delivery is circumscribed and regulated in the United States.

These and related licensure and regulatory issues are expected to remain at the fore in health personnel policy in the next decade. The regulatory process will prove particularly important as policy analysts relate its decisions to broader issues of quality of care, distribution of providers, and the cost of utilizing services.

THE FEDERAL ROLE IN POLICY

The active role of the federal government in health personnel development is a relatively recent phenomenon and roughly parallels federal participation in the health care system in general. Prior to World War II, primary concern at the national level had been with general public health issues such as sanitation, epidemic control, and quarantining those suspected of transmitting diseases. Although beginning in the 1930s there was limited federal support for doctors, nurses, and other clinicians who wished to return for additional training in public health, total expenditures were minimal and were not viewed as part of an overall strategy to meet the nation's needs for health personnel.

World War II brought immediate recognition of the importance of adequate numbers of health care providers, and the following years generated increased discussion of an expanded federal role to meet the health needs of a nation returning to normal. The passage of the Hospital Survey and

Construction Act of 1946, P.L. 79-725 (Hill-Burton), its expansion in 1949, and further amendments during the next three decades, were major steps in providing support for communities experiencing shortages of hospitals, physicians, and related health services. Although the act was seen primarily as a facilities measure, the construction of new hospitals also was viewed as an attempt to attract health providers to areas in need of service.

Nevertheless, direct federal intervention in the training and utilization of health care personnel was not to occur for another 15 years. During the 1950s, the federal government looked at apparent shortages of physicians, dentists, nurses, and allied health personnel. The Surgeon General's Consultant Group on Medical Education found the existing ratio of physicians to population only "a minimum essential to protect the health of the people of the United States" (Surgeon General, 1959).

The Kennedy Administration in 1961 proposed a program of new construction for schools of medicine, dentistry, and public health, along with a program of scholarships for health science students. Two years later Congress passed the Health Professions Education Assistance Act of 1963 (P.L. 88-129), landmark legislation that took the federal government directly into the process of increasing the supply of health care providers. For details of that act and a number of related measures (discussed next) see Exhibit 11-1.

Federal support for allied personnel came somewhat later than aid for the other health professions, following increasing awareness of an imbalance in the supply and demand for a much broader array of professionals. President Johnson, in his Health Message to Congress in January 1965, recognized the situation when he stated:

> We must look forward to the future in planning to meet the health manpower requirements of the nation. . . . If we are to meet our future needs and raise the health of the nation, we must (1) Improve utilization of available health personnel . . . (2) Expand the use and training of technicians and ancillary health workers . . . (3) Expand and improve training programs for professional and supporting health personnel . . . (4) Plan ahead to meet requirements for which the lead time is often 10 years or more (Lewis, Fein, & Mechanic, 1976).

The Allied Health Professions Personnel Training Act of 1966, P.L. 89-751, was the first legislation specifically directed at increasing the numbers of such practitioners and improving and expanding their health education and training. It authorized grants for schools offering programs to a wide range of professions not included in the 1963 legislation.

Exhibit 11-1 U.S. Health Professions Legislation, 1963–1976

Title of Act	Construction	Student Loans	Capitation	Special Projects
Health Professions Educational Assistance Act of 1963 (P.L. 88-129)	• Provided $175 million to pay for construction of teaching facilities for medicine, dentistry, osteopathy, public health, optometry, pharmacy, podiatry, nursing • Terms: up to two thirds of the cost of new facilities; one-third of the cost of renovation	• Set these terms: 90 percent federal contribution, 10 percent match; student could borrow a maximum of $2,000 per year, repayable in ten years • Designated as eligible disciplines: medicine, osteopathy, dentistry		
Nurse Training Act of 1964 (P.L. 88-581)	• Liberalized construction grants to include collegiate nursing schools and schools offering diplomas and associate degrees; change from 1963 Public Law 88-129 that had limited construction grants to schools that led to a baccalaureate or graduate degree	• Established nursing student loan program	• Change to capitation based on number of federally supported students and increase in student enrollments over 1962–1964 levels	• Offered grants to schools for improving training programs • Established traineeships to prepare clinical nursing specialists

Allied Health Professions Personnel Training Act of 1966 (P.L. 89-751)	• Authorized but did not appropriate construction grants	• Based on increase in enrollment • Grants made available to the schools of public health for first time	• Funded special projects for experimentation, demonstration, and improvement in the training of allied health personnel • Provided traineeships for advanced training • Created public health traineeships
Health Manpower Act of 1968 (P.L. 90-490)	Changes from 1963: • Provided assistance to multipurpose facilities • Aided facilities for advanced training • Increased federal share	Changes specified in more detail the use of grants: • Included schools of pharmacy and veterinary medicine • Revised formulas so all schools received $25,000 • Distributed 75 percent of remaining money on basis of increases in enrollment and 25 per-	• Increased emphasis on impact of funding on quality of programs, curriculum, teaching methods

Exhibit 11-1 continued

Page 320 — POLICY ISSUES IN PERSONAL HEALTH SERVICES

Title of Act	Construction	Student Loans	Capitation	Special Projects
			cent on basis of increases in graduates • Limited total costs to no higher than prior three years	
Nurse Training Act of 1971 (P.L. 92-158)	Change from 1963: • Moved from support of institutions to interest in output of grants • Raised maximum federal share for expansion from two-thirds to 80 percent		Change from 1964: • Became first nurse personnel bill to actually fund capitation • Provided extra amounts to encourage expansion of enrollment and training of nurse practitioners	• Established educational programs and aimed to improve, expand, and strengthen program effectiveness • Set up separate authority for schools in financial distress • Provided for special projects to bring students with exceptional ability and financial need into nursing
Comprehensive Health Manpower Training Act of 1971 (P.L. 92-157)	Change from 1963: • Raised federal share from two-thirds of cost to 80 percent • Covered acquisition of existing buildings and cost of providing interim facilities	• Extended loans under Health Professions Educational Assistance Act of 1963 (HPEA) • Increased loan maximum • Changed loan cancellation policy: up to 85 percent could be cancelled by three-year	Change from 1963: • Amended base grant from $25,000 to $50,000 per year • Changed eligibility to schools of medicine, osteopathy, dentistry that had fewer than 50 first-year students	• Established National Health Manpower Clearinghouse • Continued aid to financially distressed schools Change from 1963: • Created new program of Health Manpower Edu-

		practice in shortage area. • Provided government would repay loans of low-income and/or minority students who did not complete training	• Provided payments ranging from $6,000 per graduating physician to $320 per enrollment bonus student at schools of optometry	cation Initiative Awards to improve distribution, supply, utilization, and efficiency of health personnel and delivery system—used to fund Area Health Education Centers (AHEC) • Awarded hospitals grants for family medicine residencies • Set up new advisory council of health professions educators
Health Professions Educational Assistance Act of 1976 (P.L. 94-484)	Change from 1971: • Cut back construction grants	• Extended loans and scholarships to those with exceptional need and increased amount available in a given year	Change from 1971: • Tied capitation support to quotas for primary care residencies; required all schools to meet certain percentages of first-year residencies: 25% in 1977 40% in 1978 50% in 1979	• Tied federal scholarship program more closely to National Health Service Corps • Limited influx of Foreign Medical Graduates (FMGs) • Continued AHEC program with stricter criteria

The Health Manpower Act of 1968 (P.L. 90-490) made several changes in the program of institutional aid to health science schools and incorporated nursing and the allied health professions into several major provisions. The most important changes in the construction program were provisions for assistance to multipurpose training facilities, support for building facilities for advanced training, and increases in the federal share of such costs where special circumstances warranted it.

The 1968 act clearly provided for an expanded federal role in health professions education and for continued government monitoring of changes in the supply and demand for health professionals. For the first time, greater emphasis was placed on the impact of such federal aid on enrollments, the quality of educational programs, and the curriculum and teaching methods employed.

The Comprehensive Health Manpower Training Act of 1971 (P.L. 92-157) extended and expanded the 1963 health manpower legislation and added a series of new programs geared to eliminating physician shortages. The most important difference was that the 1963 act supported institutions rather than concerning itself directly with their output. The 1971 act made clear the government's interest in the production of health professionals—the emphasis was on the product, not the physical plant. For example, the new capitation grant program (for schools of medicine, osteopathy, dentistry, veterinary medicine, optometry, pharmacy, and podiatry), based on the number of students enrolled, replaced funding to construct facilities as the primary source of monies to the schools after the first two years.

Legislation in nursing has been, by and large, separate from that of other health professionals. Much like federal involvement with other professions, the government's role during the 1950s was limited to surveys of nursing personnel and their utilization with the exception of traineeships for nursing teachers, administrators, and supervisors.

The Nurse Training Act of 1964 (P.L. 88-581) was an important development in the history of federal assistance to schools of nursing. The act provided funding for a comprehensive program of traineeships as well as capitation grants based on the number of federally supported students in the program and increases in enrollment from 1962 to 1964. The Nurse Training Amendments of 1968 extended and liberalized the construction grants, special projects grants, traineeships, and loan programs through fiscal year 1971. Funds were authorized to conduct research into better ways to educate nurses, help schools in financial distress, expand enrollment, and achieve accreditation. A scholarship program for nursing students also was funded.

The Nurse Training Act of 1971 (P.L. 92-158) extended the 1964 act, authorized money for construction of facilities, and raised the maximum federal share for construction costs or expansion of existing facilities. Special projects to allow schools of nursing to establish educational programs and to expand, improve, and strengthen program effectiveness were approved.

Previous health professions bills (Nurse Training Act of 1964 and Health Manpower Act of 1968) had authorized special grants to nurse training programs but these never were funded. The 1971 act was the first bill to fund capitation grants with extra amounts to encourage expansion of enrollments and the training of nurse practitioners. Finally, the act extended scholarship aid and funded special projects designed to assist schools in financial distress and to bring students with exceptional financial need who had demonstrated abilities into nursing.

The Health Professions Educational Assistance Act of 1976, P.L. 94-484, was the first such major legislation since 1971 and further extended the federal role in all areas of health professions training and development (again, see Exhibit 11-1). Although construction grants to medical and other health professional schools were reduced, there were substantial increases in the loan and scholarship programs for health professions students, tying them more closely to service obligation in the National Health Service Corps (PHS, 1980a). Capitation support was continued, but tied closely to increased training in primary care. Finally, authorization for area health education centers (AHECs) was continued with much stricter legislative direction of criteria for operating such programs. In virtually all major aspects, the 1976 act sought to focus federal efforts much more closely on problems of specialty and geographic maldistribution. Increasingly aware of the fact that increasing the supply of health providers would not fully address distribution problems, Congress specifically tied federal support to efforts at improving the number of primary care providers and provided strong incentives to increase the supply of such individuals in areas of greatest need.

Although health professions legislation to replace the 1976 act was proposed in 1980 and again in 1981, no significant bills were likely to be considered seriously for several years. The combination of impending surpluses of physicians and other providers, with the serious budget shortfalls faced by the federal government, made early passage of new legislation unlikely. Nevertheless, discussions on new legislation indicated it would reflect the concept that significant federal institutional support for health professions schools no longer was necessary from a policy standpoint. Interventions to improve geographic and specialty distribution were likely to be continued at reduced levels along with some efforts to aid students with exceptional financial need. The direction of such legislation could have significant policy consequences well into the 1980s.

PERSONNEL SUPPLY AND DISTRIBUTION INTERVENTIONS

For some years, particularly during the 1970s, several major federal initiatives sought to improve the supply and distribution of health professionals in general, and primary care providers in particular. A number of these initiatives were based on earlier efforts at the state level or on relatively small-scale pilot projects. The next sections describe some of the more important interventions, with particular focus on their benefits and their outlook for long-term impact. Since federal support for most of these programs was reduced substantially in the early 1980s, their future viability depended in part on the degree to which Congress and others in health policy roles were convinced that these efforts represented cost-effective responses to personnel shortages in the health field.

Loan Forgiveness Programs

Loan forgiveness programs have received considerable attention in recent years as a means of encouraging physicians and other health care personnel to locate their practices in underserved areas. While millions of dollars have been committed to this purpose, the few studies of program impact that have been undertaken have shown mixed results (Mason, 1971; Lewis, Fein, & Mechanic, 1976). These studies are discussed later in this section.

Loan forgiveness programs consist of two parts: (1) loans are granted to students who agree to practice for a specified length of time in a shortage area; (2) all or part of the loans are forgiven in exchange for the fullfillment of that practice obligation. It is important to note that almost all of the programs have a buy-out option. Students can decide that rather than fulfill the practice obligation they can opt out by repaying the principle, plus interest and any penalties.

Programs vary in their sponsorship, amount that can be borrowed, penalties for buying out, and terms for forgiveness. Several state-sponsored programs have been in operation since the 1940s, largely in midwestern and southern states with sizable rural populations. The terms of the loans are one year of practice for each 10 percent to 25 percent of the amount forgiven, depending on the program. Most of the state programs have a buy-out option. They have been sponsored by the state medical society or the state government, or both (Lewis, Fein, & Mechanic, 1976).

Federal support of loan forgiveness began in 1965 when the Health Professions Educational Assistance Act of 1963 was amended to include a provision that up to 50 percent of an HPEA loan could be forgiven—10 percent for each year of practice in a federal designated scarcity area. The Allied Health Personnel Training Act of 1966 increased forgiveness of 10 to 15 percent for each year of service. The Comprehensive Health Manpower Training Act of 1971 allowed forgiveness of up to 85 percent of any educational loan (not only HPEA) for three years of practice in a federally designated shortage area. The terms of the loan were that 60 percent would be forgiven for the first two years of practice and 25 percent for the third year.

There are few published evaluations of these programs. Mason (1971) reviewed 11 state programs in 1970 and 1971, ten of which incorporated a loan forgiveness provision. He found that only one state program was successful (Kentucky) and that if a state had 60 percent of the physicians fulfill their obligations it was doing relatively well (Table 11-11).

In 1972, CONSAD Research Corporation, under contract to the Office of the Secretary, Department of Health, Education, and Welfare evaluated the short-term impact of loans granted between 1960 and 1965 by ten state programs and of existing federally supported loan forgiveness programs through 1972.

While nothing in the Mason study explained the variations in practice, repayment, and buy-out rates, the CONSAD study suggested two factors that could be associated with success or failure:

1. The total dollar amount of the loan available to each borrower during professional school—if more money was available, then the larger the potential loan and the larger the amount to be forgiven through practice or to be repaid if the borrower decided to buy out; the assumption was that the larger the loan available, the higher the rate of practice repayment.
2. The stringency of the loan forgiveness provision—a program requiring at least three years of practice before each annual loan could be cancelled at the rate of one year of practice for each annual loan is tougher than one that merely requires a year of practice for each annual loan (CONSAD Research Company, 1973).

However, one rather detailed study of state loan programs that related borrowers who elected to fulfill their practice obligation to the total amount of money available for loans showed little relation between the two variables (Lewis, Fein, & Mechanic, 1976). The study's authors concluded that loan forgiveness was a rather weak incentive to practice commitment. They said most practicing physicians found the amount borrowed to be a small barrier to buying out. There also was likely to be a relationship between the affluence of the medical student and the effectiveness of the program. Others have found that students who did not already have a strong interest in practicing in an underserved area would be unlikely to

Table 11-11 Experience of 11 State Practice Agreement/Loan-Forgiveness Programs

(Borrowers Available to Practice by 1970)

State	Number of Borrowers	Borrowers Available to Practice by 1970 (%)	Physicians Repaying Loan with Rural Practice[1] (%)	Physicians Buying Out of Practice Commitment (%)	Physicians in Default of Payment (%)	Borrowers Unavailable to Practice for Other Reasons (%)
Arkansas	96	57.2	32.8	56.4	10.9	0.0
Georgia	639	45.2	50.2	49.8	0.0	7.0
Iowa	62	4.8	66.7	0.0	33.3	0.0
Kentucky	331	61.0	96.0	0.0	4.0	11.5
Minnesota	22	54.5	66.7	25.0	8.3	0.0
Mississippi	611	93.6	74.4	25.5	0.0	6.4
North Carolina	301	47.5	58.0	42.0	0.0	4.3
North Dakota	40	35.0	71.4	28.6	0.0	0.0
South Carolina	160	37.5	66.7	33.3	0.0	0.0
Virginia	291	83.8	44.7	55.3	0.0	3.4
West Virginia	22	27.3	66.7	33.6	0.0	0.0
Total	2,575	Average: 62.0	63.0	34.1	2.0	5.7

1. The base number for percentage is the total number of borrowers available to practice by 1970. It includes borrowers fulfilling their practice commitment in 1970 and those who had completed either the entire commitment or the portion for which they were legally liable before buying out of the remainder.

Source: Reprinted with permission from *A Right to Health: The Problem of Access to Primary Medical Care* by C.E. Lewis, R. Fein, and D. Mechanic, John Wiley & Sons, Inc. © 1976. Source adapted from Mason, H.R. "Effectiveness of student aid programs tied to a service commitment." *Journal of Medical Education,* 1971, *46,* p. 581.

choose the loan forgiveness option. The data on the federal forgiveness programs also indicate that the existence of the loans themselves is more attractive than the forgiveness options. In 1965 and 1966, of 3,800 HPEA borrowers graduating from medical school, only 42 physicians had cancelled their loans by shortage area practice by November 1972.

The 1980 GMENAC report recommended that governmentally sponsored loan and scholarship programs be catalogued and evaluated to determine their effectiveness. The report noted that there had been little research in this area. It also recommended that future loan forgiveness programs be modeled after those that had been successful in attracting physicians to underserved areas.

The National Health Service Corps Scholarships Program attempted to learn from these prior experiences in setting policies for its program. As noted in the next section, NHSC provisions called for payback at three times the amount borrowed and within one year if the student completed the degree and did not select the service option. This provision combined with the rapidly rising amounts borrowed led many policy makers to believe that the service obligation would be honored by high proportions of the borrowers in the educational system in the early 1980s.

National Health Service Corps

The National Health Service Corps was created by the Emergency Health Personnel Act of 1970 (P.L. 91-623). The legislation authorized establishment within the U.S. Public Health Service of an administrative unit to improve the health care provided underserved communities throughout the nation. Physicians and other providers were to be assigned to areas designated by HEW (later HHS) as having critical shortages of health personnel. However, formal requests for placement had to come from a state or local health agency or nonprofit private health organization. Persons receiving services were to be charged at rates established by the agency but provisions were made for providing care free or at a reduced rate if sufficient need on the part of recipients could be established.

The scholarship program was established by the Emergency Health Personnel Act Amendment of 1972. The initial source of entrants in the corps had been volunteers but the scholarship program quickly became the major entry track. To be eligible, an individual had to be enrolled as a full-time student in a program leading to a degree in medicine, dentistry, or other health-related specialty, as determined by HEW, and eligible for appointment to the corps.

Each participant received an annual scholarship during each year of training (not to exceed four years) that included tuition, other educational expenses, and a living allowance. In return, recipients were obligated to serve as members of the NHSC following completion of their academic training on the basis of one year of service for each year of scholarship aid. Service could be postponed pending completion of an internship or residency program.

The initial penalty for failure to complete the required service was to repay scholarship funds received plus interest to the federal government within three years. The program's early experience was similar to that of other loan forgiveness activities for physicians in that a relatively high proportion of recipients chose to repay the loans rather than serve in a shortage area. For that reason, the Health Professions Educational Assistance Act of 1976, P.L. 94-484, which authorized continuation of the corps and scholarship program, imposed serious penalties on students who received scholarship funds beginning in fiscal year 1978 and who chose not to serve in the corps: a student who obtained a professional degree must repay in one year triple the amount of the total award plus interest at the maximum allowable rate; if no degree was obtained, the student had two years to repay the scholarship funds without interest. This debt could not be discharged through bankruptcy for five years from the date when the payment was due.

At the same time, P.L. 94-484 made the service obligation somewhat more flexible by allowing HHS to release an individual from service in the corps on the basis of an agreement to enter private practice in an underserved area. The individual also had to agree to charge fees at the prevailing level in the area, provide indigent care, and agree to accept Medicare and Medicaid patients.

Although the private practice option always was available, it never was given serious attention until about 1980. Starting in 1981 and 1982, the number of federally supported sites was being reduced rapidly to the point where it was projected that by 1985 all corps placements would be in private practice settings. As of 1982, Congress capped the federally supported sites at 2,500, yet that many scholarship recipients were coming out of training in that year alone.

Such a policy shift was criticized as placing too great a burden on the individual recipient to locate a private practice option. Nevertheless, it appeared that there would be little turning back to substantial federally assisted delivery systems (e.g., rural clinics and health centers) for scholarship recipients in the near future.

Funding for the National Health Service Corps rose rapidly during the 1970s. Scholarship program appropriations grew from only $3 million in FY 1974 to some $75 million in 1979. After slight increases in 1980 and 1981, its appropriations were curtailed in 1982 and no new scholarships were awarded. The Reagan budget for 1983 funded the corps at approximately $100 million, which provided for no new scholarships, and a $9,000 bonus that had been paid to NHSC recipient physicians was eliminated.

Although the vast majority (more than 80 percent) of all awards were in medicine and osteopathy, increasing numbers of dental, nursing, and other students received scholarships in recent years. A breakdown of new awards for the years 1973–1974 through 1978–1979 school years is shown in Table 11-12.

Scholarship recipients began entering their service obligations in 1976 when 47 physicians and 28 dentists went on active duty. The number entering each year rose steadily to approximately 2,500 in 1981, and the output of the program was not expected to peak until the mid-1980s. With the cutbacks in new scholarships, however, that peak number could be smaller than anticipated and could be reached sooner. For example, the number of new awards rose to 1,500 in 1980, then fell to 500 in 1981 and to 0 in 1982.

Scholarship recipients contributed about 32 percent of the field strength of the corps in 1978. The other 68 percent consisted of volunteers but their percentage fell steadily as the output from the scholarship program increased.

Evaluating the effectiveness of the NHSC in overcoming the maldistribution of health care providers was difficult from the outset. Part of the problem lay in deciding whether or not the corps should be viewed as a short-term intervention (with success being defined in terms of care for underserved communities) or a more long-term one where retention in the community after completion of the corps obligation was the criterion of accomplishment. A 1978 report by the General Accounting Office leveled several criticisms at the corps, not the least of which was its very low retention rate up to that point (U.S. General Accounting Office, 1978).

Defenders of the corps pointed out that long-term outcomes would not be available to measure until well into the 1980s. The corps also noted that its practitioners had served more than 1.3 million persons in 1980, and that this number was expected to grow as the output increased. Communities served by the corps also, by definition, were historically underserved and thus likely to be unattractive or infeasible for private practitioners without the subsidy of the NHSC or other public-assisted programs. Nevertheless, the assignment process and the corps's inability to consult with local communities in determining need and seeking the best match of practitioner to community were criticized. Several states increased their involvement in the placement process in order to correct some of these problems.

The corps was the linchpin in the federal government's active role in alleviating health personnel shortages in the 1970s and faced careful reviews in coming years. With the supply of M.D.s and other health practitioners

Table 11-12 NHSC Scholarship Awards 1973–1974 through 1978–1979 School Years

School Year	1973–74	1974–75	1975–76	1976–77	1977–78	1978–79	Total
New Awards	372	1,498	871	885	2,089	3,346	9,061
M.D. and D.O.	372	1,498	823	835	1,834	2,702	8,064
Medicine	343	1,327	714	729	1,595	2,388	7,096
Osteopathy	29	171	109	106	239	314	968
Dent stry	—	—	48	50	99	387	584
Nurs ng	—	—	—	—	40	160	200
Other	—	—	—	—	116	97	213

Source: Unpublished data from the Department of Health, Education, and Welfare, U.S. Public Health Service, Health Resources Administration, Division of Manpower Training Support, 1981.

increasing rapidly, policy makers must determine whether an aggressive program of such scope and size still was warranted or whether those illusive market forces finally would begin to force health care providers into underserved areas in sufficient numbers.

Support for Family Medicine

Earlier data in this chapter documented the historical decline in general or family practitioners in the United States, both in absolute terms and as a proportion of the total physician supply. By the late 1960s, the number of physicians in general practice was decreasing by approximately 2,000 per year.

In the late 1950s and early 1960s, efforts were made to upgrade the traditional one-year general medicine internship, the historical track for graduates choosing general practice. With the approval of the AMA House of Delegates, 20 programs throughout the country sought to upgrade the internship to a two-year family practice residency on a pilot basis. These programs never generated the support required from the health science centers or medical communities and had considerable difficulty in attracting students. Most programs were less than half filled and gradually were phased out in the late 1960s.

Renewed efforts were made, starting in the mid-1960s, to develop well-planned residency training in family medicine that could compete with the established specialties for faculty, resources, and students. A host of national studies and conferences produced, among other documents, the 1966 report of the AMA Council on Medical Education's Ad Hoc Committee on Education in Family Practice, better known as the Willard Report. The passage of Medicare and Medicaid created much more demand for primary services by populations that had been largely underserved by the medical system at that time. With these and a variety of political forces moving toward support of this new grouping, family practice was formally recognized as a medical specialty field by the AMA's House of Delegates in February 1969. In 1971, the American Academy of General Practice became the American Academy of Family Physicians.

With AMA approval and interest running high in this new specialty, many states moved to establish residency programs in family practice. It had long been recognized that there was a close association between specialty choice and practice location, and thus many states viewed increases in primary care training as a means to increase the number of physicians settling in rural and other underserved areas as well. Family practice residency programs thus were started at many major medical centers. Larger community hospitals in some states also made efforts to establish residencies as well but found it difficult to generate the resources necessary to operate the programs effectively.

For this reason and to encourage expansion of family practice training opportunities, the Comprehensive Health Manpower Training Act of 1971 (P.L. 92-157) authorized federal support for developing or expanding residency programs in family medicine. Funds were made available for a broad array of uses including faculty, support personnel, travel, student stipends, and so forth.

Although the dollars available to support such programs were small at first, the federal support totalled more than $150 million from 1972 to 1980 and was set at some $30 million for 1982. The level of support was expected eventually to fall somewhat although family medicine fared well in light of the major federal cuts made in most other health professions training programs.

Although many family practice residency programs were just reaching full output capacity by 1982, indications were that they were an important tool in increasing the supply of physicians in traditionally underserved rural areas and small towns. The total number of family practice residents had grown to nearly 6,000 by 1982, with roughly 2,000 graduating each year and entering practice. From 1976 on, the declines in family and general practitioners for the previous several decades finally were reversed and showed a steady increase once again.

Data from the American Academy of Family Practice that was cited in a 1978 GAO Report indicated more than half of the family practice graduates were locating in towns of less than 30,000 population (GAO, 1978). Figures from at least one state, North Carolina, also showed favorable retention rates for family practitioners trained there. The proportion staying in the state and going to towns under 10,000 population was much higher for those in family practice than in other specialties.

Despite these favorable trends, several key policy issues remained for the family practice movement. Where federal support for physician training programs was cut, family medicine departments were particularly vulnerable because of the ambulatory nature of their practice. Surgical specialties and medical subspecialties were better able to generate support through patient fees than were primary care programs.

Reductions in medical school enrollments and residency positions, if implemented, would hit family medicine particularly hard. Since they were the newest residency programs in most medical centers and hospitals, pressure could be brought to bear for them to take an inordinate share of any cuts in residency positions. Nevertheless, the GMENAC Report did project family practice as one of the few specialties that would be roughly in balance between supply and requirements in 1990. (It should be noted, however, that its report was issued in September 1980, before the Reagan victory, and thus could not take into consideration the budget-cutting program he introduced.) Any significant cuts in the number being trained could lead to a shortfall in primary care providers, a situation federal policy makers might well not want to encourage, given the level of investment in family practice.

New Health Practitioners

Interest in the training of nurse practitioners (N.P.s) and physician's assistants (P.A.s) began in the middle to late 1960s, largely as a response to physician shortages that were particularly acute in rural areas and inner cities. Other factors contributing to the interest in expanding the role of the nurse and creating the new function of physician's assistant were:

- the large numbers of veterans returning from the Vietnam War with experience in the medical corps but with no similar role on their return to civilian life
- the increasing professionalism of nurses coupled with their increasing dissatisfaction with the limited role of the hospital/office nurse
- the rising cost of medical care and journal articles by those in the academic community envisioning a system of delivering primary health care services to all in a cost-effective manner

The first training program for physician's assistants was begun in 1965 at Duke University as a response to some of these forces and the first program for nurse practitioners was started at the University of Colorado in the same year. Programs began to develop nationwide modeled on these two but it was not until the 1970s that federal interest focused on the potential of these new health professions to ameliorate the maldistribution and shortage problems.

In his Annual Health Message of 1971, President Nixon recognized the value of physician's assistants and nurse practitioners in increasing the availability of primary care services. His proposal to fund the training of nurse practitioners was realized through the passage of the Nurse Training Act of 1971 (P.L. 92-158). Physician's assistants were included in this support in the Comprehensive Health Manpower Training Act of 1971 (P.L. 92-157).

Federal support for education and training of these two groups continued over the years with enactment of such bills as the Nurse Training Act of 1975 (P.L. 94-63), and the Health Professions Educational Assistance Act of 1976 (P.L. 94-484). The Rural Health Clinics Service Act of 1977 assured reimbursement under Medicare and Medicaid for medical services provided by an N.P. or a P.A. in a rural clinic. This act also authorized funds for demonstration projects that paid for the services of nurse practitioners and physician's assistants under Medicaid and Medicare in inner-city areas.

The nurse practitioner programs vary in terms of: (1) whether they grant a degree or simply a certificate, (2) their duration, (3) whether they require a preceptorship or rely solely on formal didactic classroom training, and (4) the level of specialization (e.g., family nurse practitioner, geriatric, pediatric, etc.).

Where nurse practitioner programs grew out of an interest in expanding nurses' roles in primary care settings, physician's assistant programs evolved to train P.A.s as practitioners working for and under the supervision of a practicing physician. This difference is evident in the curriculum of all P.A. programs, with most being located within medical schools and thus having more ties to a medicine curriculum. Nevertheless, programs for training physician's assistants vary along parameters similar to those of the N.P. programs, with three major types predominant:

1. The Medex program, originally designed for ex-medical corpsmen (from which it took its name), requires 12–15 months of study, including 3 months of didactic work in basic and clinical sciences at a university medical center followed by a preceptorship with a practicing physician for 9–12 months. The student, upon completion, receives a certificate.
2. The university medical center P.A. program consists of a two-year program beginning with 9–12 months didactic work in basic and clinical sciences followed by 12–15 months of various clinical rotations in tertiary care settings and preceptorships in private practice settings. Upon completion, students receive a certificate and/or baccalaureate degree.
3. The college or university program in a nonmedical school setting requires about two years of training, beginning with 9–12 months of clinical didactic work followed by 10–15 months of clinical rotations in an affiliated teaching hospital and local community-based preceptorships. These programs may lead to a certificate, an associate or baccalaureate degree. (Fisher & Horowitz, 1977)

Curricula for all programs have been developed around five basic functions of the new health practitioners, namely, their ability: "(1) to elicit a comprehensive health history, (2) to perform a comprehensive physical examination, (3) to perform simple diagnostic laboratory determinations, (4) to perform basic treatment procedures for common illnesses, (5) to make an appropriate clinical response to commonly encountered emergency care situations '' (Fisher & Horowitz, 1977).

Many studies have been conducted to determine the economic effectiveness of new health practitioners, although this is difficult to judge because of the problems of deciding how to measure productivity. Three studies of California family nurse practitioners and primary care physician's assistants demonstrated that these health practitioners were economically feasible in private practice and in a county-based hospital family practice program (O'Hara-Devereaux, Dervin, Andrus, & Judson, 1977). Other studies demonstrated that physician extenders increased both M.D. productivity and income in a cost-effective manner (Nelson, Jacobs, Cordner, and Johnson, 1975).

In a study that compared the cost-effectiveness of an FNP-staffed rural clinic with one staffed entirely by M.D.s, Siegal, Jenson, & Coffee (1977) found that the former was less expensive to operate, costing approximately $50,000 a year, as against $68,000 for the latter.

The evidence on quality of care is extensive and universally favorable to the new health practitioners. Several studies have shown that when patients are seen by N.P.s or P.A.s and later by physicians, the diagnosis and treatment almost always is in substantial agreement. Physicians associated with new health practitioners report that the quality of care they provide is either better than, or at least comparable to, that of M.D.s. Studies show that N.P. and P.A. adherence to established protocols is as good as or better than that of physicians. And finally, patient management by M.D.s and new health practitioners has been judged to be roughly equal by third party physician review (Bliss & Cohen, 1977).

In a paper in conjunction with the National Information Program on Rural Health Center Development, DeFriese and Bernstein (1979) reported on the results of the first nationwide longitudinal survey of rural health centers staffed by new health practitioners. Their study demonstrated that the rural center staffed by the new health practitioners was an important strategy to provide quality primary care services to underserved areas. The study found that even though the nation's medical schools were increasing their output of primary care physicians, the assumption that large numbers of doctors would migrate to rural areas was erroneous. The report cited as evidence for this conclusion the fact that increases in the volume of physician supply were not a sufficient force to overcome the many social, cultural, technological, and professional inducements to locate in suburban and urban areas.

The Institute of Medicine also studied new health practitioners in developing a health professions policy for primary care. The IOM study recommended that the number of new health practitioners being trained should remain at about 1980 levels. The study cited the continued importance of utilizing new health practitioners to provide high-quality economical services in rural areas, to augment and improve access to primary care in urban areas, and to serve as patient educators.

While the quality issue was largely resolved and questions of productivity were not unfavorable to these new practitioners, several key questions regarding their future in the health care system remained. With more than 20,000 nurse practitioners and physician's assistants in practice, and this number projected to grow as high as 40,000 by 1990, many policy makers felt the issue of competition with their physician colleagues could not be avoided much longer. There is a potential problem because the licensure of both groups depends on the concurrence of boards of medical examiners in most states. Many believed that organized medicine would attempt to disallow practice by the new groups as they had been functioning in the 1970s. Nevertheless, others pointed to the fact that nurse practitioners, and P.A.s to a somewhat lesser extent, continued to practice in many underserved areas unable to attract physicians. These issues no doubt could be expected to be the focus of considerable policy debate as the nation moves further into the 1980s.

Area Health Education Centers (AHECs)

The area health education centers (AHECs) program was an attempt to develop decentralized systems for educating health personnel so as to aid in the recruitment of health providers into high-need areas. In addition, the program was intended to build permanent regionally based education support systems to improve the retention of both new and existing health personnel in underserved areas and to ensure the continued offering of high-quality services.

The Carnegie Commission on Higher Education (1970) proposed development of a system of AHECs to address issues of maldistribution of the supply of health professionals. The Comprehensive Health Manpower Training Act of 1971, P.L. 92-157, the congressional response to the Carnegie report, was designed to encourage diverse experimental initiatives to promote improved distribution and increased access to care.

Specifically, the act encouraged the establishment or continuation of programs to alleviate shortages of health personnel in facilities located in designated high-need areas. This section of the law became the enabling legislation for the AHEC program. In the summer of 1972, funds were made available for the first 11 projects through five-year, incrementally funded, cost-shared contracts.

From 1972 to 1977, these 11 projects were the only ones supported by the Bureau of Health Professions, although several states started their own AHEC programs without federal funds. Under the 1976 Health Professions Educational Assistance Act, much stricter definitions of what constituted an AHEC project were written into law and funds to support development of new ones were made available. Since 1977, 12 new AHEC contracts have been awarded, and a total of 21 projects were operating in 1982.

Although from its inception the AHEC program was characterized by a considerable diversity of projects as each state sought to respond to local needs and priorities, the shared overall goals of the program were to:

- improve the geographic and specialty distribution of health care providers in rural (and now, urban) underserved areas
- improve the retention of health care providers in shortage areas
- improve the quality, utilization, and efficiency of health professionals in shortage areas

As an educational intervention, the AHEC program emphasizes primary care while maintaining a multidisciplinary focus. Undergraduate, graduate, and continuing education for health professionals takes place in AHEC regional centers on the premise that changing the educational process can provide effective incentives and support systems to encourage practitioners to locate and remain in underserved areas. With increased exposure to community practice, students not only are made more aware of the needs of underserved areas but also are trained in skills more relevant to those needs.

Although each regional center varies, even within the same state, most have the following types of educational programs:

- Undergraduate health professions education: P.L. 94-484 requires that 10 percent of the clinical educational experiences of medical students take place in a community setting apart from the university. Most programs have students in one or more of the following disciplines as well rotating to regional sites: nursing, pharmacy, dentistry, public health, or allied health.
- Primary care residency training: Most AHECs have either a free-standing family practice (or other primary care) residency program or receive residents on rotation from a university-based residency. These residencies have been the foundation for many AHEC programs, since

evidence is mounting that residents trained at a regional center are more likely to remain in the geographic area, and go to smaller towns in the region, than those trained at a university medical center. Given the political attention focused on the need to improve the supply of primary care physicians in underserved areas, residency training has been the most visible aspect of AHECs in many states.

- Continuing education and technical assistance: AHEC faculty and staff do extensive continuing education programming for health professionals in the region. These programs are conducted not only at the main center but also throughout the region. Before the development of AHECs, continuing education for many health practitioners, particularly in the allied health fields, generally was not available in the region where they worked. AHEC faculty and coordinators also provide considerable technical assistance to colleagues in hospitals and other health agencies in their region. Both the continuing education and technical assistance are designed not only to raise the quality of practice in community hospitals and health agencies but also to reduce isolation and thus improve the likelihood of retaining practitioners in smaller and more rural towns.

- Nurse practitioner or physician's assistant training: All AHECs started after 1976 are required to have an association with a midlevel primary care practitioner training program. Many of the original projects have them as well, for there is evidence that nurse practitioners or physician's assistants trained in regional sites show the same high retention rates as their physician colleagues and are willing to practice in many rural areas where physician private practice is not economically viable.

As of 1982, 21 of the 23 AHEC projects that had received federal funding remained active. These 21 operated 48 regional centers, with more than 30 additional centers planned by the newer projects.

Cost-sharing has been a federal requirement for AHEC projects from the outset, with each program required to pay a minimum of 25 percent of total contract expenses. This cost-shared support is provided in several ways, including indirect costs, direct state appropriations for the AHEC program (North Carolina, North Dakota, Colorado), state appropriations for educational components established under the project (South Carolina, Illinois, California), and private foundation monies (Navajo Indian and West Virginia). From 1972 to 1980, the total federal investment in the AHEC program reached $127 million, amounting to two-thirds of the total negotiated program cost of $190 million.

Several national studies have sought to evaluate the impact of the AHEC program in relation to its long-term goals of improved quantity, quality, and distribution of health practitioners. Since this is only one of a host of state and federal initiatives with similar long-term goals, and programmatically it is well integrated into other educational components, sorting out its specific effects has been difficult. Frequently, AHECs have had to rely on reporting educational accomplishments such as more primary care residency training, increased undergraduate medical education off-campus, or additional continuing education opportunities for health professionals.

Nevertheless, two national studies reported some clear evidence of AHEC's early impact on health professionals supply and distribution. The U.S. Department of Health, Education, and Welfare, in a 1978 report to Congress on assessment of the national AHEC program, presented the following findings:

- Physician supply in AHEC target counties grew 12.2 percent from 1972 to 1976, compared to an increase of 7.1 percent in similar counties throughout the United States without AHEC activities.
- The dentist-to-population ratios improved in the same years in AHEC target counties at a faster rate relative to non-AHEC counties.
- Graduates of medical schools with AHEC programs were more likely collectively to choose primary care residency positions than were graduates of medical schools without AHEC programs (PHS, 1979).

Although these data were for only the earliest years of the program when many AHEC activities still were getting organized, figures from specific states for more current years confirmed these trends. In North Carolina, for example, primary care residents trained at an AHEC center were much more likely to remain in the state to practice than those trained at a university medical center.

With the AHEC program in its second decade, several important issues must be faced:

- Will the lingering problems of maldistribution continue to provide sufficient justification for a relatively expensive educational intervention at a time of impending surpluses of physicians and some other health professionals?
- Will more direct interventions such as the National Health Service Corps appear to be more cost-effective to policy makers?
- Can local and state support for AHECs be sustained as the federal role in health professions training is diminished?

- Can AHEC programs be developed in urban settings with the same success as some of the earlier rural efforts?
- Will concerns for health professionals other than physicians (e.g., nurses and allied health) provide community-based programs such as AHEC a raison d'être?

These and similar policy questions must be addressed if AHEC is to maintain itself as a strong and viable option for long-term solutions to shortages and maldistribution of primary care and other health providers.

CONCLUSION

This chapter has reviewed historical trends in the supply and distribution of health professionals in the United States, in light of current and future demand for their services. Most of the critical policy questions concerning health personnel center on the issue of the appropriate level of continued federal support for health professions training and development.

If it were determined that the success of prior interventions, along with current market forces, was assuring the availability of well-trained health care providers to meet the nation's needs, the federal role in this area would continue to diminish. However, history has shown that certain underserved populations and regions are extremely difficult to serve equitably without active involvement by a variety of special programs designed to meet their needs. The rest of the decade of the 1980s is likely to see new policy directions that attempt to balance these somewhat divergent forces.

REFERENCES

Bliss, A.A., & Cohen, E.D. *The new health professionals: Nurse practitioners and physician's assistants.* Germantown, Md.: Aspen Systems Corporation, 1977.

Carnegie Commission on Higher Education. *Higher education and the nation's health: Policies for medical and dental education.* New York: McGraw-Hill, 1970.

CONSAD Research Corporation. "An evaluation of the effectiveness of loan forgiveness as an incentive for health practitioners to locate in medically underserved areas." (ASPE-73-4) NTIS No. PB 231 244/5.

DeFriese, G., & Bernstein, J. *Longitudinal study of the use of new health practitioners in rural health clinics.* Unpublished manuscript, 1979.

Dolan, A.K. *Occupational licensure and the obstruction of change in the health care delivery system: Some recent developments.* In R.D. Blair & S. Rubin (Eds.), *Regulating the professions: A public policy symposium.* Lexington, Mass.: Lexington Books, D.C. Heath and Company, 1980.

Fisher, D.W., & Horowitz, S.M. The physician's assistant: Profile of a new health professional. In A. Bliss & E.D. Cohen (Eds.), *The new health professionals: Nurse practitioners and physician's assistants*. Germantown, Md.: Aspen Systems Corporation, 1977.

Friedman, M. *Capitalism and freedom*. Chicago: The University of Chicago Press, 1962.

Friedson, E. *Professional dominance: The social structure of medical care*. New York: Atherton Press, 1970.

Galambos, E.C. *Supply and demand for registered nurses in the south, 1985*. Atlanta: Southern Regional Education Board, 1979.

Institute of Medicine. *A manpower policy for primary health care*. Washington, D.C.: National Academy of Sciences, May, 1978.

Lewis, C.E., Fein, R., & Mechanic, D. *A right to health: The problem of access to primary medical care*. New York: John Wiley & Sons, Inc., 1976.

Mason, H.R. Effectiveness of student aid programs tied to a service commitment. *Journal of Medical Education*, 1971, *46*, 577–583.

National Commission on Nursing. *Initial report and preliminary recommendations*. Chicago: The Hospital Research and Educational Trust, December 1981.

Nelson, E.C., Jacobs, A.R., Cordner, K., & Johnson, K.G. Financial impact of physician's assistants on medical practice. *The New England Journal of Medicine*, 1975, *293*, 527–530.

O'Hara-Devereaux, M., Dervin, J.V., Andrus, L.H., & Judson, L. Economic effectiveness of family nurse practitioners' practice in primary care in California. In A.A. Bliss & E.D. Cohen (Eds.), *The new health professionals: Nurse practitioners and physician's assistants*. Germantown, Md.: Aspen Systems Corporation, 1977.

Siegal, B., Jenson, D.A., & Coffee, E.M. Cost effectiveness of FNP versus MD-staffed rural practice. In A.A. Bliss & E.D. Cohen (Eds.), *The new health professionals: Nurse practitioners and physician's assistants*. Germantown, Md.: Aspen Systems Corporation, 1977.

Sorkin, A.L. *Health manpower: An economic perspective*. Lexington, Mass.: Lexington Books, D.C. Heath Company, 1977.

Surgeon General's Consultant Group on Medical Education. *Physicians for a growing America*. (Department of Health, Education, and Welfare, U.S. Public Health Service, Publication No. (PHS) 709). Washington, D.C.: U.S. Government Printing Office, 1959.

U.S. General Accounting Office. *Progress and problems in improving the availability of primary care providers in underserved areas*. (HRD 77-135). Washington, D.C.: U.S. Government Printing Office, 1978.

U.S. Public Health Service. *Training health manpower for underserved areas: A report to the people on the National Health Service Corps scholarship program* (Department of Health, Education, and Welfare, Health Resources Administration, Publication No. (HRA) 79-58). Washington, D.C.: U.S. Government Printing Office, 1980. (a)

U.S. Public Health Service. *Health United States, 1980* (Department of Health and Human Services, Publication No. (PHS) 81-1232). Hyattsville, Md.: 1981.

U.S. Public Health Service. *Summary report of the graduate medical education national advisory committee,* Vol. 1 (Department of Health and Human Services, Health Resources Administration, Publication No. (HRA) 81-651). Hyattsville, Md.: September 1980. (b)

U.S. Public Service. *Report of the graduate medical education national advisory committee*. Vol. 3, Geographic distribution technical panel (Department of Health and Human Services, Health Resources Administration, Publication No. (HRA) 81-653). Hyattsville, Md.: September 1980(c).

U.S. Public Health Service. *Supply and characteristics of selected health personnel* (Department of Health and Human Services, Health Resources Administration, Bureau of Health Professions, Publication No. (HRA) 82-20). Hyattsville, Md.: June 1981. (a)

U.S. Public Health Service. *The recurrent shortage of registered nurses* (Department of Health and Human Services, Health Resources Administration, Bureau of Health Professions, Publication No. (HRA) 81-23). Hyattsville, Md.: September 1981. (b)

U.S. Public Health Service. *An assessment of the national Area Health Education Center program* (Department of Health, Education, and Welfare, Health Resources Administration, Bureau of Health Manpower). Hyattsville, Md., November 9, 1979.

Western Interstate Commission for Higher Education. *Analysis and planning for improved distribution of nursing personnel and services* (Department of Health, Education, and Welfare, U.S. Public Health Service, Health Resources Administration, Bureau of Health Manpower, Publication No. (HRA) 79-16). Hyattsville, Md.: December 1978.

Chapter 12

Policy Issues in Dental Health

R. Gary Rozier

Several different dental delivery systems have been identified in the United States. Approximately 90 percent of personal dental health care is provided through only one of these—the private practice dental delivery system. The implied goal of each system is the maintenance of oral health status through the prevention of dental disease and resolution of explicit needs. Indicators of oral health status suggest that this goal is being achieved for only a limited number of people. While improvements are evident, dental disease or its sequelae continues to be the most prevalent health problem in the country. Dental disease annually takes its toll in terms of economic, social, and health consequences.

This chapter focuses on delivery of personal dental care, its impact on oral health, and alternatives for maximizing the level of oral health in the nation. This involves three components:

1. a description of the dental delivery system—the people and their needs; the providers and their services; and the administrative arrangements, such as financing, under which care is provided
2. a discussion of selected issues that have a direct and substantial impact on health
3. a presentation of alternatives for improved dental health

The terms personal dental health care and dental health services, while often used synonymously, imply different types of activities:

- Personal dental health care involves the preventive, diagnostic, or restorative services provided by a health professional on a one-to-one basis. The term is limited primarily to services provided in a clinical setting by a dentist or an auxiliary.

- Dental health services, on the other hand, imply a broader concept. They are services provided on a group or community basis, including primary preventive activities such as fluoridation of community water supplies, fluoride mouthrinse programs, and health education.

Any analysis of alternatives to the current delivery system must consider the role of both dental care and dental services in promoting and maintaining adequate oral health levels.

THE DENTAL CARE DELIVERY SYSTEM

The Nature of Dental Disease

About 265 categories of diseases or conditions involving the lips, oral cavity, and pharynx have been identified (WHO, 1978a). Diagnostic, preventive, and treatment services provided by dental personnel are related almost entirely to three of these conditions and their sequelae: dental caries, periodontal disease, and malocclusions. Therefore, this review deals only with these conditions.

Dental caries (tooth decay) is the most common disease known to humankind. The etiology of the disease is complex. A chain of events must occur before the carious process begins and progresses. Plaque (bacteria) on the teeth must ferment components of the diet (primarily sugars) to produce acid. The strength and duration of the acid attack are balanced by the resistance of the tooth. When that resistance is overcome by the acid challenge, demineralization of the tooth occurs. Given sufficient time for the process to occur repeatedly, demineralization to the point of a clinical cavity occurs.

Periodontal disease is a collective term used to denote one of several clinical entities affecting the supporting structures of the teeth. Like dental caries, the disease is bacterial in origin. Unlike dental caries, however, the progress of the disease is much more chronic, and obvious clinical signs most often go unnoticed by the individual. In its early inflammatory stages, referred to as gingivitis, the disease can be controlled without leaving permanent damage. Untreated, the disease usually progresses into periodontitis, which produces irreversible damage to the supporting tooth structures.

Both dental caries and periodontal disease lead to the loss of a staggering number of teeth in the population.

The relative importance of dental caries and periodontal disease in dental morbidity and tooth mortality varies during the life cycle of an individual.

Trend lines indicating how one example—the North Carolina population—is affected by dental caries and periodontal disease starting at age 5 are depicted in Figure 12-1.

Dental caries is a disease of major concern in children, adolescents, and young adults. Teeth are affected quickly by dental decay soon after they erupt into the mouth. After adolescence, there is a steady decline in the

Figure 12-1 Dental Morbidity and Tooth Mortality in North Carolina, 1976–77

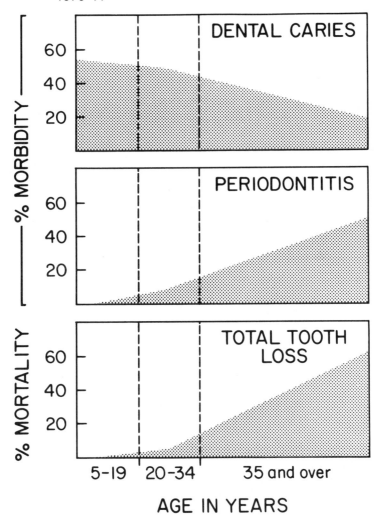

prevalence of decayed teeth. On the other hand, severe, destructive periodontal disease afflicts adults. Very few children suffer irreversible damage, but, with increasing age, more and more adults are affected with more periodontal disease in general as well as more of its severe forms. The cumulative result of dental disease is the increase in tooth loss in the adult population.

The third area of concern is dental occlusion, or the relationship of the teeth when the jaws are closed. A number of genetic or environmental factors acting alone or in combination may result in various degrees of deviation (called malocclusion) from the ideal occlusal state. Malocclusion is defined subjectively and depends on the amount of departure from an ideal occlusion that the individual is willing to accept.

Health Status Indicators in Dentistry

Over the years, dental epidemiologists have developed reliable and valid clinical indicators of the major conditions. Dental caries is universally measured by the DMF Tooth (T) or Surface (S) Index (Klein, Palmer, & Knutson, 1938). Each of the 32 permanent tooth spaces are scored as to whether they are normal or ever diseased. If ever diseased, the tooth must exhibit one of three conditions: (1) it may be untreated (*D*ecayed), or (2) show evidence of surgical treatment (*M*issing) or restorative treatment (*F*illed). The DMFT Index for an individual is the sum of these three conditions and can range from 0 to 32.

Periodontal disease is most commonly measured in prevalence surveys according to Russell's Periodontal Index (PI) (Russell, 1956). Criteria have been developed to classify the supporting structures of each tooth in the mouth as normal, having reversible disease (gingivitis), or having advanced, destructive disease (periodontitis). Disease prevalence and severity for a group can be quantified as (1) the percent of individuals with each condition or (2) an overall score derived by averaging individual tooth scores weighted according to the severity of conditions.

The Treatment Priority Index (TPI) describes the occlusion of the teeth (Grainger, 1967). Several characteristics of occlusion are used to derive a weighted score. Occlusal status may range from ideal occlusion (a score of 0) to very severe malocclusion (10 or more).

Oral Health Status

Dental Caries

Seven surveys of the oral health status of probability samples representing large noninstitutionalized populations have been conducted. National estimates are available from three cycles of the National Health Examination Survey (NHES I-III) conducted in 1960–1970 in which adults (Kelly, Van Kirk, & Garst, 1973), children (Kelly, Sanchez, & Van Kirk, 1973; Kelly & Scanlon, 1974), and youths (Kelly & Harvey, 1974; Kelly & Harvey, 1977) were examined clinically. The National Health and Nutrition Examination Survey (NHANES I) of 1971-1974 provided a second national estimate of oral health status and includes ages 1 through 74 years (Kelly & Harvey, 1979; Harvey & Kelly, 1981).

The National Institute of Dental Research (NIDR) completed the National Dental Caries Prevalence Survey (NDCPS) in 1979–1980 (U.S. PHS, 1981a). This included about 38,000 school children ages 5 to 17. Dental health estimates are available for one state, North Carolina, at two points in time (NC I and NC II) that are 13 years apart (Fulton, Hughes, & Mercer, 1965; Hughes, Rozier, & Ramsey, 1982).

Estimates for the mean DMFT scores and components per child 6 to 17 years of age obtained in each of the six surveys that included that age group are displayed in Table 12-1. If the NDCPS and the NC II are compared to earlier national and state data, respectively, an improvement in dental health is evident. For example, the national estimates indicated that for the age group 6 to 11 years, the occurrence of dental caries (mean DMFT scores) declined 35 percent and for the age group 12 to 17 years, 26 percent. In North Carolina, improvements of approximately 18 percent were evident.

Concurrent with the decline in dental caries were increases in restorative care and decreases in extractions of teeth. These improvements in dental health are supported by local surveys (DePaola, Soparkar, Allukian, DeVelis & Resker, 1981; Glass, 1981; Zacherl & Long, 1979). These trends result in large measure from increases in public preventive programs such as fluoridation and increased utilization of preventive and restorative care.

The NDCPS indicated that in 1979–1980, the 45.3 million school children aged 5 to 17 years had 4.77 DMFS and 2.91 DMFT per child. DMF teeth were distributed in the following manner: O DMFT, 36.6 percent; 1 to 4 DMFT, 39.8 percent; 5 to 8 DMFT, 15.9 percent; and 9 or more DMFT, 7.7 percent. The prevalence of DMFT was found to: (1) increase with age; (2) be slightly higher in females than males; (3) be lower in urban than in rural areas; and (4) vary regionally, with caries being highest in the Northeast and Far West, lowest in the Southwest, and intermediate in other areas.

The level of restorative care in school children was high. The Restorative Index (RI), or F/F + D percent, provided a rough estimate of the extent to which dental decay needs were being met (Jackson, 1973). While the RI in Table 12-1 varies considerably from survey to survey, the 1979–1980

Table 12-1 Average Number of DMFT, DMFT Components, and RI per Person

U.S. and North Carolina Children and Youths, 1960–80

Study	Year of Survey	Age Group	D	M	F	DMFT	RI
NHES II[1]	1963–1965	6–11	0.5	0.1	0.8	1.4	61.5
NHES III[2]	1966–1970	12–17	1.7	0.7	3.8	6.2	69.1
NHANES I[3]	1971–1974	6–11	0.7	0.1	0.8	1.7	53.3
		12–17	1.8	0.6	3.7	6.2	67.3
NC I[4]	1960–1963	6–11	1.0	0.2	0.5	1.7	33.3
		12–17	3.3	0.9	2.7	6.9	45.0
NC II[5]	1976–1977	6–11	0.7	0.1	0.7	1.4	50.0
		12–17	1.8	0.7	3.0	5.6	62.5
NDCPS[6]	1979–1980	6–11	0.3	0.0	0.8	1.1	72.7
		12–17	0.8	0.1	3.4	4.6	81.0

Sources:

1. *Decayed, Missing, and Filled Teeth Among Children: United States,* by J.E. Kelly and J.V. Scanlon, U.S. Department of Health, Education, and Welfare, Publication No. (HRA) 74-1003, Vital and Health Statistics Series 11, No. 106, U.S. Government Printing Office, May 1974.

2. *Decayed, Missing, and Filled Teeth Among Youths 12–17 years: United States,* by J.E. Kelly and C.R. Harvey, U.S. Department of Health Education, and Welfare, Publication No. (HRA) 75-1626, Vital and Health Statistics Series 11, No. 144, U.S. Government Printing Office, October 1974.

3. *Basic Data on Dental Examination Findings of Persons 1–74 years: United States, 1971–1974,* by J.E. Kelly and C.R. Harvey, U.S. Department of Health, Education, and Welfare, Publication No. (PHS) 79-1662, Vital and Health Statistics Series 11, No. 214, U.S. Government Printing Office, May 1979.

4. *The Natural History of Dental Diseases,* by J.T. Fulton, J.T. Hughes, and C.V. Mercer, University of North Carolina, School of Public Health, Department of Epidemiology, 1965.

5. *The Natural History of Dental Diseases in North Carolina, 1976–1977,* by J.T. Hughes, R.G. Rozier, and D.L. Ramsey, Carolina Academic Press, 1982.

6. *The Prevalence of Dental Caries in United States Children, 1979–1980: The National Dental Caries Prevalence Survey,* U.S. Department of Health and Human Services, National Institute of Dental Research, National Caries Program, Publication No. (NIH) 82-2245. Washington: December 1981a.

NDCPS indicated that between 73 percent and 81 percent of children's needs were being met.

Periodontal Disease

Periodontal disease is widespread. Information collected by the World Health Organization (1978b) from 35 countries indicated a very high prevalence (more than 75 percent) among persons aged 35 to 44 years in seven countries, a high prevalence (40 to 75 percent) in 13 countries, and a moderate prevalence (less than 40 percent) in 15 countries. According to the NHANES I, of the 41.2 percent of the United States population 6 to 74 years of age who had periodontal disease, 16.6 percent had one or more teeth with advanced disease.

Table 12-2 displays the percent distribution of persons in the NHANES I and the NC II 18–74 years of age according to a three-way classification: (1) without disease, (2) with disease but having gingivitis only, and (3) with advanced disease. Nationally, the percentage free of disease decreased from 56.5 percent at 18 to 44 years of age to 36.3 percent at 65 to 74 while the presence of destructive disease increased from 14.8 percent in the youngest group to 50.2 percent in the oldest.

Based on these estimates, about 54 million of the adult population at risk—the 110 million men and women with at least one permanent tooth—had periodontal disease. Of those affected, about 28 million had reversible disease only and 26 million had advanced, destructive disease. These estimates were conservative because diagnoses were made without a full complement of diagnostic aids. Moreover, they probably were biased

Table 12-2 Periodontal Disease in U.S. and North Carolina Adults

By Age Group

Study	Year of Survey	Age Group	Without Periodontal Disease (%)	With Periodontal Disease	
				Gingivitis (%)	Periodontitis (%)
NHANES I[1]	1971– 1974	18–44	56.5	28.7	14.8
		45–64	43.4	19.9	36.6
		65–74	36.3	13.5	50.2
NC II[2]	1976– 1977	18–44	37.9	50.5	11.6
		45–44	29.6	36.3	34.2
		65–74	25.2	30.6	43.9

Sources:

1. *Basic Data on Dental Examination Findings of Persons 1–74 Years: United States, 1971–1974,* by J.E. Kelly and C.R. Harvey, U.S. Department of Health, Education, and Welfare, Publication No. (PHS) 79-1662, Vital and Health Statistics Series 11, No. 214, U.S. Government Printing Office, May 1979.

2. *The Natural History of Dental Diseases in North Carolina, 1976–77,* by J.T. Hughes, R.G. Rozier, and D.L. Ramsey, Carolina Academic Press, 1982.

downward because of selective tooth survival. Many of the teeth lost might have had periodontal disease.

An alarming trend in periodontal disease has been occurring in North Carolina. The prevalence in children of all races and in nonwhite adults has increased since 1963, although the rise in children is primarily of the reversible type. However, in nonwhite adults, the increase in both gingivitis and periodontitis has been dramatic. The percent of at-risk teeth with pockets (Table 12-3) increased 2.6 times in nonwhite males and 1.7 times in nonwhite females between 1960 and 1977.

The prevalence of periodontal disease showed dramatic differences according to race and socioeconomic subgroups of the population. For example, in the NHANES I, blacks had 41 percent more disease than whites for ages 6 to 74. Periodontal disease was inversely related to income and education. In NHES I, almost three times more adults in the highest income group were without disease compared to the lowest group. These differences tended to disappear when groups were balanced by age and oral hygiene status. One epidemiologist suggested that about 90 percent of the variance in periodontal disease (as quantified by the PI Index) could be explained by these two variables—age and oral hygiene (Russell, 1963).

The impact of periodontal disease is significant in terms of both morbidity and socioeconomic consequences. An ad hoc scientific evaluation panel at the National Institute of Dental Research (U.S. PHS, 1976) estimated the annual cost of treatment at $1.5 billion for the 27 percent of the population seeking care. The cost of treatment for those having disease and not receiving care was put at billions more. Periodontal disease represents a significant health problem that has been ignored by the public and by health professionals. As of this writing, no geographic or political

Table 12-3 Percent of At-Risk Teeth with Advanced Disease

By Race and Sex, North Carolina 1960–1963 and 1976–1977

		% At-Risk Teeth with Pockets	
Race	Sex	1960–63	1976–77
White	Male	6.7	6.3
	Female	4.5	5.0
Nonwhite	Male	6.4	16.9
	Female	6.6	11.3

Sources: The Natural History of Dental Diseases in North Carolina, 1976–77, by J.T. Hughes, R.G. Rozier, and D.L. Ramsey, Carolina Academic Press, 1982.

jurisdiction had a policy for the prevention and control of periodontal disease.

The significance of the problem can be expected to increase in the future. As tooth decay continues to decline and fewer teeth are lost in children and young adults, more teeth will be at risk to disease. The social importance of disease is influenced by the perceived seriousness of other illnesses and problems. As the impact of tooth decay and the pain and discomfort that result from it lessen over the next decade, periodontal disease is most likely to assume more significance as a social and health problem.

Tooth Loss from Caries and Periodontal Disease

Dental caries and periodontal disease contribute about equally to tooth loss, together accounting for about 80 percent of the total. However, the significance of these two diseases varies by age. Dental caries is the most important determinant before age 30. During the span from 30 to 40, extractions because of periodontal disease increase rapidly and exceed those caused by caries for the remaining years. Approximately 20 percent of teeth are lost or absent because of accidents or congenital or prosthetic reasons (Waerhaug, 1966).

Partial and total tooth loss (edentulousness) represents a significant problem in the adult population. Among those 18 to 74 with one or more remaining teeth, 43.8 percent of DMFT were missing. Tooth loss was linearly related to age. By 45 to 54 years, more than half of DMFT and almost one-third of all teeth were missing. By ages 65 to 74, 68.5 percent of DMFT were missing. In general, blacks had more missing teeth than whites (Harvey & Kelly, 1981).

In the 1971–1974 span, approximately one out of four (23.9 percent) persons 18 to 74 years of age were edentulous in one or both arches. For the group 65 to 74, about two of three were edentulous in one or both arches (60.9 percent) (Harvey & Kelly, 1981).

Greene and Suomi (1977) estimated the economic impact of edentulousness in 1977 dollars to be about $5 billion for the population already having purchased dentures. It would have cost individuals or society about $1.5 billion for the 10 percent needing dentures, excluding treatment necessary before constructing dentures, repairing and refitting of ill-fitting ones, and time lost from work because of disease or treatment.

Malocclusion

Estimates from NHES I and II provided an indication of children's occlusal status. In those 6 to 11 years of age, 24 percent had normal occlusion, 39 percent had only minor manifestations, and 36 percent had definite malocclusion. The prevalence of malocclusion tended to be higher in those 12 to 17 than in the younger age group because of the larger number of teeth erupted. In the 12-to-17 age group, only 11 percent were normal according to the TPI, 35 percent had minor occlusal manifestations, and 54 percent had definite malocclusion. There were no differences in occlusal status associated with sex, race, family income, education, or geographic region.

Population Dental Care Needs

Spencer (1980) defined the need for dental care as "that quantity of dental health care which expert opinion judges ought to be consumed over a relevant time period, in order for people to remain or become as dentally healthy as is permitted by existing knowledge." Estimates of disease and its required treatment are necessary for planning and allocation of resources, priority setting, and evaluation. Yet the science of obtaining large population estimates of dental needs is not well developed. Research in this area is complicated by a number of factors, including the following:

- Treatment planning in a clinical setting requires assimilating relatively large volumes of data from sources including the physical examination, diagnostic and laboratory tests, and the medical history into a logical sequence of interrelated treatment events. Treatment planning in population-based surveys, or in nonclinical (field) settings must be done in a relatively short period of time using limited data. These survey conditions encourage independent considerations of conditions and their treatment rather than interrelationships of conditions.
- The limited data available to the diagnostician in the field result in pathology's going undetected. The degree to which field evaluations underestimate dental care needs has not been determined.
- Provider-defined treatment needs are influenced to a large degree by the training, experience, and attitudes of the provider. Dentists' decision-making processes in deciding on treatment are poorly understood and standardization of data collection efforts is difficult.
- Diagnostic and preventive services are associated more with a philosophy of care than with actual oral pathology. These services are subject to more variability than therapeutic needs.
- Most surveys of large populations must be cross-sectional because of the expense of longitudinal surveys. Therefore, only needs that exist at the time of the survey can be estimated; incremental ones cannot be.

Dental epidemiologists must seek solutions to these complex problems so that the limited data presented next can be expanded.

The NDCPS (Miller, Brunelle & Smith, 1982) emphasized the extensive need for treatment for children's dental caries despite the apparent improvements in oral health status. Based on these survey results, it was estimated that of children 5 to 17 years old:

- 37 percent needed some form of dental treatment
- more than 21 million primary tooth surfaces needed new or replacement fillings
- 3 million primary tooth extractions were required
- 1 million primary teeth required crowns
- 32 million permanent tooth surfaces needed restoration
- 1 million permanent tooth extractions were required
- 1.3 million crowns were required on permanent teeth
- 2 million permanent teeth needed replacement
- 1 million permanent teeth needed treatment for nerve damage.

The NHANES I indicated that in addition to these restorative needs, 6.4 percent of children 6 to 11 and 7.1 percent of those 12 to 17 needed treatment for severe malocclusion.

In the adult population, 61 to 73 percent needed at least one of nine specific dental services identified in NHANES I (Table 12-4). The largest percentage of persons 18 to 44 years needed decay treatment, followed by fixed bridges and/or partial dentures, and removal of debris and calculus. The largest number of 45-to-64-year-olds, like young adults, needed decay treatment and fixed bridges and/or partial dentures, but 19 percent in this range needed periodontal disease care, the most of any age group. In the 65-to-74 group, the largest percentage needed full dentures, followed by decay treatment and periodontal disease treatment.

Demand for Dental Care

Young and Striffler (1965) identified three subgroups of the population, each with a different level of "demand" for dental care:

1. those who had the desire to get care and the ability to do so; this is "effective demand" and usually is equated with utilization
2. those who also desired care but did not have the ability, financial or otherwise, to obtain it; this is referred to as "potential demand"
3. those who, even though they might recognize a health need, did not desire care and thus there was no demand

Table 12-4 Percent of Persons Aged 18–74 with Specific Dental
Treatment Needs

By Age, United States, 1971–74

Specific Dental Treatment Needed	Age		
	18–44	*45–64*	*65–74*
General (at Least 1 of the Following):	72.7	67.5	61.0
Removal of Debris and Calculus	22.4	13.5	8.4
Gingivitis Treatment	13.8	6.9	3.5
Periodontal Disease Treatment	12.2	19.3	15.4
Severe Malocclusion Treatment	0.9	—	—
Decay Treatment	49.3	30.1	17.9
Extractions, Any Reason	5.8	8.4	9.8
Fixed and/or Partial Bridges	25.3	23.3	8.5
Repair Denture or Bridge	1.9	6.7	7.7
Construct Full Denture	4.2	15.6	24.8

Source: Basic Data on Dental Examination Findings of Persons 1–74 Years: United States, 1971–1974, by J.E. Kelly and C.R. Harvey, U.S. Department of Health, Education, and Welfare, Publication No. (PHS) 79-1662, Vital and Health Statistics Series 11, No. 214, U.S. Government Printing Office, May 1979.

One comprehensive review of the literature identified 16 different measures of utilization in 44 different studies (Bauer, Pierson, & House, 1978). Utilization most commonly is measured as the annual number of visits per person; the second most common measure is the percentage of the population visiting a dentist on an annual basis. This section examines the population in terms of (1) the proportion of the population and characteristics of those using dental services, (2) the average number of visits per person, and (3) the types of services used.

While improvement was evident, utilization of dental services remained relatively low in the United States. During the years between 1963 and 1979, those with no dental visits in the previous year declined from about 58 percent of the population to about 50 percent. Similarly, the proportion who had never visited the dentist declined and, in 1979, was at about 9 percent. Aggregate utilization of services per person remained constant. Over that same 1963–1979 span, the annual number of dental visits per person varied very little from 1.6 per year (Wilder, 1982). Utilization of services was localized in a small segment of the population—in 1974, 25 percent of the population accounted for 75 percent of all dental visits (Newman & Larsen, 1980).

Newman and Larsen analyzed data from two national surveys in terms of utilization according to characteristics of the population and what changes occurred during the decade 1964–1974. Characteristics considered as explanatory variables were demographic (age, sex, race, family size, and life cycle), social structure (occupation and education of household head), family resources (family income, ability to pay, and dental insurance coverage), community resources (region and community type), and self-perception of need (perceived condition of teeth and perceived need for dental care). The effects of some of these variables as determined in their study are summarized:

Age: Utilization by age was lowest in the extremes of the life cyle, with the highest in the 14-to-24 group. Differences in use by age declined somewhat over the decade.

Sex: Females averaged more visits than males in 1974, 1.8 to 1.5 per year.

Race: Utilization on the basis of race was strikingly different. In 1974, whites had 1.0 more visits per year than nonwhites, a differential that had not changed in ten years.

Education of Household Head: There was a direct relationship between education and number of dental visits. As the education of the head of the household increased from eight years or less to college graduate, mean visits increased from 0.8 to 2.7.

Occupation of Household Head: There was an association between occupation of household head and utilization. Professional-managerial and clerical-sales categories evidenced the highest utilization, 2.3 visits per person, with the lowest utilization, 1.0 visits per person, among laborers. The other categories were intermediate at 1.2 to 1.4.

Family Income: Income was related to utilization but the relationship most likely was not linear. An income threshold appeared to distinguish low users from high users. In 1974 this threshold was about $8,000; families with incomes below $8,000 had mean visits of 1.0. For those with incomes of $8,000 or above, use increased with income, reaching 3.1 visits per person in families with incomes of $25,000 or more. The effect of family income still was evident when age, sex, and race were controlled.

Region and Community Type: In 1974 the Northeast had the highest utilization, followed by the West, North Central, and the South. The differential between the lowest and highest was 1 visit. Urban residents had a higher utilization than rural residents but the differential improved during the decade.

Newman and Larsen (1980), analyzing the relative importance of these variables in explaining utilization of dental services, reported family resources (insurance coverage and family income) to be the most important. Community resources were found to have a low predictive value. Demographic (age and race, in particular), social structure (education and occupation), and perceived need (perceived condition of teeth and need for care) were of medium importance in relation to the other variable groups.

Table 12-5 shows the proportion of persons provided with different types of dental services in 1963–1964 and in 1971, classified as follows: examinations, cleaning teeth, fillings, denture work, extractions, straightening teeth, and gum treatment. In general, the distribution of services changed between 1963 and 1971 as preventive care increased while therapeutic and rehabilitative treatments decreased. The number of visits for examination, cleaning, or straightening teeth increased, those for filling or extraction declined, and those for denture work or gum treatment remained virtually the same.

After analyzing data from a 1977 practice-based survey, Douglass and Cole (1979) suggested that an important trend could be occurring in the kinds of services being provided. They identified crown and bridge services as the primary reason for 13.5 percent of all visits. These services represented a significant proportion of dentists' time (20 percent) and charges

Table 12-5 Percent Distribution of Dental Visits by Type of Service 1963–1971

| | Percent Distribution | |
Type of Service	1963–64[1]	1971[2]
Examination	21.1	23.8
Cleaning Teeth	13.6	17.8
Fillings	37.8	29.7
Denture Work	13.2	13.3
Extractions	15.0	12.3
Straightening Teeth	5.8	8.5
Gum Treatment	3.6	3.3

Sources:
1. *Volume of Dental Visits, United States, July 1963–June 1964,* U.S. Department of Health, Education, and Welfare, National Center for Health Statistics, PHS Publication Series 10, No. 23), U.S. Government Printing Office, October 1965.
2. *Current Estimates from the Health Interview Survey, United States, 1971,* U.S. Department of Health, Education, and Welfare, National Center for Health Statistics, PHS Publication Series 10, No. 79, U.S. Government Printing Office, February 1973.

(32 percent). Such visits were the third most frequent, behind those for fillings and for examinations and x-rays.

Supply of Dental Personnel

Dentistry ranks fourth among the health professions in the number of trained personnel, behind nursing, medicine, and pharmacy. The dental work force consists of five types of providers:

1. Dentists, who represent about 35 percent of the work force, are responsible for diagnosis and prescription of treatment and drugs and provide most of the care.
2. Dental hygienists also provide direct patient care but it is limited to the primary prevention of dental caries and periodontal disease.
3. Dental assistants aid dentists and hygienists at chairside and represent the largest proportion of the work force. In some states a specially trained dental assistant, an expanded function dental assistant (EFDA), is allowed to perform direct patient care, primarily reversible procedures, under the direct supervision of dentists.
4. Technicians assist the dentist through the fabrication of intraoral appliances such as dentures. Most technicians work outside the dental office in commercial laboratories and have little if any patient contact.
5. The denturist, the newest member of the dental work force, has been legally recognized in four states. Denturists are permitted in those states to perform direct intraoral procedures necessary for denture care.

Dentists

In 1979 there were 117,223 professionally active dentists, or one dentist for every 1,858 persons in the country. This total included clinical practitioners, dental school faculty or staff, dentists in the armed forces or public health field, members of hospital and health organization staffs, graduate students, and those involved in residency programs. The American Dental Association (ADA) estimated that there were 2,076 people in the United States for each dentist involved directly in delivering personal dental health care. The overwhelming majority of active dentists were in general practice (ADA, 1979a).

The ADA recognizes eight dental specialties—oral and maxillofacial surgery, endodontics, orthodontics, pedodontics, periodontics, prosthodontics, oral pathology, and public health. Specialization grew rapidly during the 1960s and 1970s, increasing by 500 percent from 2,751 in 1955 to 16,595 in 1979. However, the number of specialists represented only about 13 percent of active dentists. Based on new enrollment slots in education programs, specialization seemed to be leveling off. Six of ten specialists were either orthodontists (39 percent) or surgeons (23 percent). The remaining 38 percent was composed of periodontists (13 percent), pedodontists (12 percent), endodontists (7 percent), prosthodontists (5 percent), oral pathologists (1 percent) and public health dentists (1 percent) (AADS, 1980).

The supply of dentists was unevenly distributed throughout the United States. More than 80 percent of the country's counties had dentist-to-population ratios less favorable than the national average. The distribution of professionally active general practitioners and dental specialists in 1979 in the nine regions defined by the United States Census is presented in Table 12-6. The lowest population figures per dentist, for both general dentists and specialists, were in the Middle Atlantic, Pacific, and New England areas. The East South Central region, composed of Alabama, Kentucky, Mississippi, and Tennessee, had the largest number of people per generalist or specialist in the nation.

The supply of dentists was limited by the capacity of dental schools to train them. Under national legislation, the number of schools and the size

Table 12-6 Number of Active Dentists and Population per Active Dentist

By Region and Practice Type, 1979

	Number of		Population/Active	
Geographic Area	General Practitioners	Specialists	General Practitioner	Specialist
New England	6,599	1,137	1,867	10,836
Middle Atlantic	20,526	2,958	1,818	12,614
South Atlantic	13,484	2,323	2,568	14,907
East South Central	4,625	675	3,009	20,615
East North Central	17,793	2,360	2,314	17,447
West North Central	7,464	929	2,280	18,318
West South Central	7,739	1,155	2,815	18,864
Mountain	4,924	711	2,070	14,333
Pacific	16,287	2,711	1,807	10,859
U.S. Total	99,441	14,959	2,190	14,559

Source: Reprinted from *Distribution of Dentists in the United States by State, Region, District, and County,* by permission of American Dental Association, Bureau of Economic and Behavioral Research, © 1979.

of graduating classes increased substantially starting in 1965. As a result of the Health Professions Educational Assistance Act (HPEA) of 1963, dental school enrollments increased from 14,020 in 1965 in 49 schools to 21,510 in 1977 in 59 schools (Ake & Johnson, 1979).

By 1970, the dentist-to-population ratio that had steadily worsened since the 1950s began to improve. Using an econometric model for the dental sector, the Bureau of Health Manpower estimated that the number of dentists would increase to one dentist for every 1,366 persons in 1995 (Hixon & Mocniak, 1979). These projections were based on the assumption that the number of graduates would remain constant through 1995 but with the decline in national subsidies to dental schools, that no longer may be valid. Some schools announced reductions in class size, others were studying such moves, and a few faced closing.

Allied Dental Personnel

The supply of dental hygienists, assistants, and laboratory technicians increased substantially after 1950. These providers represented about 65 percent of the dental work force.

In 1977 there were 32,200 active dental hygienists, or 27 per 100 active dentists—a tenfold increase over the 1950 total. The geographic distribution varied from a high of 45 hygienists per 100 dentists in New England to a low of 23 per 100 in the Mountain region (Ake & Johnson, 1979). Active dental hygienists tended to be young, about half of those licensed in 1979 being under 30 years of age. About 70 percent were employed as dental hygienists and 86 percent had worked as hygienists during the 1976–1978 period. This suggested that dental hygienists might remain in the work force to a greater extent than had been thought. About 90 percent of working hygienists were employed in private practice (Malvitz & Mocniak, 1982).

There were 144,700 dental assistants in 1977, or 123 per 100 active dentists. Information was not available on the proportion of expanded function dental assistants (EFDAs); however, by 1978 there were 7,000 graduates from 61 EFDA training projects.

The number of active dental laboratory technicians in 1977 was 45,100, or 38 per 100 dentists. More than 75 percent of the technicians were employed in commercial dental laboratories (Ake & Johnson, 1979).

The Nature of Dental Practice

Dental health services are provided to the public through a number of different delivery systems. The Division of Dentistry, Department of Health,

Education, and Welfare (U.S. PHS, 1977a) identified 19 distinct systems. The agency defines such a system as "an organized group of related and interdependent activities that can be bounded because they are designed to accomplish a purposeful objective; the objective of a dental delivery system is the resolution of explicit dental needs through the delivery of the dental services."

The delivery systems defined by the Division of Dentistry include: federally sponsored programs such as the military, community health centers, Veterans Administration, the National Health Service Corps, and the Indian Health Service; state or locally sponsored efforts in health departments and in prisons and jails; educational programs; hospital, industry, nursing home, and school-based activities; dental cooperatives; health maintenance organizations (HMOs); research and demonstration projects; incremental dental care programs; philanthropic and foundation-sponsored programs; and the private practice delivery system.

The private practice system represents the predominant mode. The ADA (1979a) indicated that 88.2 percent of active dentists in the United States listed themselves as primarily private practitioners. The rest gave their practice settings as follows: 3.4 percent in the armed forces, 2.8 percent in dental schools, 1.4 percent in federal service other than the military (i.e., Veterans Administration, U.S. Public Health Service), 1.2 percent in local and state government, 1.9 percent in academic programs as residents or interns, 0.8 percent in hospitals as members of dental staffs, and 0.3 percent in other health/dental organizations. Since the great majority of dental care was provided through private practice, this description of the nature of dental practice concentrates on that type of service.

The ADA periodically surveys dentists to provide information on selected characteristics of private practice. This discussion relies on the most recent of these as of the date of writing, the *1979 Survey of Dental Practice,* the 12th in the series of such analyses (ADA, 1982).

Ownership and Practice Arrangements

Slightly more than 95 percent of the 88.2 percent cited previously own their own practices. There are a number of different ownership arrangements. These can be divided into three classifications: (1) sole proprietor, (2) shareholder-incorporated, and (3) partnership. Sole proprietor is defined as a dentist who is the only owner of an unincorporated practice; 67 percent are in this category, the great majority of them (87.5 percent) as solo practitioners. In the second group are 25 percent of the dentists, who were classified as having a sharcholdcr-incorporated ownership, i.e., owned some or all of an incorporated practice. In most states, solo practitioners are allowed to incorporate their practices, thus receiving tax benefits. The majority (60.5 percent) of dentists owning an incorporated practice were in solo practice. About 4 percent of dentists were in partnership with one or more others in which the practice was jointly owned. Most of these dentists (61.8 percent) were in partnership with only one other, 24.1 percent with two others, and 14 percent with three or more others.

Group practice has been advocated as an organizational arrangement that results in improved productivity while controlling costs and maintaining quality. Dentists showed a growing tendency to practice together. As of 1979, 27 percent of dentists were in practice with one or more others, up from 22 percent in 1977. Not all of these practices met the definition of a group practice, however. The Public Health Service (PHS) and American Academy of Dental Group Practice defined a group practice as one in which (1) three or more dentists were organized to provide dental care; and (2) the dentists operated according to a formal arrangement in which they shared patient care responsibility, professional skills, facilities, personnel, income, and/or expenses.

A 1971 PHS survey to determine the extent to which group practice had been adopted by the dental profession identified 715 groups as meeting the definition above. There were 3,148 dentists practicing in the groups, an average of 4.4 per practice. Groups ranged in size from 3 to 30 dentists. In terms of type of practice, slightly more than half were general practice groups, and 25 percent were composed of both generalists and specialists. The survey indicated that group practice was a relatively new phenomenon, with the largest number of groups being formed since 1965 (U.S. PHS, 1972a).

Utilization of Personnel

More than 94 percent of solo dentists employed one or more auxiliary persons while only 5.5 percent had none. Of solo dentists, 14 percent employed one auxiliary; 21 percent, two; 26 percent, three; and 34 percent, four or more. Very few dentists had bookkeepers (19 percent) or laboratory technicians (5.5 percent). The majority of dentists had one or more chairside assistants (88 percent) or secretaries/receptionists (75 percent). Slightly less than half of the solo dentists employed hygienists.

Working Time

Independent dentists worked an average of 46.7 weeks during 1978 in their primary practice location for an average of 43.1 hours a week. Practice activities per week were distributed as follows: 33.0 hours on treating patients, 2.5 on laboratory procedures, 1.5 on filing prepayment and/or government forms, 0.9 of an hour in bookkeeping procedures, 1.8 on professional reading; 0.8 on other activities (e.g., training employees), and 3.7 hours on personal time (lunch, etc.).

Dentists practicing alone had a median of 1,500 patients of record. They treated 59.5 patients in 70.5 visits per week. Productivity tended to increase with age, peaking at 45 to 49 years and then declining. Incorporated dentists tended to treat more patients than did sole proprietors. The median number of emergency cases seen each week for new patients was 3.0 and for patients of record was 3.4.

Referrals

Most general dentists were completely self-contained and depended very little on other facilities or resources in the community. The general professional isolation was highlighted by the number of patients whom solo dentists received on a referral basis. The median percentage of referral patients from another practicing dentist or physician for all solo dentists was a remarkably low 4.9 percent. On the other hand, about 75 percent of specialists' patients were referrals.

Factors in Practice Busyness

The ADA's 1979 Survey of Dental Practice gave three indicators of practice busyness: (1) waiting time to schedule an initial appointment for new patients and patients of record, (2) waiting time in the office for a scheduled appointment, and (3) dentists' own estimate of their busyness. The waiting time for an initial appointment in a series for patients of record was 7.1 days. In general, the median waiting time for a new patient for a nonemergency appointment was less than for a patient of record—6.6 days. The median waiting time in the office for scheduled appointments was 8.4 minutes.

Dentists' own perceptions of how busy they were was measured by asking survey participants to indicate which of the following statements most closely represented their situation: (1) too busy to treat all people requesting appointments, (2) provided care to all who requested appointments but felt overworked, (3) provided care to all who requested appointments and did not feel overworked, and (4) not busy enough and would have liked more patients.

Slightly more than half (52.3 percent) of dentists felt that they provided care to all requesting appointments and were not overworked. Another 24.8 percent were not busy enough, 14.6 percent were overworked, and 8.3 percent could not treat all patients requesting appointments. The distribution of respondents across these four categories had changed slightly since the 1977 Survey of Dental Practice (ADA, 1978a). Compared to 1978, a larger proportion of dentists had turned patients away or felt overworked in 1976 and a smaller proportion had believed they had the right number of patients or were not busy enough.

Income

Solo practitioners in 1979 reported a median gross income of $100,000 for their primary practices. The cost of operating a dental practice was high, however. Dentists netted about 42 percent of gross. More than half of overhead expense was for two items—salaries and commercial dental laboratory charges. Income was found to vary according to age, practice type, number of patient-care operatories (treatment rooms), number of auxiliaries, and geographic region. Income tended to peak at 45 to 49 years of age and was higher in specialty practice than general practice. Income increased as the number of operatories and auxiliaries increased. For example, the median net income of solo dentists with one operatory and no auxiliary was $21,988; this increased to a high of $79,500 among those with five or more operatories and zero to five auxiliaries.

Purchasing Dental Care

Health expenditures in the United States in 1980 as estimated by Gibson and Waldo (1981) totaled $247.2 billion, a substantial 15.2 percent increase over 1979. This was the largest advance in 15 years. During 1980, the overall economy grew by only 8.8 percent so health expenditures represented a greater portion of the gross national product (GNP) in that year than before, rising from 8.9 percent in 1979 to 9.4 percent in 1980.

Expenditures for the professional dental care portion of the total health bill in 1980 were estimated at $15.9 billion, or 6.4 percent. Expenditures per person were $68.42 in 1980, a gain of about $10 over 1979. The purchase of dental care traditionally has been sensitive to buying power but 1980 data indicated that this might be changing to some extent. Despite an increase in fees because of higher labor costs and gold and silver prices (the Consumer Price Index showed a 12 percent rise for dental care compared to 10.6 percent for medical services) and a slumping economy, adjusted expenditures per person increased for dental services. This increase in real expenditures in the face of rising costs and less disposable income might reflect the effect of growing dental insurance coverage. The potential for utilizing more services, as well as costlier ones, was greater if financial barriers to purchase of care were lessened or removed.

Douglass and Day (1979) estimated the type and costs of services according to three broad categories of dental care bought in 1977. Using data from a national office practice survey, they estimated that of the total expenditure of $10 billion in 1977, $769 million (7.7 percent) was for preventive services, $4,972 million (49.6 percent) for basic corrective services (diagnostic, operative, removable prosthetics, and surgery), and $4,281 million (42.7 percent) for reconstructive services (fixed prosthetics, periodontics, endodontics, and orthodontics). They also pointed out that high technology crown and bridge reconstructive services had become the nation's largest single dental expense item—about 35 percent of the total.

Dental health insurance coverage grew rapidly after 1967. In that year, there were fewer than 5 million eligible dental beneficiaries. By the end of 1980, an estimated 80.5 million persons or more than one-third of the United States population of 226.5 million, had dental expense protection (Health Insurance Association of America, 1982). A large portion of this growth occurred in the mid-1970s as a result of collective bargaining. Large numbers of individuals were covered with comprehensive plans in single negotiations. For example, a dental benefit plan negotiated in 1974 by the United Auto Workers covered about 3 million persons—union members and their families—nationwide.

Private insurance company group plans provided about 60 percent of the insurance coverage; independent plans such as dental service corporations, HMOs and union self-insurance trusts, about 30 percent; and Blue Cross and Blue Shield plans about 10 percent (Health Insurance Association of America, 1982). Three-fourths of dental insurance plans were comprehensive and included a full range of preventive, restorative, and reconstructive services. Most comprehensive plans required some out-of-pocket payments, however. Ninety percent called for one or more of three types of cost-sharing—deductibles, copayments, or maximum benefits. Copayment was the most common cost-sharing arrangement (U.S. PHS, 1981b).

Even with the rapid growth of insurance, a large proportion of total costs for dental care was paid directly by consumers using disposable income. In 1980, about three-quarters of dental care costs ($12 billion) were paid directly by consumers, about one-fifth ($3.3 billion) by private insurance, and only a very small proportion by tax dollars ($0.6 billion), primarily federal and state expenditures for Medicaid (Gibson & Waldo, 1981).

Of the $68.42 per capita dental expenditure in 1980, consumers paid $51.61 (or 75.4 percent) directly out of pocket. Expenditures for physician services were almost three times as expensive, at $201.18 per person, but consumers paid only about a third of that out of pocket. For the single most expensive personal health service item—hospital care, costing $429.80 per person—consumers paid less than 10 percent directly (Gibson & Waldo, 1981).

SOME ISSUES IN PERSONAL DENTAL HEALTH

The many policy issues in the delivery of dental care in the United States that have or will have a direct and substantial impact on all Americans include the oral health status of the people, the professional and allied personnel providing service, and the quality and financing of treatment.

Decline of Dental Caries

Dental caries was documented as early as the 1930s as the most prevalent chronic disease in the United States (Dean, 1946). A commonly accepted statistic is that 95 of 100 people are affected with dental caries at some point during their lifetimes. Many characteristics of the disease process and its diagnosis and treatment have led to an emphasis on caries in both the private and public sector:

- The magnitude of the problem and the postwar increased birth rate highlighted the issue and mobilized societal support for public programs, especially for children.
- The condition is relatively easy to diagnose by a professional and appropriate treatment consistent with the diagnosis is easily determined. Consumer self-diagnosis is possible in many cases at a stage when the tooth can be treated successfully. Consumers are oriented toward looking for defects in their teeth as children, not toward other oral health problems such as periodontal disease or oral cancer. This orientation continues into adulthood.
- Available prevention and control modalities are highly successful. The occurrence of dental caries and need for treatment can be reduced by one-half through community fluoridation. Fluoridation, combined with other preventive activities used on a regular basis—such as application of sealants, topical fluorides, and plaque control—can almost eliminate decay. Techniques are available to restore affected teeth at relatively low cost with materials that are long lasting. The effectiveness of restorative dental treatment on oral health led McKeown (1976) to suggest that if we are admitted to heaven based on our deeds on earth, obstetricians, physicians treating medical emergencies, and dentists are likely to be the first of those in the medical profession to enter.
- The disease and its sequelae are more likely to result in an acute condition requiring treatment. The public knows that pain, infection, difficulty in eating, or poor esthetics are likely to result in a relatively short period of time if dental caries are not treated. On the other hand,

periodontal disease can be present for years before it becomes serious enough to be considered by the public as an "acute" condition. Periodontal disease manifests itself at an age at which the public has come to expect dental, as well as other health problems associated with aging, to manifest themselves.

As documented earlier, the patterns of dental disease are changing. A decline in national caries rates is well documented. A similar trend in other developed countries is evident and has been referred to as the "rise and fall of dental caries" (Heloe & Haugejorden, 1981). Combined with declining birth rates and an increase in supply of personnel and treatment, dental caries is becoming less of a problem. On the other hand, periodontal disease continues to be highly prevalent and there is some indication that it may even be increasing in blacks (Hughes et al., 1982).

The implications of this decline in caries are far reaching and can impact on other oral diseases. Dubos (1960) suggested that an ideal health state was a mirage. As basic biological research and/or clinical practice masters any one disease in human populations, another will come to the forefront. Thus, complete health is an ideal state that can never be achieved. As caries is prevented and tooth mortality resulting from it is reduced, other dental conditions are likely to surface or become defined by society as a greater problem. Even without an increase in periodontal disease, its prevalence may increase by virtue of the fact that more teeth are available to be affected. Since teeth are retained through childhood and periodontal disease occurs in adulthood, recession of supporting structures will occur, exposing tooth roots. Roots are less resistant to tooth decay than the coronal structure and thus root decay will become a problem.

The increase in tooth retention and consequent growth in root caries and periodontal disease risks may apply to only younger and middle-aged adults, however. The reduction in dental caries may not translate into significant gains in tooth retention in older adults. Given the current dental behavior of the public and the small amount of periodontal treatment being provided, tooth mortality rates may remain the same for this age group. Teeth may be being preserved in children and young adults only to be lost to periodontal disease later in life. Studies indicate that fluoridation is truly a preventive measure and does not merely delay the onset of dental caries (Jackson, 1974).

The analogy can be made between death rates resulting from infectious and chronic diseases and tooth mortality rates attributable to dental caries and periodontal disease. Death rates have declined significantly since the early 1900s. In 1900 a newborn was expected to live to age 47. In 1977 the life expectancy at birth had increased 26 years to 73 years. During that same period, the life expectancy of the average 45-year-old increased only five years, presumably because of the unchanging influences of chronic diseases over that time (U.S. PHS, 1979a). The argument can be made that fluoridation programs, despite their effectiveness in reducing the prevalence of dental caries, will not impact significantly on tooth mortality—that, as noted, teeth of children and young adults are being preserved, only to be lost to other causes as those individuals grow older.

In the private practice sector, the trend in dental disease could have a tremendous impact on both traditional delivery systems and the justification for alternative systems. Dentists traditionally have practiced according to the medical model, with emphasis on restorative or reparative dentistry. More than 75 percent of general dentists' time is devoted to diagnosis of dental caries problems and restorative and reconstructive treatment of this one disease process and resulting conditions. For example, decayed and broken teeth are "cured" by replacing the diseased structure with very durable materials and missing teeth are supplanted by prosthetic appliances.

A reduction in the need for these curative services can reduce the providers' workload and reduce "busyness." To maintain workloads, dentists will have to expand the scope of their practices by treating more complex problems, increasing the number of periodontal services, or expanding patient flow. Some of these new areas, especially periodontal disease, require different skills and, above all, different concepts of prevention and treatment. Prevention and treatment of periodontal cases requires an understanding of the behavioral model of disease causation in which such factors as life style and individual behaviors (e.g., eating too many sweets) are the primary cause of the disease. Dentistry's traditional orientation to acute disease management and the philosophy that a patient is either cured or diseased fails to recognize the etiology of periodontal disease and the various degrees of remission after therapy.

Certain dental specialists also may be affected by the decline in caries rates. Most noticeable in the short term will be pedodontists who spend more than half of their time just in treatment of dental caries. There already are discussions in the profession that pedodontics should be combined with orthodontics as a single specialty.

The increasing significance of periodontal disease in the face of declining caries rates should stimulate experimentation with alternative delivery systems. Dental hygienists who are trained in the primary and secondary prevention of periodontal disease are suggesting that access to their services, and thus improvement in periodontal health, can be effected through changes in supervision clauses of dental practice acts. By allowing them to work under general supervision or even in independent practice, hygienists would be able to serve in remote private or public sector settings and thus increase the supply of services.

Unless reductions in caries are combined with increased efforts in prevention, costs for dental care can be expected to increase. Improvements in tooth mortality rates should result in people's having dentitions that require maintenance for longer periods of time. As teeth are retained, shifts toward complex, highly technological restorative procedures and periodontal services can occur unless rigorous preventive activities are maintained throughout life. Prevention and control of periodontal disease is very personnel-intense. Research has shown that control can be achieved through frequent (every two to three months) professional tooth cleanings (Axelsson & Lindhe, 1981).

Changing disease patterns will affect predoctoral education and continuing education of practicing professionals. Dental education is structured much like private practice in that it is oriented in didactic and clinical time and in philosophy toward the medical model. An overwhelming percentage of dental curricula are focused on diagnosis of dental caries and its cure through alternative restorative and reconstructive treatment modes. Dental schools are experiencing a shortage of teaching patients just as private practitioners are facing a shortage of patients. More basic questions in dental education are raised as to the amount of curriculum time that should be devoted to the restorative and reconstructive disciplines such as operative, prosthetics, and pedodontics relative to periodontics, orthodontics, oral medicine, oral pathology, and behavioral factors, given the epidemiology of dental disease.

Public programs also may feel the effects of changes in disease patterns. As dental caries becomes less of an issue, feasible, practical, and effective ways of dealing with what now is the major public health problem— periodontal disease—must be found. Difficult but important policies must be developed at local, state, and federal levels.

Are educational programs directed at changing behavior and placing responsibility for health on the individual to be encouraged? In many cases, the resources involved in controlling periodontal disease will have to be in addition to those being used for other preventive programs such as fluoridation. If caries prevention programs are discontinued, caries rates will rise.

Societal values have placed great emphasis on treatment programs for children. Is society willing to shift values to the control of periodontal disease? Horowitz (1981) suggested that the reduction in caries might have a backlash effect on public programs. As dental caries becomes less of a problem, the public may be less inclined to accept programs that are offered because of a perception that they no longer are needed.

Appropriateness and Necessity of Care

In little more than a decade there has been an explosion of interest in quality assurance. Health planners, administrators, and researchers all have been involved in defining issues and their resolution in this relatively new area of health care delivery. The national policy on quality of health care was expressed first in the 1972 federal legislation creating professional standards review organizations (PSROs). This stimulated research and demonstrations designed to develop practical and scientifically sound quality assurance mechanisms.

The initiative for research in this area was assumed first by the federal government and later transferred largely to the private sector when, in 1976, the W. K. Kellogg Foundation allocated $2.5 million for a research program in dental quality assurance. The American Fund for Dental Health administered the Kellogg funds through a National Dental Quality Assurance Advisory Committee and supported 13 projects over three and a half years. In 1981, the ADA established an office of quality assurance to coordinate professional activities in this area (Quality Assurance, 1982).

For several reasons, data needed for defining the many and complex policy issues in dental quality assurance were not available or were severely limited as of this writing. What information existed was not focused and tended to be unrepresentative in nature. Demonstration and research projects had concentrated on development of methods for quality assurance and their feasibility, costs, and professional acceptability. Congressional legislation was concerned mainly with institutional care and with services reimbursed under federal programs. Almost all dental care was provided in ambulatory settings, no services were reimbursed through Medicare, and only a small amount of total dental expenditures were covered by Medicaid. Finally, quality assurance activities at the federal level and in private insurance were focused primarily on cost control first and quality second. The assumption was that large Medicare and Medicaid expenditures resulted from unnecessary care. Thus, pretreatment authorization was the primary method used in quality control systems.

Support for PSROs later waned because they were perceived as being ineffective in controlling costs. The PSRO legislation, however, set in motion forces that should continue to make quality of dental care a major issue. Issues such as peer review, the effect of continuing education and relicensure on quality, standards of quality, the best quality assurance systems and their effect on dentists' behavior, dental health status and dental curricula, patients' roles, the federal function, and the voluntary nature continue to be discussed (Quality Assurance,   1982).

Bailit (1980), in discussing the major issues on development of policies for regulating quality of care in the private dental sector, identified the following as important: (1) the quality of care, (2) the relationship between quality and oral health, and (3) cost/benefit and cost-effectiveness of quality assurance. The discussion focuses next on the first of these.

Quality of Care

Quality of care usually is thought of as involving one of three areas: (1) the technical aspects of care, (2) the personal interactions of patients and providers, or (3) the necessity and appropriateness of the treatment.

Little information was available in the literature on consumers' perceptions of the quality of dental care; they appeared to be pleased with the service they received. The technical quality of care generally was adequate. A posttreatment clinical evaluation of 11,000 Medicaid patients in New York State indicated that 81.2 percent were treated satisfactorily (Cons, 1973). In a study of military dental patients, Ryge and Snyder (1973) found that less than 2 percent of newly placed amalgam restorations needed replacement, although 35 percent had defects that needed observation. Grasso, Nalbandian, Sanford, and Bailit (1979) examined several studies and found that the great majority of amalgam restorations were adequate. In addition, unacceptable restorative work appeared to be concentrated in a small percentage of the population. Milgrom, Weinstein, Ratener, Read, and Morrison (1978) found generally high levels of care in private practice.

The necessity and appropriateness of dental care provided to the American public is less clear, however. A particular treatment is necessary if "a condition exists that requires a professional dental service" (AFDH, 1980, p. 10) and the treatment is appropriate if "the service being provided is suited for the condition that is present" (p. 6). Both are important concepts in quality of care and refer to the level of treatment, number of services, and the extent to which they are consistent with the diagnosis.

The biggest question is the quality of periodontal care. The widespread nature of periodontal disease has been noted. Practice-based surveys have documented a low level of treatment for it. These two facts are not sufficient evidence, however, to substantiate undertreatment of periodontal disease in general dental practices. The level of such treatment is very complex and is poorly understood. Both population and provider variables impact on the level of services provided. Dentists cannot be held account-able for services that they recommend but that patients do not accept.

One study provided empirical evidence of the quality of periodontal services. It compared the need for periodontal services determined by an independent investigator and based on a radiographic and clinical exami-nation of patients with treatment plans of dentists submitting claims to insurance carriers. Only 21 percent of needed services were requested on these claims (Bailit, 1980). The necessity and appropriateness of perio-dontal services must receive the attention of policy makers in the future if dental health is to be improved.

The appropriateness of fixed prosthetic services is more difficult to assess. More persons are receiving treatment as insurance coverage increases, and the care received often is more comprehensive than might have been sought or received without coverage. Dentistry is entering an era of high-cost, highly technological care.

An example from the fee-basis Veterans Administration (VA) dental program illustrates the point. In fiscal year 1977, the VA spent approxi-mately $4.4 billion for health services, $117 million of which was for dentistry—approximately $67 million for staff-provided care and more than $50 million for fee-for-service dentistry (Schonfeld, 1979). In a pilot study, treatment plans for 46 patients—22 veterans from a VA service area with plans prepared by private dentists and 24 dental school patients with student-prepared and faculty-approved plans—were compared. Each of these 46 also received a standard epidemiological examination to deter-mine oral health status. The two samples were similar in terms of age and oral health status. The number of teeth with untreated carious lesions was almost identical in the two patient populations (2.3 and 2.5 teeth per person, but the proposed treatment differed dramatically. Dental school patients were more likely to have a tooth restored (restorative and fixed prosthodontics). However, when a dentist made the decision to treat a tooth, VA patients were three times more likely than dental school patients to receive full crown coverage (Rozier, Kelly, & Slome, 1981).

Research by Bailit and Serling (1979) suggested that few dentists con-sciously either provided restorative treatment that was unnecessary or inappropriate or tried to maximize income. The real issue is the added oral health benefits that result from the complex prosthetic treatment that is becoming the most expensive single item in dentistry. Are patients health-ier as a result of more expensive treatment plans and, if so, are the benefits worth the increased costs? The answer lies in the area of public policy debate.

Supply of Dental Personnel

Stimulated by declining dentist-to-population ratios in the 1950s and by results of empirical studies projecting a shortage of dental personnel in the 1960s and beyond, the federal government initiated a number of programs in the 1960s to increase both dental supply and productivity. The Health Professions Educational Assistance Act of 1963 (P.L. 88-129) provided support for increasing the number of dental schools and enrollment in existing ones. These programs were supplemented with a series of initiatives to increase productivity of professional and allied personnel. The programs dealt with training of (1) dental students in the efficient use of auxiliaries (Dental Auxiliary Utilization Program—DAU) and management of the total dental team (Training in Expanded Auxiliary Management—TEAM) and (2) a pool of auxiliaries in expanded functions such as restoring teeth (Expanded Function Dental Auxiliary—EFDA). By 1976, the Health Professions Educational Assistance Act (P.L. 94-484) still was tied to increases in supply. One criterion for receiving federal funds (capitation) was to increase class size. However, the criterion also could be met through activities directed at the problems of geographic maldistribution and the growing numbers of specialists.

By the mid-1970s there was a growing feeling that increases in personnel supply and productivity, changes in disease patterns, and the general state of the economy were beginning to have an impact on dentists' busyness. The number of dentists needed to meet future demands had become a major policy issue. Several empirical studies addressed this issue.

Policy decisions on dental personnel traditionally used to be based on studies using the ratio approach—either dentist-to-population or utilization. More recently, estimation of personnel requirements involved the use of more sophisticated economic approaches, including both supply-demand projections and economic forecasting. This effort was stimulated by research by the staff of the Division of Dentistry, Bureau of Health Manpower (BHM), and other organizations under contract to that division (Brown & Winslow, 1981). These efforts provided useful information for defining national manpower issues.

Two reports by the BHM are discussed next. Both used national models of the supply and demand of dental services to predict the degree to which the future stock of dentists would meet the requirements for services. The two studies differed in the technical aspects of the modeling effort. The first was based on a projection technique that assumed that what had occurred in the past would continue in the future. The second was based on a forecasting technique that attempted to predict future changes based on knowledge of cause-and-effect relationships.

The 1977 Projections

The 1977 report, titled *Projections of National Requirements for Dentists, 1980, 1985, and 1990,* provided estimates of needs based on an aggregate supply-and-demand model of the private dental care sector (U.S. PHS, 1977c). The long-run relationships between supply and demand and the variables that bring them into balance were estimated using historical time-series data from the period 1950–1970. Variables used to estimate demand for services were (1) population size, (2) personal disposable income, and (3) extent of dental insurance. Variables used in estimating supply of dental services were (1) the national stock of dentists and (2) technological advances. The analysis projected demand for dental services and the number of dentists needed to meet it according to historical long-run trends in utilization of services. The adequacy of dental personnel through 1990 was assessed by comparing the projected number of dentists needed to meet demand with the projected output of practitioners and allied persons.

Several assumptions in the model are important when results are evaluated. First, the model and its interpretation assumed that there was a long-run historical trend in the balance of supply and demand and that this trend should continue into the future with only slight inflation of real prices of dental care. The report took the position that some short-term fluctuation around this trend line was to be expected and did not call for any policy decisions. Within a range of fluctuation, it said demand would be met by changes in prices, employment of auxiliaries, queuing of patients, delegation of tasks, and hours worked. Stated another way, demand would and could be met within a wide range of personnel. Only extreme fluctuations in supply and demand required action.

A second assumption related to the growth of dental insurance. The report assumed that insurance would continue to grow at a rapid rate but because of the uncertainty of the precise rate at which that rise would occur, it used two estimates to project increases in demand. The lower estimate assumed that the proportion of the population included in dental prepayment benefits would reach 43 percent, the higher estimate, 50 percent.

A third assumption was that the historical rate of technological progress would be maintained in the future through the employment of EFDAs.

The results of the study projected a slight national surplus of dentists (about 2,000) in 1990, given the conservative estimates of insurance growth. With higher estimates of insurance growth, supply was expected to about equal demand. This surplus was within the range in which market forces would balance supply and demand through the end of the project period.

However, the trend in dentist requirements was toward a surplus beyond 1990, given the leveling off in the growth of dental insurance projected for that decade.

The 1979 Forecasts

The BHM report titled *Forecasts of Employment in the Dental Sector to 1995* represented an extension of the analysis discussed above (Hixon & Mocniak, 1979). The report did not address requirements for dentists directly but discussed the implications that projected increases in supply might have on their future workloads and on the employment of dental auxiliaries. The model predicted conditions of the dental care market based on economic growth, population changes, and growth of dental prepayment plans. The model was very complex, with almost 200 equations expressing variable interrelationships.

The model forecast increasingly tight economic conditions for dentistry. It said demand for services would continue to rise because of the increase in population, growth in the economy, and expansion of the proportion of the public covered by dental insurance. However, increases in the supply and productivity of dental manpower were projected to be more than adequate to meet the demand. Additional competitive pressures in the form of marketing of dental services and perhaps the practice of dentistry by denturists and independent hygienists all would discourage fee increases and inefficient practices while costs of maintaining a dental office would be rising.

For example, the model expected real wages of dental auxiliaries to follow the general trend of economic growth and predicted the rate of price increases would be less than that of overall economic growth. To accommodate the increasingly difficult economic conditions, the model suggested that dentists work longer hours and assume a greater responsibility of patient care by substituting their own time for that of auxiliaries.

While not speaking directly to the issue of personnel requirements, this study suggested that there would be a surplus of dentists for the rest of the century.

This analysis had an important bearing on another important issue, that of cost containment. It suggested that increasing prices should not be an issue, assuming that dentistry did not become a component of an extensive financing scheme such as national health insurance.

The Health Needs Approach

In one state—North Carolina—dental personnel planning was approached from another perspective, that of health needs (Bawden & DeFriese, 1981).

In this analysis, personnel requirements were based on a determination of the staffing required to treat the prevalence and incidence of diseases and conditions as diagnosed by professional judgment. This approach was attractive and logical since it started with the disease and resulting conditions in the population, then translated those conditions into required services and finally into need for personnel. A focus on diseases and conditions would allow for categorical planning for different health services—preventive, diagnostic, and treatment—and the kinds and numbers of personnel required for providing each. Furthermore, requirements could be calculated in a variety of service time measures such as per visit, per hour, or per service that a practitioner should spend in providing "good" care.

Many personnel policy decisions are best based on categorical disease. For example, if resources appeared to be adequate or more than adequate for a condition that consumed a large proportion of practitioners' time, and yet another prevalent disease persisted with a large need-supply gap, personnel policies should be directed toward closing that gap. Forecasts based on need without reference to demand in most cases would provide ideal upper limit boundaries of personnel requirements.

The health needs approach to planning is exemplified by the Graduate Medical Education National Advisory Committee (GMENAC) in which national specialty-specific physician requirements for each of 23 medical specialties were estimated (Donaldson, Jacoby, & Wills, 1981). In North Carolina, the number of general dentists required in 1976 to treat several major dental conditions was estimated. These two studies differed from classical needs-based approaches in that various data sources were adjusted to reflect realities of provider and consumer behavior. In the North Carolina Dental Manpower Study (NCDMS), health needs were adjusted downward by estimates of demand.

The types of data necessary to use the health-needs approach involve (1) the number of persons in the population who have certain conditions and/or should receive certain types of services, (2) the number and type of services required for these conditions, and (3) the number and type of services that the average practitioner can provide. Given these data, it is possible to calculate the total number of providers required, now or in the future. The calculation is done by multiplying the number of individuals in the population by the total number of diseases or conditions and the services required per disease or condition, then dividing this product by the average or desirable workload of each practitioner.

Data to complete these calculations for major dental conditions in the NCDMS were obtained from five study components:

1. A statewide prevalence survey: the prevalence and incidence of the most common dental conditions were obtained from a household survey of approximately 3,500 individuals.
2. Estimation of treatment needs: treatment needs in terms of visits, procedures, or hours were estimated using these epidemiological data and normative professional standards.
3. Treatment capacity of the private, general practice system: procedure-specific data were obtained from a random sample of 240 dental offices in the state.
4. Dental personnel supply and distribution: these figures were obtained from the computerized license renewal files of the North Carolina State Board of Dental Examiners.
5. Estimation of consumer demand: a collaborative effort with the Michigan Health and Social Security Research Institute, an affiliate of the United Automobile Workers union in Detroit, provided estimates of probable bounds for effective demand.

The results of the NCDMS are summarized in Table 12-7. Treatment services for the four disease conditions represent 80 percent or more of care provided by dental general practitioners. The population in the state needing different types of treatment, the treatment needed according to professional judgments in units of visits, services, or hours, and the annual number of treatment units provided by general dentists at the time of the study are listed.

Of most interest are Columns 4 and 5. Column 4 provides information on the residual or unmet need in the North Carolina population. Of importance is the great variability by condition. For example, at 1976 levels of productivity, general dentists in the state could treat either 30 percent of the existing backlog or 100 percent of the annual occurrence of dental caries, given the then-existing pattern of dental care delivery. Full denture services also seemed to be adequately met. A large gap existed, however, between the need for treatment and actual treatment received for periodontal disease and diagnostic/preventive services. For example, almost eight times more periodontal disease existed than general practitioners could treat at 1976 supply levels. The need-supply ratios had important implications for public policy but must be interpreted in terms of effective demand when estimating personnel requirements.

Column 5 displays effective demand as a proportion of need. These estimates were used as guidelines in adjusting need downward to reflect actual consumer behavior more closely. Generally, these percentages indicated that utilization of dental services was at a low level in North Carolina. The highest demand involved utilization of prosthetic services or replacement of missing teeth (47.3 percent), with the demand for periodontal

Table 12-7 Treatment Needed and Supplied, and Their Relationship
North Carolina, 1976

Condition	Number Needing Treatment (in 1,000s) (1)	Treatment Needed (in 1,000s) (2)	Treatment Provided (in 1,000s) (3)	Need/Supply Ratio (4)	Percentage Supply/Need (5)
Diagnosis and Prevention					
Periodic Examination	5,216	9,774 visits	1,518 visits	6.4	
Prophylaxis	4,558	9,116 visits	1,904 visits	4.8	19.1
Fluoride Treatment	4,558	9,116 visits	1,929 visits	4.7	
Dental Caries					
Backlog	5,046	9,930 services	3,027 services	3.3	23.0
Annual Occurrence	5,046	3,244 services		1.1	
Periodontal Disease					
Backlog	351	117 hours	15 hours	7.8	12.5
Annual Occurrence	10	3 hours		0.2	
Edentulousness					
Backlog	72	288 visits	159 visits	1.8	47.3
Annual Occurrence	41	162 visits	237 visits	1.0	
Denture Adjustments and Repairs	194	388 visits		1.6	

Source: Adapted by permission from *Planning for Dental Care on a Statewide Basis: The North Carolina Dental Manpower Project,* J.W. Bawden and G.H. DeFriese, editors, The Dental Foundation of North Carolina, © 1981.

services the lowest (12.5 percent). Demand for treatment of dental caries (23.0 percent) or for diagnosis and treatment (19.1 percent) was intermediate.

Based on the low level of demand and the increasing supply of dentists (rising at an average net rate of 4 percent a year while the state's population was growing at only 1 percent a year) the study reported that the supply of dental personnel was adequate at the time of the survey.

In other conclusions, the study suggested that (1) access to dental care in the state was improving because of increased supply and a more favorable geographic distribution, (2) dentists could respond to fairly large growth in demand through changes in staffing patterns, and (3) trained dental assistants were in short supply.

Requirements for Specialists

There have been few attempts to disaggregate dental personnel into generalists and specialists and to estimate requirements for each. In 1978 the American Association of Dental Schools (1980) in cooperation with the American Dental Association Council on Dental Education convened a task force to explore problems in advanced dental education and suggest solutions. A portion of this effort involved an estimate of the need for specialties through the year 2000.

In 1979 there were 445 specialty programs with 1,237 first-year positions. All but 46 of these positions were for the six clinical specialties. In aggregate, both the number of programs and first-year positions remained fairly constant during the 1970s.

Specialization in dentistry is a relatively recent phenomenon. In the quarter-century between 1955 and 1979, the absolute number of active specialists increased from 2,751 to 16,595, a gain of more than 500 percent. The number of specialists per 100,000 population rose from 1.6 to 7.5. During this same period, the number of active dentists increased by 46 percent.

While specialty training positions did not increase in the 1970s, the supply of dentists kept increasing. Given 1979 enrollments, the task force estimated that the supply of specialists would increase by 72 percent in the ensuing 20 years, reaching 28,540 in the year 2000. The number of specialists per 100,000 population was projected to rise from 7.5 to 10.9. The panel expected the relative numbers of orthodontists would decrease and endodontists, periodontists, and prosthodontists would grow but the remaining specialty areas would not change relative to the other specialties.

Using the 1979 clinical specialist-to-population ratio of 7.4 per 100,000 as a normative standard for planning, the task force estimated that 19,347 clinical specialists would be needed in 2000. Compared with projections of 27,924 active clinical specialists, a surplus of nearly 50 percent would exist at the turn of the century.

The increasing number and proportion of specialist dentists, combined with the potential adverse effects of an oversupply of specialists, a lack of evidence of substantial increase in demand, the absence of sufficient data to accomplish more sophisticated econometric forecasts on personnel, and guided by the philosophy that general practice had been and should continue to be the major source of dental care, the task force recommended that first-year positions in advanced programs for the six clinical specialties be reduced by one-third from the 1979–1980 level of 1,191.

Redefining Roles of Paradental Personnel

Expanded Functions for Dental Auxiliaries

The policy issue concerning the expansion of the role of dental auxiliaries is primarily one of ensuring the supply and efficiency of care through dentists' offices rather than one of improving access to care through remote-site practice of auxiliaries. A redefinition of the traditional roles of dental auxiliaries in the United States has paralleled that of medical auxiliaries.

In the mid-1960s, academic institutions, the National Center for Health Services Research, and the federal government through personnel legislation (Nurse Training Act of 1971, P.L. 92-158, and the Comprehensive Health Manpower Training Act of 1971, P.L. 92-157) began experimentation with the concept of expanding the roles of allied health personnel to include certain aspects of physicians' traditional roles. Documented benefits of physician extenders, as they were called, included an increase in the productivity of medical practice; an improvement in access to care through existing practices and newly established ones, especially in rural, underserved areas; and the potential for containing costs.

Internationally, the use of auxiliaries for providing oral health services began in New Zealand with the School Dental Service in 1921. Specially trained dental nurses there began providing a range of therapeutic services to school children on the school grounds. By 1977, New Zealand had 1,373 clinics providing routine care at six-month intervals as requested for 622,000 children 2 ½ to 13 years of age. Radiographs and extractions of permanent teeth were the only routine procedures they did not perform. They no longer provided extractions because the need had fallen to such a low level that such training was inefficient financially. These dental nurses worked under remote supervision of district dentists and dental nurse supervisors. The dental profession played an important role in instigating the program (Logan, 1978).

The dental nurse concept has spread to other countries, including Australia, England, the provinces of Saskatchewan and Manitoba in Canada, and a number of Latin American nations. The rationale for this approach to dental care delivery was the high prevalence of disease combined with a shortage of care. Faced with a similar situation in the United States, ADA policies in the 1960s reflected the position that the supply of dental services could be increased through more efficient utilization of dental auxiliaries and it advocated evaluation of expanding their functions.

A number of studies subsequently did evaluate the practicality of training auxiliaries in expanded functions and the quality of care they provided. With few exceptions, the auxiliary chosen to perform intraoral functions was the dental assistant rather than the hygienist. Dental practice acts rarely limit the assistant to specific procedures. The transition for the assistant rather than the hygienist seemed more logical since this auxiliary was involved chairside with the dentist in therapeutic procedures and would be more familiar with restorative functions. The assistant could enter the work force after a shorter training period. When the dental hygienist was trained and used in expanded functions, the role was oriented primarily toward restorative work. Only two of the studies redefined the traditional role of dental hygienists to examine the feasibility of their performing expanded preventive and periodontal functions (Ancell, 1972; Sisty, Henderson, Paule, & Martin, 1978).

Research studies on expanded functions reviewed by Douglass and Lipscomb (1979) and by Sisty, Henderson, and Paule (1979) indicated that expanded duty dental assistants (EFDAs) with a few months of additional training could provide intraoral procedures at a level of quality comparable to dentists. The studies also indicated that productivity in diverse settings such as public health clinics, university settings, military clinics, and private practice could be increased.

Computer-assisted mathematical modeling also demonstrated productivity benefits from the use of EFDAs. While positive in all settings, productivity benefits generally were greatest in modeling experiments, with public settings ranked second and private practice third. Modest improvements in private practice experiments depended heavily on the dentist's management skills, supervision, and philosophy toward delegation of duties.

The success of the EFDA concept in all settings depends on nonrestrictive state dental practice acts, a large patient demand and favorable attitudes, a population needing restorative care, adequate facilities, and enough supporting staff for the dentist and the auxiliary. These conditions limit the general applicability of the diffusion of this concept into both public and private practice. For example, demand for services might not be great enough in the private sector for EFDAs to be effective. The case mix also could be changing from fewer restorative to more preventive cases and to periodontal needs. Many public settings have inadequate facilities or cannot provide adequate assistance to both dentists and EFDAs. The U.S. Air Force discontinued its EFDA program when it was unable to replace assistants who were moved up to EFDAs (U.S. GAO, 1980).

The restrictiveness of state dental practice acts and the political reactions to expanded roles of dental auxiliaries, among other reasons, have limited the degree to which auxiliaries have been used in dental care delivery. In 1977, only ten states allowed dental auxiliaries to perform restorative functions such as placing, shaping, and finishing restorations. Most dental laws, rules, or regulations in state acts have been changed since, however, to permit expanded functions. Most states now permit hygienists and assistants to perform limited functions within the mouth, including reversible procedures that can be corrected without harm to the patient.

Permissible procedures vary considerably from state to state. For example, a 1977 study showed more than half of the states allowed assistants to expose radiographs, take impressions for study casts, remove periodontal and surgical dressings, remove sutures, apply topical anesthetic agents, apply topical fluorides, place and remove rubber dams and matrices, and remove excess cement from the coronal tooth surfaces. Ten or fewer states allowed EFDAs to place and contour restorative materials. Only a few states permitted nonreversible procedures such as administering local anesthetic agents and soft tissue curettage (ADA, 1977).

The Council of State Governments National Task Force on State Dental Policies suggested that state practice acts should be written to allow dentists to delegate functions for which auxiliaries were trained and the dentists were willing to take responsibility (Council of State Governments, 1979).

Research has shown that auxiliaries can be trained to provide quality care that is acceptable to the patient, thus reducing costs per unit of service in public and private settings. To the extent that private providers are willing, savings can be transferred to patients through a reduction, or smaller increases, in fees, thus controlling costs.

The policy issues related to the role of paradental personnel in the delivery of personal health services seemed to be changing, with the focus of the controversy shifting from "what" auxiliaries could do, which had been well established by research and demonstration, to "where" the service could be provided. Decreasing demand for services in the private sector and the apparent trend toward fewer restorative needs would point toward a reduced need and acceptance for EFDAs in private practice.

The private sector argued that increased productivity and access through the use of EFDAs no longer were needed because there were enough dentists. Official ADA policy reflected this position. An ADA House of Delegates resolution adopted in 1975 called for the "termination of research in expanded functions and a return to traditional roles and responsibilities of dental auxiliaries" (ADA, 1975). It seemed that use of EFDAs in private practice had become a dead issue with the ADA since demand could be met within the existing delivery system using auxiliaries with traditional functions. The ADA felt that expanded functions were no longer necessary and should no longer be encouraged.

Public clinical programs such as state and local health departments, the military, Veterans Administration, the National Health Service Corps, and federal, state, and local prisons and jails constantly face excess demand for services and limited resources. EFDAs' use in those settings should provide benefits according to the original concept. The American Public Health Association in 1981 adopted a policy statement in conflict with the ADA position and in support of the use of EFDAs in federal, state, and local public dental programs. The official statement "encourages and urges all public agencies at state and local levels providing care to populations which do not have access to dental care in the private sector to make maximum use of EFDAs whenever feasible" (APHA, 1982).

Supervision of Auxiliaries

Another issue related to roles of paradental professionals involved dental hygienists and the degree of supervision required by a dentist. A movement, led primarily by the dental hygiene profession, sought to change practice acts to reduce supervision. This issue in most cases was completely separate from that of auxiliaries' scope of practice discussed earlier.

Dental hygienists were not challenging the functions they are allowed to perform under the dental practice act but were disputing the "over-the-shoulder" supervision clauses that require dentists to prescribe treatment, see that it is accomplished, and be available on-site during the treatment. With less supervision, the proponents argue, hygienists would be less restricted in where they practice, thus increasing public access to preventive services.

No state dental practice act allows hygienists to practice without supervision of a dentist and most require direct supervision. Private practice options and supervision for hygienists were summarized by Bean (1981):

1. Hygienists could be employed by dentists and work under their supervision as defined by the dental practice act.

2. Hygienists could be self-employed as independent contractors and work under dentists' supervision in accordance with the dental practice act. As such, they could either work in dentists' offices, in which case they would rent the space and make business decisions pertaining to such things as hours, fees, and purchasing of supplies, or maintain a separate office with no financial ties to the dentists.
3. Hygienists could be independent practitioners without supervision of dentists. That is illegal in every state but was tested in the courts in at least two states, Pennsylvania and North Carolina.

Few hygienists are self-employed independent contractors. A few states allow them to provide preventive services under general supervision in public programs.

Several organizations have criticized dental practice acts as too restrictive, thus preventing the optimum use of auxiliaries and experimentation with alternative delivery systems. A task force of state and local officials appointed by the Council of State Governments in 1979 studied the regulation of dental providers and produced a suggested dental practice act.

The proposed legislation and background papers reflected the view that state acts were unnecessarily restrictive. Supervision clauses prevented the optimum use of dental hygienists and restricted access to their services. Hygienists through their education and experience possessed skills and knowledge in the primary and secondary prevention of dental disease at both the individual and community levels. Their training and philosophy were directed toward education, motivation, and counseling in nutrition, plaque control, fluoride therapies, application of sealants, prophylaxis and therapies for control of periodontal disease, maintenance of restorations (polishing), examination, screening, and referral.

If hygienists were allowed to practice these activities under general supervision of dentists, access to care would be improved, the report said, suggesting that practice under these conditions raised only marginal questions of public safety. The author of one background paper commented that "in the name of delivering a single best standard of care, none at all is delivered to millions of young, isolated, or disabled Americans" (Council of State Governments, 1979, p. 61).

The Federal Trade Commission (1980) also investigated state rules on the supervision of hygienists to determine whether those practicing independently would provide greater access to care at lower costs. The study found four basic questions, whether:

1. hygienists had sufficient and proper training to ensure quality of care
2. fragmentation of preventive and therapeutic services would result

3. hygienists were able to treat medical emergencies
4. the practice mode would be economically feasible.

In 1980 the FTC discontinued the investigation, stating that it had found insufficient evidence as to the quality of care hygienists might provide independently.

Unlike the expanded function issue, the effect of general or no supervision of hygienists is not known. Research and demonstrations must be conducted to determine whether public health and safety are jeopardized, what training is needed, the effect on demand for care, fragmentation of care, access, and disease levels.

The Emerging Paradental Professional

Accomplishment of intraoral procedures for the prosthetic replacement of missing teeth has been restricted by state dental practice acts to dentists. Fabrication of dentures involves a radiographic and physical examination of the mouth, correcting or treating any areas that would contradict denture use, making impressions of the mouth, determining how the jaws should relate to each other, fitting the denture, and providing postdelivery care— all intraoral procedures. The laboratory technician, usually employed by a commercial laboratory and following a written work order from the dentist, provides custom-made materials to be used by the dentist when performing intraoral procedures and makes the dental appliance.

Four states—Arizona, Colorado, Maine, and Oregon—have given dental professionals other than dentists legal status to provide intraoral functions. This probably is only the beginning of a movement that has come to be called denturism—efforts by dental laboratory technicians, called denturists, to be recognized as licensed professionals who can independently provide prosthetic services directly to the public. In three of these states, the denturist functions as an auxiliary under the supervision of a dentist. However, in Oregon, the denturist practices independently of the dentist and is required only to have a certificate of oral health from a dentist or physician in order to provide all denture services. The 1978 Oregon referendum that legalized denturism passed with 78 percent of the vote (Oregon Lesson, 1979).

The emergence of this public policy issue has been painful. As physicians attempted to limit the development of separate professions such as podiatry, optometry, and chiropractic, the dental profession has openly opposed denturism. The ADA defines the movement as the "unqualified as well as illegal practice of dentistry in any form on the public" (ADA, 1976).

The issue in the minds of the public and elected officials is primarily economic. Sixty-one percent of the adult population 65 to 74 years of age is edentulous in at least one arch. It is estimated that Americans spend a billion dollars on dentures each year, or about 10 percent of expenditures for dental care (Douglass & Day, 1979). Edentulousness is more prevalent in the aged poor. It has been estimated that 825,000 persons among the poverty stricken and working poor need prosthetic care.

However, the dental profession has viewed the issue as a health threat in which public health and safety are imperiled. The major position for each side has been summarized by Rosenstein, Joseph, Mackenzie, and Wyden (1980).

Dentists make the following major points:

1. Only dentists have the basic knowledge to diagnose pathological conditions before denture insertion or the need for denture adjustments as a result of injury.
2. The need for dentures is declining because people are keeping their teeth longer as a result of public and private prevention efforts. It also has been suggested that the denturism movement might detract from the preventive movement (Council of State Governments, 1979).
3. Initial savings to the consumer would disappear once denturists became established.
4. There are no standards for training of denturists so quality control is not possible.

The major points made by denturists are as follows:

1. It is feasible to train denturists to provide dentures without a knowledge of other facets of dentistry. The concentration in one area is, in fact, an advantage in that the denturist becomes more skillful than the dentist. Fee (1974) reported that denturist students at Northern Alberta Institute of Technology in Canada received 1,334 curriculum hours of complete denture construction, compared to only 600 hours for complete and removable dentures by dental students at the University of Alberta.
2. Removing denture construction from the scope of dentists' practices would give dentists more time to perform procedures requiring their training and would result in a more efficient use of personnel.
3. Denturists have lower overhead and thus can provide dentures at a lower cost to the public. Barone (1974) suggested that in providing services directly to the public, the denturist eliminated the middleman (dentist), so costs could be lower.
4. Denturists can be licensed and standards established to ensure quality. The standards would include educational requirements and a

provision similar to that in Canadian provinces in which the patient must receive a certificate of oral health from a dentist or physician before dentures are made.

5. Patients would be given a freedom of choice as to where to get dentures.

Dentistry recognized the issue as an economic one and responded with that in mind. The ADA appointed an Ad Hoc Committee for the Delivery of Quality Prosthetic Care for the Financially Disadvantaged that issued a report indicating ways in which low-cost, quality prosthetic dental care could be provided ("Final Report", 1977). The methods suggested for controlling denture costs included:

- use of modest and simple office equipment and furnishings
- use of standardized and efficient denture construction techniques
- provision of a limited number of treatment options to the patient
- use of sound business principles
- purchase of materials and supplies in large quantities
- in-office denture construction or negotiated reduced fees with commercial laboratories

Unmet Dental Needs

While the dental health of many Americans is improving, there still are population subgroups (defined by certain demographic, socioeconomic, physical, and legal characteristics) with high levels of untreated disease. The dental care system dominated by autonomous, fee-for-service, individualistic practices provides care to only a small proportion (20 percent) who realize the need for care and effectively demand it.

The poor, minorities, institutionalized, handicapped, young, and old all are characterized by low levels of treatment.

The Ten-State Nutrition Survey (U.S. PHS, 1972b) documented the oral health status of the young, minorities, and lower socioeconomic groups in the Southeast United States in 1968-1970. The TSNS is relevant to this discussion because of the volumes of data it provides on those disadvantaged groups. More than 10,000 individuals 5 to 20 years of age were examined. Their treatment needs were substantial and greater than those of advantaged groups. The two sex and three ethnic groups (white, black, and Hispanic) in the low-income states had 24 percent to 60 percent more decayed teeth in need of treatment than comparable groups in the high-income states. Blacks had 12 percent to 36 percent more decayed and untreated teeth than whites.

Sixty-one percent of the elderly population in the United States was found edentulous in a 1971-1974 study. An average of 15.2 teeth per person were missing in individuals with some natural teeth remaining. Sixty-four percent of those with at least one tooth had periodontal disease and more than half had one or more periodontal pockets (Kelly & Harvey, 1979). Edentulousness was concentrated in low-income groups. In 1977, 11.6 million elderly persons were estimated to be edentulous, 7 million of them with incomes below $5,000 (ADA, 1978b). While the percentage of the elderly needing dental services generally was no greater than in other age groups, the type and mix of services and medical problems tended to make treatment—consisting of restorative, periodontal disease, and denture services—more complex and costly.

The 33 million handicapped individuals in the United States have not been surveyed systematically but studies indicated that they had poorer oral health than nonhandicapped persons and were more likely to receive less care. The care that the handicapped received also was more likely to be of the symptomatic type. Periodontal disease, as a result of poor oral hygiene practice, was a common problem. In one study of mentally retarded adults aged 17 to 43, 97 percent of those surveyed were in need of treatment for dental caries (Rosenstein, Bush, & Gorelick, 1971). In a community treatment program for handicapped children and adults, an average of more than 10 restorations and extractions per person were needed (Horowitz, Greek, & Hoag, 1965).

Institutionalized groups demonstrate high treatment needs. Normally, their care is provided by dentists who use facilities in the institution. However, resources are extremely limited. A dental survey of 762 inmates in the Michigan Department of Corrections illustrates the backlog of need in these populations. All of the women and 96 percent of the men examined needed dental treatment. Treatment needs by type of service were as follows: 80 to 90 percent, restorations; 33 to 37 percent, extractions; and 50 to 60 percent, periodontal disease. Of those with full denture units, 80 to 90 percent needed repair or replacement (Office of Health and Medical Affairs, 1975). Other institutional settings such as nursing homes and hospitals for mentally retarded have documented high dental needs.

Rational policies for improving the oral health status of these disadvantaged groups must be based on a consideration of factors that are predictive of disease levels. Three general areas must be considered: (1) exposure to preventive measures, either individual or community, that would affect disease prevalence; (2) the level of demand for care, primarily asymptomatic care; (3) barriers that prevent or hinder utilization of dental services.

There are indications that one reason for the poor health of these groups is their low level of self-care practices. Oral hygiene practices are related to the prevalence of dental diseases. One study found that oral hygiene indicators were 40 percent worse in blacks than in whites. Oral cleanliness steadily worsened with age: in the 65-to-74-year-old age group, hygiene indicators were 48 percent worse than in those 6 to 11 (Kelly & Harvey, 1979). The National Survey of Personal Health Practices and Consequences (NSPHPC), a panel study conducted in 1979 and 1980, provided data on health habits and practices for adults 20 to 64 years of age. It found individuals in lower educational groups were much less likely to report brushing their teeth at least twice a day than those with higher educational attainment (Danchik, Schoenborn, & Elinson, 1981).

A second reason for high disease levels in these groups appeared to be related to their low level of utilization. Aggregate demand for dental services was discussed earlier. Utilization rates from the 1978–1979 National Health Survey specific to the groups with high need were:

- 74.3 percent of children under 6 years of age had never seen a dentist
- 32.5 percent of persons 65 years and older had not had a dental visit in the preceding year and an additional 44.0 percent had not visited a dentist in the past five years or more
- 45.0 percent of those retired at age 45 or older for health reasons had not made a visit in the past five or more years
- 62.2 percent of minority races had not had a visit within a year
- 60.5 percent or more of those with a family income below $10,000 had not had a visit in the preceding year (Wilder, 1982).

Utilization rates of poor and nonpoor have not converged in dentistry as they have in medicine. The type of services utilized by the disadvantaged is more symptomatic than that of other groups. As income and education rise, the number of basic preventive services (cleanings and restorations) increases while extractions decrease.

Significant barriers to utilization of health services exist for these groups. Certain groups such as the institutionalized and mentally and physically handicapped face unique access problems. Those for the handicapped arise from the fact that dental professionals:

- lack basic knowledge regarding special patients and appropriate physical and/or psychological management
- lack experience in treating these patients
- presume that such individuals will disrupt the usual office routine
- presume these persons need special facilities and equipment
- consider the possibility of receiving inadequate compensation for the increased time involved in treatment (Gurney & Alcorn, 1979).

Access to care in correctional facilities is severely constrained by custody policies and regulations.

Barriers to the utilization of dental health services from a more general perspective are listed in Table 12-8. The list is a compilation of barriers identified by three task forces composed of dental practitioners, educators, hygienists, assistants, researchers, lawyers, social workers, and economists (U.S. PHS, 1979b). Some of these constraints are analyzed next in relation to the disadvantaged groups under discussion in order to identify those that may be responsible for their low level of health.

A study a year earlier indicated that knowledge appeared to bear little relationship to individuals' attitudes and behaviors (Frazier, 1978). This might be expected because of the substantial difference between what people know to be good dental health behavior and how they actually react to that knowledge.

Psychosocial factors have been considered extensively in explanatory research on dental care utilization. A majority (63 percent) of Americans felt no need to go to the dentist (ADA, 1979b). Most perceived themselves as being susceptible to dental disease but did not consider the problem serious (Kegeles, 1961).

Attitudes varied by age and socioeconomic groups. For example, the young were more likely to mention fear as a reason for not going to the dentist. Elderly persons were more likely than other age groups not to feel

---

Table 12-8 Barriers to the Utilization of Dental Health Services

Consumer Factors	*Delivery System Factors*
• Orientation toward symptomatic care • Lack of knowledge and motivation • Inappropriate attitudes • Fear and anxiety	• Restrictive regulations/legislation • Inappropriate utilization of dental personnel • Availability of care • Monolithicity of system • Disease orientation • Resistance to change • Deficiencies in professional education process • Lack of national policy for dentistry • Fragmentation of public health strategy

Source: Adapted from *Barriers to Attaining an Effective Dental Health System,* Proceedings of the Region IX Dental Conference. U.S. Department of Health, Education, and Welfare, U.S. Public Health Service, Pacific Grove, California, August 30–September 1, 1979b.

a need to seek dental care, perhaps perceiving their loss of teeth as an inevitable part of growing old (Dworkin, Ference, & Giddon, 1978).

Kegeles (1974) summarized research on social and psychological factors and their relationships to asymptomatic dental care, pointing out the following factors as among those studied in attempting to explain utilization behaviors:

- perceived susceptibility to disease
- belief that preventive dental visits would reduce the likelihood of having serious dental problems
- perceived importance of dentistry
- fear of pain
- anxiety about dental care
- costs of care
- perceived characteristics of dentists

Of these factors, Kegeles concluded that only the first two consistently differentiated between those who routinely used dental care and those who did not. On the other hand, Kriesberg and Treiman (1962) concluded in a study limited to teenagers that neither knowledge, beliefs, nor values about teeth explained preventive dental behavior. Whether youths' attitudes had changed in the years since had not been surveyed.

Costs represent a barrier to these groups. For example, the National Health Care Expenditures Study estimated that 93 percent of charges for dental visits for ages 65 and over were paid out of pocket. This figure was higher than the national all-age average of 77 percent (Rossiter & Lawson, 1980).

Economists generally view costs as the major barrier to utilization of dental services. There are indications that when the cost barriers are removed, utilization will increase but not as high as might be expected. Utilization under insurance plans in which the cost barrier has been removed is not substantially higher than by the population in general. The experience of the UAW dental benefit plan illustrates this point. The percentage of its subscribers using services during the three and a half years the plan was studied differed little from that before the program went into effect. Other factors such as perceived need and value of care seemed to be important in utilization patterns. Lower socioeconomic groups continued to be more oriented toward emergency treatment than check-up visits after benefits were instituted (Bawden & DeFriese, 1981).

It seems that there is a very complex interplay of psychosocial factors and barriers under which utilization of dental services occurs. Consumers must want care and must not be faced with significant barriers. Removing cost and structural barriers can improve utilization somewhat.

TOWARD A RATIONAL POLICY FOR IMPROVED ORAL HEALTH

> There is a curious irony in our lives . . . we are conquering ever more disease and training more and better physicians, dentists, nurses, and pharmacists—and yet the quest for health remains as elusive as the quest for the Scarlet Pimpernel. We are doing better but feeling worse (Nikiforuk & Nikiforuk, 1979, p. 147).

Aspects of the dental health of the American people have never been better. The nation is witnessing a decline in the prevalence of dental decay, the most common health problem. Aided by increases in dental personnel and insurance coverage, Americans are receiving more treatment for their dental disease than ever before. Yet issues in the delivery of personal dental health services remain, issues that must be resolved through public policy if significant additional gains are to be made.

However, while dental caries is declining, periodontal disease remains highly prevalent and possibly is even increasing, with resulting tooth loss a continuing major problem. Significant segments of the population are untouched by the delivery system or are provided only symptomatic care for relief of pain. The dental profession is struggling with the evolution of paradental personnel and the effects that alternative delivery approaches might have on the traditional system. It appears that increases in third party coverage may be affecting the increases in the price of dental services through removal of the usual market forces (Gibson & Waldo, 1981).

The United States does not have a clearly defined national dental health policy. Policy issues are discussed most often in isolation without extensive debate, and resulting decisions are fragmented. There has been no conscious, systematic examination of the issues, no identification of alternatives, and no selection of other means of guiding dental service delivery. A serious information deficiency has hampered this process. Policies that have evolved often are the result of decisions made in other health areas. Federal initiatives to increase the supply and distribution of health personnel are examples. As a result of these factors, legislation has evolved piecemeal. In 1976, more than 100 health-related legislative programs affected dentistry (U.S. PHS, 1979c).

Public policy has concentrated on supply-side issues and how resources should be developed and distributed. The number of providers, where they are located, how efficiently they work, how they are organized, and how they are paid all were issues addressed by federal legislation during the 1960s and 1970s. This approach was not entirely satisfactory because the focus was not on health. It was based on the assumption that personal care was the main approach to improving health status. Efficient and available health care is a desirable aspect of public policy but is not the only approach and, at this point, not the preferred one for resolving issues that would lead to improved oral health.

Policy analyses should consider health problems and other population-side issues when identifying alternative strategies. Those ultimately adopted must bear a direct relationship to improved health. A comprehensive approach should involve a combination of strategies involving personal dental health care, dental health services, and the generation and dissemination of information. A framework for consideration of policy initiatives is presented in Table 12-9.

Dental Health Services

Policies directed at the public consisting of various activities in health promotion and disease prevention should be given a high priority. The magnitude of dental disease suggests that prevention is the most efficient strategy. The declining public support for primary care programs that traditionally have provided services for certain segments of the population suggests the need for more emphasis on prevention in the future. For dental caries, highly cost-effective and acceptable community interventions are available. The changing pattern of dental disease requires, however, that the strategy be broadened to include behavioral as well as environmental interventions to combat the most pressing dental public health problem existing today—periodontal disease.

Prevention of Tooth Decay

Dental caries is multifactorial in etiology and prevention strategies have included both environmental and behavioral interventions. Efforts to control decay have been directed at lowering the amount of refined sugar in the diet and the potential of bacteria to produce acids by removing plaque from the mouth through brushing and flossing. In public health almost all educational efforts to change behaviors have been directed toward school populations.

Fluorides in various modalities have been used to help reduce the prevalence of dental decay. Systemic fluorides present in community and school water systems and fluoride tablets help develop resistance by the

Table 12-9 A Framework for Improved Oral Health

Targeted System Component	Strategy	Goals
Dental Health Services	Health Promotion and Disease Prevention	With Respect to Individual Behavior • Increase knowledge • Raise norms for oral health status • Direct attention to periodontal disease prevention and treatment • Encourage proper brushing and flossing of teeth • Reduce sugar exposures • Increase use of fluoride tablets, mouthrinse, and dentifrices • Increase utilization of asymptomatic care With Respect to Environmental Factors • Increase community water fluoridation • Increase school water fluoridation • Promote availability of oral hygiene products • Promote restrictions on advertising of sweets
Personal Dental Health Care	Predoctoral and Continuing Professional Education	• Promote positive attitudes toward prevention, periodontal disease, role of auxiliaries, and community involvement • Encourage early detection, treatment, and referral
	Develop Alternative Delivery Systems and Financing Mechanisms	• Assure accessibility of care
	State Licensure Boards and Dental Practice Acts	• Emphasize periodontal treatment • Remove restrictions that do not relate to safety and welfare of public nor permit maximum utilization of personnel
Information	Research and Demonstrations Formation of Commission on Dental Health Policies	• Increase availability of information for health policy • Debate public policy issues • Plan for improved oral health

enamel when the fluoride ion is incorporated into the developing structure of the tooth and promote remineralization of decalcified enamel.

These preventive methods can reduce the occurrence of dental caries by 40 to 80 percent. Self-administered fluoride mouthrinse in school dental programs can lower the prevalence of decay by 25 percent. Very favorable cost-benefit ratios for each of these methods have been reported: public water fluoridation, 1:50; school water fluoridation, 1:5.3; and fluoride tablets administered at school, 1:17.5 (Burt, 1978).

In 1975, 49.4 percent of the total United States population and 60 percent of those with community water systems were drinking community fluoridated water (U.S. PHS, 1977b). Emphasis on this highly cost-effective method received renewed, but short-lived, emphasis in 1979 when Congress appropriated $1 million for the Dental Disease Prevention Activity of the Centers for Disease Control (CDC) in Atlanta. Another $11 million was appropriated through fiscal year 1981 to help communities implement or upgrade community and school water fluoridation through categorical grants to states. During those three years, 765 additional community and 108 school water systems serving a combined total of 11.24 million persons were fluoridated (ADA, 1981).

The Reagan administration's 1981 switch from the categorical grant program to a block grant program was expected to reduce the use of preventive funds for fluoridation because of the competition with other health programs. Emphasis on fluoridation must continue for the favorable trends in dental caries to continue. Data from North Carolina, as an example, emphasize both the success of fluoridation and the impact yet to be made through its wider diffusion. In 15 years, dental caries declined 15 to 20 percent in the state. On the other hand, only about a third of the state population in 1976 had exposure to fluoride during the first eight years of life in which the permanent teeth were developing—a period thought to be most critical in developing resistance to decay (Hughes et al., 1982).

A Strategy for Periodontal Disease Prevention and Control

The etiology of periodontal disease requires a different strategy. Prevalence, cohort, and experimental studies implicate bacteria (in plaque) as the primary etiological agent in periodontal disease. Extensive epidemiological research into factors correlated with the occurrence of periodontal disease consistently identifies only two factors—age and oral hygiene. The experimental work of Loe, Theilade, and Jensen (1965) demonstrated conclusively that if plaque were allowed to build up on the teeth, gingivitis would result. When plaque was removed, the gingivitis disappeared. Only after the disease progresses to the more serious stages (periodontitis) is self-care no longer entirely effective in reversing problem levels. Long-term preventive trials demonstrated that periodontal disease could be prevented and controlled through plaque removal (Jackson, 1979).

So it appears that the primary risk factor in the initiation and progression of periodontal disease is poor oral hygiene. No method other than scrupulous, mechanical removal of plaque through brushing and flossing by an individual on a frequent basis, supplemented with professional prophylaxis, is available.

There was some dissatisfaction with the long-term effectiveness of school-based plaque control programs. They were doomed to failure for certain segments of the population because they dealt with only one member of the family, and the least influential one at that. Any strategy for dealing with this widespread disease must involve a broad, community-based intervention, including education and prevention, based on sound theoretical principles of behavioral change.

No comprehensive periodontal community intervention had ever been attempted as of this writing. Other health interventions can be used as a model for dealing with this problem. Despite its bacterial origin, periodontal disease is similar in many important respects to chronic and degenerative diseases such as cardiovascular ailments. For example, the high-risk groups defined by age, race, and sex are similar; both diseases are asymptomatic in their early stages; secondary treatment can be time consuming and expensive; and both require high levels of commitment to life style changes by the affected individuals. These similarities suggest that effective cardiovascular intervention models might serve as a useful guide for developing others for periodontal disease.

Only a few attempts have been made to plan and develop broad-scaled community interventions for cardiovascular disease, most health promotion activities being directed toward individuals. The North Karelia Project was one community effort that provided evidence that control of chronic disease was feasible through health promotion (McAlister, Puska, Salonen, Tuomilehto & Koskela, 1982). The project produced a number of examples of behavior change with broad application to reducing risk factors in dentistry. North Karelia is a rural county of about 180,000 in Eastern Finland. Its complex public health intervention was aimed at improved detection and control of hypertension, reduced smoking, and lowered intake of saturated fats. The program included education; preventive services; persuasion; training of health personnel, volunteer workers, community leaders, and the public; environmental changes; and community organization.

The Role of Education

Education of the public about periodontal disease is an important component of any intervention. Frequent and simple sources of information can have a large impact on public knowledge about any condition. Given the nature of periodontal disease occurrence and progression, public knowledge and attitudes about its etiology, symptomatology, prevention, and treatment are extremely important. Periodontal disease is a chronic malady that is relatively symptom free and painless. Its development is so gradual that affected persons usually do not know that they have the disease. Only in advanced stages does it become bothersome, with loosening and drifting teeth, abscesses, bad breath, and, finally, loss of teeth.

Little is known about public awareness of periodontal disease. One survey of a national sample of adults conducted for the American Academy of Periodontology indicated that several important misconceptions were widely held among those who never had been treated for it (Market Facts, 1980):

- an unclear understanding of bleeding gums as a warning sign
- underestimation of the importance of frequent flossing as a preventive measure
- underestimation of the role of plaque as a cause
- erroneous belief in the effectiveness of drugs or a controlled diet as treatment
- resistance to acceptance of a diagnosis of periodontal disease when the ailment is asymptomatic

Another example of the limited public awareness came from a group of first-year dental students who responded to questions on dental disease at the beginning of their studies. While all students had some basic knowledge of cavities, none of those who, it was found, had periodontal disease (87 percent of those surveyed) were familiar with its symptoms or etiology (Hangorsky, 1981).

Increasing public awareness toward periodontal disease should receive priority in national health policy. The public then must be persuaded to use the knowledge. Dentists must become involved in communicating and disseminating information about prevention and control to decision makers and the community at large. As discussed later, dentists must be prepared through continuing education and professional education to assume this role.

Preventive Services

Improved preventive services also should be made available to the entire public, not just the proportion that uses (demands) services. Private and public sectors must work together to promote the availability of screening, detection, and referral for periodontal disease. The detection and referral must involve a community approach. The many patients outside the dental care system, public or private, must be identified and, depending on their financial resources, fed into either of the two systems.

The program can best be coordinated and implemented by a public health hygienist based in the local health department who coordinates screening clinics conducted by private dentists in each community. Screening and referral clinics should be held where people work, shop, and play. The public health hygienists also should function in the school system, where frequent prophylaxis for high-risk groups should be made available. Research has shown that with frequent services, caries and periodontal disease can essentially be eliminated in children.

Training, Environment, and Community

These activities also must be supplemented by training of groups and individuals in the community in self-care practices and should include guides and increasing independent practice, feedback, and reinforcement.

To increase the potential for success, environmental changes must be made. Examples include: restrictions on the availability of sweets that tend to promote plaque, increases in the availability of oral hygiene products in stores, restrictions on advertising of sweets, and financing mechanisms that can support periodontal disease prevention and control.

All of these elements can be accomplished only through community organization. The community must be mobilized to facilitate adoption of the health promotion and disease prevention activities as well as to help carry them out.

Dramatic improvements will not come quickly. However, a national strategy should be adopted that will impact on societal norms concerning dental health in general and periodontal disease specifically, then transfer these intervention proposals into actions. Communities must be encouraged to adopt these activities. Sufficient knowledge exists about the etiology of periodontal disease and how individuals can prevent and control it. This knowledge is not being applied by individuals, or either the public or private sectors. Drawing from the theoretical basis of behavioral science and the clinical and epidemiological knowledge of periodontal disease, the potential exists for controlling this malady through dental health services.

Personal Dental Health Care

If significant improvements are to occur in the nation's health, changes in the system through which services are delivered must be made, in addition to population interventions discussed earlier. A major change must occur in attitudes of the profession and its practices. As noted, dentists are repair oriented. They devote major amounts of their practice time to diagnosis and treatment of diseases and conditions that are subject to rehabilitation or repair through well-defined and highly effective procedures. They concentrate on disease and its treatment rather than on health and its maintenance. This orientation toward treatment, and primarily toward care and rehabilitation of dental caries, reinforces the attitude that dental diseases can be cured. A diseased tooth can be treated or repaired and may need no further treatment for many years.

Periodontal disease does not fit readily into the curative model. True prevention probably is not practical, given the state of knowledge about the disease, its prevention, and its treatment. Control requires a lifetime commitment on the part of both patients and providers. Periodontal disease thus more easily fits the behavioral model of disease prevention.

Professional attitudes are formulated initially in dental education. Therefore, progress in changing those attitudes must begin with predoctoral dental education and be reinforced with appropriately designed continuing education. The structure of dental education promotes the curative model of practice. Dental curricula begin with the study of the anatomy and physiology of the body and oral cavity but quickly turn to pathology, diagnosis, and treatment. Clinical experiences are oriented toward disease and procedure, with a lack of emphasis on prevention and control. Students must acquire patients with disease who can be treated to fulfill graduation requirements.

Dental decay provides good teaching material. It is diagnosed easily and effective treatment can be accomplished in short order without medical or dental complications. Other treatment areas such as the replacement of missing teeth also have most of these characteristics of the reparative model. Periodontal disease treatment does not fit easily into this area.

Student evaluation is difficult at times since successful treatment requires a behavioral commitment on the part of the patient. Treatment often is protracted. Since patients "belong" to the student rather than to the institution, the full sequence of diagnosis, treatment, and follow-up cannot be accomplished within the available curriculum time. Specific periodontal treatment procedures are not as effective or have not been evaluated as thoroughly as has treatment for other conditions. Faculty attitudes also reflect the reparative model.

Thus, for a number of reasons, periodontal disease receives less emphasis than it should. The competition between preventive/periodontal and other clinical departments for scarce instructional time is most often won by reconstructive departments other than periodontics. A survey indicated that less than 2 percent of total dental school curricula in the United States were devoted to either didactic or clinical instruction in preventive dentistry. The majority of these experiences were in the first two years of study (Ayers, Williams, & Lausten, 1979).

Dental hygiene curricula also are deficient in preventive instruction in periodontics. Because of the crucial role dental hygienists play in the delivery of care, preventive periodontics should receive emphasis in educational programs. A 1978 national survey of dental hygiene education programs provided information on the type and amount of instruction in preventive periodontics in curricula. While the majority of schools required students to probe periodontal pockets (the main tactile diagnostic procedure available to identify periodontal disease) only about a third of the institutions mandated that this information be recorded for each patient in a periodontal chart. Eighty-one percent of the schools taught root planing procedures for only one term, 61 percent required only one semester of didactic courses in periodontology, and only 2.5 percent required a two-year sequence in periodontics. The instruction in two-year programs offering certificates or diplomas—programs that prepared the majority of hygienists in private practice—seemed to have the lowest emphasis on preventive periodontics (Odrich, 1979).

Periodontal education involves didactic and clinical goals almost exclusively, with few objectives directed toward influencing attitudes. Proper attitudes on periodontal disease prevention and treatment, an active involvement in community activities, and the role of auxiliaries all should be developed.

Attitudes toward oral health become imbedded in professionals during their dental education. Curricula should refocus on oral health and on procedures for maintaining it. The medical model that views disease etiology from the microbiological perspective must be replaced by one that focuses more on the ecological and behavioral perspective. Only by focusing on people, where they live, and how they live, can health be maintained.

Important public attitudes, values, and beliefs such as perceived need for dental care and its effectiveness can be improved through health promotion activities. These improvements may not increase utilization of dental services by some socioeconomically disadvantaged segments of the public, even when successful in motivating them to seek care, if barriers are not removed. Two such barriers are (1) financial resources and (2) characteristics of providers and how they are organized to deliver care.

The United States is the only major developed country that does not have a significant program for either reducing or eliminating the financial barriers to dental care. Financial resources should be available to the extent that all Americans who want care are able to obtain it from both public and private sources. Inclusion of dental care under Medicaid is elective and not all states so choose. In many of the states that do make provisions for care, coverage is limited.

Priority should be given to lowering or eliminating the financial barrier to everyone through a combination of private insurance and public programs. These programs must contain incentives for preventive care that have demonstrated effectiveness. For example, most private insurance plans provide for one to two preventive visits for prophylaxis each year. Scientific evidence indicates that preventive visits on a more frequent basis may be necessary to control disease (Axelsson & Lindhe, 1981). In some patients, especially those prone to the incidence and progression of periodontal disease, preventive visits on a three-month cycle are required for control. Effective quality control and utilization review mechanisms must develop concurrently with increased funding.

Dentist members of state and regional examining boards reflect in general the curative orientation of practitioners and educators. This orientation affects the nature of licensure examinations. All of these consist of a clinical component in which examinees are required to perform certain clinical procedures on patients with certain diseases and/or conditions. Most required procedures are oriented toward treatment of dental caries and its sequelae.

Some state licensure examinations do not contain any clinical testing in periodontology. This gap on examinations certifying qualifications for entry into the profession is yet another example of periodontal disease's apparently being assigned a low priority. Only when periodontology pervades the thinking and practice of all segments of the dental care system—professional education, professional certification and regulation, financing mechanisms, consumers, and dental research—will the situation be totally conducive to controlling this problem.

Quantity and Quality of Information

Extensive high-quality information is necessary for identification of issues in the public and private sectors, debate over strategies for these issues, and formulation of rational policies that will impact on health. The information base in dentistry upon which policy makers can rely is seriously deficient, especially so in some geographic areas. Many policy decisions are difficult at the local level, for instance, because the information needed to define the issues can not be disaggregated from state or national data.

Many important questions need more complete definitional and evaluative information so that policy might evolve along lines that will improve oral health. Within the issues identified and discussed in this chapter, some of the macrolevel questions that need addressing include the following:

- What effect would remote-site practice of dental hygienists have on the availability of care and on the safety and welfare of the public?
- What would be the impact of increasing dental insurance coverage on demand for care, costs of care, case mix of dental services, and oral health of the public?
- What would be the cost-effective and acceptable method for increasing the demand for asymptomatic dental care and how should the supply of personnel be balanced with projected demand?
- How much would utilization of asymptomatic dental services be increased and oral health improved if alternative delivery systems were available?
- What are the most effective strategies for changing the orientation in dental education, dental practice, and consumer demand from the medical model of dental etiology, prevention, and treatment to the behavioral model in which the ecological and behavioral factors of disease causation are emphasized?

The list could include many more broad public policy questions that need debate in the public and private arenas but require additional information to enable policy makers to reach rational decisions. To the list could be added many microlevel questions.

Research to generate the types of necessary data is needed critically. Biodental, clinical, and health services research all are important in providing these data. It is to be hoped that biodental and clinical experimentation can provide a periodontal breakthrough in the years to come. Experimentation with chemical control of dental plaque was in progress in the early 1980s but private and public funding for training of investigators and for conducting health services research was at a critically low level. As a result, a large gap existed between the information available for public policy decisions in dentistry and what was available for other health professions, such as medicine.

The beneficial impact that funding can have on stimulation of research and on providing needed information is demonstrated by programming at the W.K. Kellogg Foundation in the 1970s. It funded major dental projects involving resource planning, quality assurance, national health insurance, use of expanded functions, and regulation of care. It produced volumes of information that could prove invaluable to the public, dental profession, and elected officials for years (W.K. Kellogg Foundation, 1979).

The lack of a systematic examination of dental health policies was mentioned earlier as a contributor to fragmentation in the formation of those principles. Policies are made without consideration of all aspects of the dental care system. Decisions in education concerning the required number of general dentist graduates are made without consultation with those planning community preventive health services that will have a substantial impact on dental needs and thus on the demand for practitioners.

Dental curricula are designed without a consideration of the major oral health problems of the people. Public programs are planned without input from practicing professionals. Services for disadvantaged groups are provided by different public programs and are not coordinated.

A mechanism is needed through which dental policy issues can be identified, examined, and monitored continuously. The mechanism should allow for:

1. planning for meeting the dental health needs of the people,
2. providing public debate on major dental health policies, and
3. providing visibility to dentistry.

A national commission with state affiliates having representatives from the public, education, government, and dental profession could serve as this mechanism. The commission should be a private organization independent of government and professional or private entities.

REFERENCES

Ake, J.N., & Johnson, D.W. *Dental manpower fact book* (U.S. Department of Health, Education, and Welfare, Health Resources Administration, DHEW Publication No. (HRA) 79-14). Washington, D.C.: U.S. Government Printing Office, March 1979.

American Association of Dental Schools. *Advanced dental education: Recommendations for the 80s.* Final report of the Task Force on Advanced Dental Education of the American Association of Dental Schools. September 1980.

American Dental Association. *Report of the meeting of the House of Delegates, annual session.* Chicago: Author, 1975.

American Dental Association, Bureau of Economic Research and Statistics. *Denturism: The illegal and unqualified practice of dentistry.* Chicago: Author, December 1976.

American Dental Association. *Legal provisions for delegating expanded functions to dental hygienists and dental assistants.* Chicago: Author, October 1977.

American Dental Association, Bureau of Economic Research and Statistics. *The 1977 survey of dental practice.* Chicago: Author, 1978. (a)

American Dental Association, Bureau of Economic Research and Statistics. *Utilization of dental services by the elderly population.* Chicago: Author, 1978. (b)

American Dental Association, Bureau of Economic and Behavioral Research. *Distribution of dentists in the United States by state, region, district, and county.* Chicago: Author, 1979. (a)

American Dental Association, Bureau of Economic and Behavioral Research. *Dental habits and opinions of the public: Results of a 1978 survey.* Chicago: Author, July 1979. (b)

American Dental Association. Expiring fluoridation program success despite short lifespan. *ADA News,* November 23, 1981.

American Dental Association, Bureau of Economic and Behavioral Research. *The 1979 survey of dental practice.* Chicago: Author, 1982.

American Fund for Dental Health, National Dental Quality Assurance Advisory Committee. *Dental quality assurance terminology: A glossary.* Chicago: Author, April 1980.

American Public Health Association. Employment of expanded function dental auxiliaries in public dental care programs: Policy statement 8121. *American Journal of Public Health,* February 1982, *72*(2), 202–203.

Ancell, M.Z. *The dental hygienist as a periodontal cotherapist.* Paper presented to the Section on Dental Hygiene Education at the annual session of the American Association of Dental Schools. Las Vegas, Nev., March 21, 1972.

Axelsson, P., & Lindhe, J. Effect of controlled oral hygiene procedures on caries and periodontal disease in adults: Results after 6 years. *Journal of Clinical Periodontology,* June 1981, *8*(3), 239–248.

Ayers, C., Williams, D., & Lausten, L. A survey of prevention in dental education. *Journal of Dental Education,* August 1979, *43*(9), 515–516.

Bailit, H.L., & Serling, J.M. The development of dental treatment planning criteria. In M.K. Hine (Chair), *Proceedings of a Workshop on: Dental Quality Assurance.* Workshop held by National Dental Quality Assurance Advisory Committee, American Fund for Dental Health. Denver, June 29, 1979.

Bailit, H.L. Issues in regulating quality of care and containing costs within private sector policy. *Journal of Dental Education,* September 1980, *44*(9), 530–536.

Barone, J. Know your foe—"the denturist." *Journal of the American Dental Association,* April 1974, *88*(4), 678–679.

Bauer, J.C., Pierson, A.P., & House, D.R. *Factors which affect the utilization of dental services* (U.S. Department of Health, Education, and Welfare, Health Resources Administration, Publication No. (HRA) 78-64). Washington, D.C.: U.S. Government Printing Office, May 1978.

Bawden, J.W., & DeFriese, G.H. (Eds.). *Planning for dental care on a statewide basis: The North Carolina dental manpower project.* Chapel Hill, N.C.: The Dental Foundation of North Carolina, 1981.

Bean, S. Options in dental hygiene practice. *Dental Hygiene,* May 1981, *55*(5), 29–34.

Brown, L.J., & Winslow, J.E. (Eds.). *Proceedings of a conference on modeling techniques and applications in dentistry* (U.S. Department of Health and Human Services, Health Resources Administration, Publication No. (HRA) 81-8). Washington, D.C.: U.S. Government Printing Office, 1981.

Burt, B.A. (Ed.). The relative efficiency of methods of caries prevention in dental public health. *Proceedings of a Workshop at the University of Michigan,* June 5–8, 1978. Ann Arbor, Mich.: The University of Michigan, 1978.

Cons, N.C. The clinical evaluation of Medicaid's patients in the State of New York. *Journal of Public Health Dentistry,* Summer 1973, *33*(3), 186–193.

The Council of State Governments, National Task Force on State Dental Policies. Issues in dental health policies. *Journal of Dental Education,* Special Issue, October 1979, *43*(11), 1–100.

Danchik, K.M., Schoenborn, C.A., & Elinson, J. *Highlights from Wave I of the national survey of personal health practices and consequences, United States, 1979* (U.S. Department of Health and Human Services, U.S. Public Health Service, National Center for Health Statistics, Series 15, No. 1, Publication No. (PHS) 81-1162). Washington, D.C.: U.S. Government Printing Office, June 1981.

Dean, H.T. Epidemiological studies in the United States. In F.R. Moulton (Ed.), *Dental caries and fluorine.* Washington, D.C.: American Association for the Advancement of Science, 1946.

DePaola, P.F., Soparkar, P., Allukian, M., DeVelis, R., & Resker, M. Changes in caries prevalence of Massachusetts children over thirty years. *Journal of Dental Research,* March 1981, *60* (Special Issue A), 360 (Abstract No. 200).

Donaldson, W.F., Jacoby, I., & Wills, J. *Report of the graduate medical education national advisory committee to the Secretary, Department of Health and Human Services: Vol. II. Modeling, research, and data technical panel* (U.S. Department of Health and Human Services, Health Research Administration, Publication No. (HRA) 81-652). Washington, D.C.: U.S. Government Printing Office, 1981.

Douglass, C.W., & Cole, K.O. Utilization of dental services in the United States. *Journal of Dental Education,* April 1979, *43*(4), 223–238.

Douglass, C.W., & Day, J.M. Cost and payment of dental services in the United States. *Journal of Dental Education,* June 1979, *43*(7), 330–348.

Douglass, C.W., & Lipscomb, J. Expanded function dental auxiliaries: Potential for the supply of dental services in a national dental program. *Journal of Dental Education,* September 1979, *43*(10), 556–567.

Dubos, R.J. *The mirage of health.* London: George Allen and Unwin, Ltd, 1960.

Dworkin, S.F., Ference, T.P., & Giddon, D.B. *Behavioral science and dental practice.* St. Louis: The C. V. Mosby Company, 1978.

Federal Trade Commission. *Commission statement upon closing the dental hygienist portion of its investigation of dental industry practices.* File No. 772,3020, 1980.

Fee, A.D. The dental mechanics of Canada. *Journal of Prosthetic Dentistry,* January 1974, *31*(1), 10–21.

Final report from the Ad Hoc Committee for the Delivery of Quality Prosthetic Care for the Financially Disadvantaged. *Journal of the American Dental Association,* November 1977, *95*(5), 1024–1038.

Frazier, P.J. A new look at dental health education in community programs. *Dental Hygiene,* April 1978, *52*(4), 176–186.

Fulton, J.T., Hughes, J.T., & Mercer, C.V. *The natural history of dental diseases.* Chapel Hill, N.C.: University of North Carolina, School of Public Health, Department of Epidemiology, 1965.

Gibson, R.M., & Waldo, D.R. National health expenditures, 1980. *Health Care Financing Review,* September 1981, *3*(1), 1–54.

Glass, R.L. Secular changes in caries prevalence in two Massachusetts towns. *Caries Research,* 1981, *15*(5), 445–450.

Grainger, R.M. *The orthodontic treatment priority index* (U.S. Department of Health, Education, and Welfare, U.S. Public Health Service, National Center for Health Statistics,

Publication No. (PHS) 1000, Series 2, No. 25). Washington, D.C.: U.S. Government Printing Office, December 1967.

Grasso, J.E., Nalbandian, J., Sanford, C., & Bailit, H.L. The quality of restorative dental care. *Journal of Prosthetic Dentistry,* November 1979, *42*(5), 571–578.

Greene, J.C., & Suomi, J.D. Epidemiology and public health aspects of caries and periodontal disease. *Journal of Dental Research,* October 1977, *56* (Special Issue C), C20–C26.

Gurney, N.L., & Alcorn, B.C. The concept of attitudes. In K.E. Wessels (Ed.), *Dentistry for the handicapped patient: Postgraduate dental handbook series* (Vol. 5). Littleton, Mass.: PSG Publishing Company, 1979.

Hangorsky, U. Early detection of periodontal disease by the general practitioner. *Oral Health,* October 1981, *71*(10), 27–30.

Harvey, C., & Kelly, J.E. *Decayed, missing, and filled teeth among persons 1–74 years: United States* (U.S. Department of Health and Human Services, U.S. Public Health Service, Publication No. (PHS) 81-1673, Vital and Health Statistics Series 11, No. 223.) Washington, D.C.: U.S. Government Printing Office, August 1981.

Health Insurance Association of America , Public Relations Division. *Source book of health insurance data: 1981–82.* Washington, D.C.: Author, 1982.

Heloe, L.A., & Haugejorden, O. 'The rise and fall' of dental caries: Some global aspects of dental caries epidemiology. *Community Dentistry and Oral Epidemiology,* December 1981, *9*(6), 294–299.

Hixon, J.S., & Mocniak, N. *Forecasts of employment in the dental sector to 1995* (U.S. Department of Health, Education, and Welfare, Health Resources Administration, Publication No. (HRA) 79-6.) Washington, D.C.: U.S. Government Printing Office, 1979.

Horowitz, H.S., Greek, W.J., & Hoag, O.S. Study of the provision of dental care for handicapped children. *Journal of the American Dental Association,* December 1965, *71*(6), 1398–1410.

Horowitz, H.S. The future for self-applied fluorides. *Journal of Public Health Dentistry,* Fall 1981, *41*(4), 255–259.

Hughes, J.T., Rozier, R.G., & Ramsey, D.L. *The natural history of dental diseases in North Carolina, 1976–77.* Durham, N.C.: Carolina Academic Press, 1982.

Jackson, D. Measuring restorative dental care in communities. *British Dental Journal,* May 1, 1973, *134*(9), 385–388.

Jackson, D. Dental caries: The distinction between delay and prevention. *British Dental Journal,* November 5, 1974, *137*(9), 347–351.

Jackson, D.B. Longitudinal studies: What has been learned about the prevention and treatment of periodontal disease. *Clinical Preventive Dentistry,* May–June 1979, *1*(3), 18–22.

Kegeles, S.S. Why people seek dental care: A review of present knowledge. *American Journal of Public Health,* September 1961, *51*(9), 1306–1311.

Kegeles, S.S. Adequate oral health: Blocks and means by which they must be overcome. In W.E. Brown (Ed.), *Oral health, dentistry, and the American public.* Norman, Okla.: University of Oklahoma Press, 1974.

Kelly, J.E., Van Kirk, L.E., & Garst, C.C. *Decayed, missing, and filled teeth in adults: United States—1960–62* (U.S. Department of Health, Education, and Welfare, Health Resources Administration, Publication No. (HRA) 74-1278, Vital and Health Statistics Series 11, No. 23). Washington, D.C.: U.S. Government Printing Office, August 1973.

Kelly, J.E., Sanchez, M., & Van Kirk, L.E. *An assessment of the occlusion of the teeth of children 6–11 years: United States* (U.S. Department of Health, Education, and Welfare,

Health Resources Administration, Publication No. (HRA) 74-1612, Vital and Health Statistics Series 11, No. 130). Washington, D.C.: U.S. Government Printing Office, November 1973.

Kelly, J.E., & Scanlon, J.V. *Decayed, missing, and filled teeth among children: United States—19* (U.S. Department of Health, Education, and Welfare, Health Resources Administration, Publication No. (HRA) 74-1003, Vital and Health Statistics Series 11, No. 106). Washington, D.C.: U.S. Government Printing Office, May 1974.

Kelly, J.E., & Harvey, C.R. *Decayed, missing, and filled teeth among youths 12–17 years: United States—19* (U.S. Department of Health, Education, and Welfare, Health Resources Administration, Publication No. (HRA) 75-1626, Vital and Health Statistics Series 11, No. 144). Washington, D.C.: U.S. Government Printing Office, October 1974.

Kelly, J.E., & Harvey, C.R. *An assessment of the occlusion of the teeth of youths 12–17 years: United States* (U.S. Department of Health, Education, and Welfare, Health Resources Administration, Publication No. (HRA) 77-1644, Vital and Health Statistics Series 11, No. 162). Washington, D.C.: U.S. Government Printing Office, February 1977.

Kelly, J.E., & Harvey, C.R. *Basic data on dental examination findings of persons 1–74 years: United States, 1971–74* (U.S. Department of Health, Education, and Welfare, U.S. Public Health Service, Publication No. (PHS) 79-1662, Vital and Health Statistics Series 11, No. 214). Washington, D.C.: U.S. Government Printing Office, May 1979.

Klein, H., Palmer, C.E., & Knutson, J.W. Studies on dental caries: I. Dental status and dental needs of elementary school children. *Public Health Reports,* May 1938, *53*(19), 751–765.

Kriesberg, L., & Treiman, B.R. Preventive utilization of dentists' services among teenagers. *Journal of the American College of Dentists,* March 1962, *29*(1), 28–45.

Loe, H., Theilade, E., & Jensen, S.B. Experimental gingivitis in man. *Journal of Periodontology,* May–June 1965, *36*(3), 177–187.

Logan, R.K. Dental care delivery in New Zealand, In J.I. Ingle & P. Blair (Eds.), *International dental care delivery systems.* Cambridge, Mass.: Ballinger Publishing Company, 1978.

Malvitz, D.M., & Mocniak, N. Profile of dental hygienists licensed in the United States. *Journal of Public Health Dentistry,* Winter 1982, *42*(1), 54–71.

Market Facts, Inc. *Developing communications themes for increasing awareness, detection and treatment of periodontal disease: A report to the American Academy of Periodontology.* Chicago: Author, September 1980.

McAlister, A., Puska, P., Salonen, J.T., Tuomilehto, J., & Koskela, K. Theory and action for health promotion: Illustrations from the North Karelia project. *American Journal of Public Health,* January 1982, *72*(1), 43–50.

McKeown, T. *The role of medicine: Dream, mirage, or nemesis?* London: The Nuffield Provincial Hospitals Trust, 1976.

Milgrom, P., Weinstein, P., Ratener, P., Read, W.A., & Morrison, K. Dental examinations for quality control: Peer review versus self-assessment. *American Journal of Public Health,* April 1978, *68*(4), 394–401.

Miller, A.J., Brunelle, J.A., & Smith, J.E. Dental restorative treatment needs of U.S. school children. *Journal of Dental Research,* March 1982, *61*, 242 (Abstract No. 574).

Newman, J.F., & Larsen, A. *A decade of dental service utilization: 1964–1974* (U.S. Department of Health and Human Services, Health Resources Administration, Publication No. (HRA) 80-56). Washington, D.C.: U.S. Government Printing Office, 1980.

Nikiforuk, G., & Nikiforuk, M. Health for and by the people. *Journal of Dental Education,* March 1979, *43*(3), 147–152.

Odrich, J. Preventive periodontics in the dental hygiene curriculum: Results of a nationwide survey. *Journal of Dental Education,* August 1979, *43*(9), 506–509.

Office of Health and Medical Affairs. *Key to health for a padlocked society: Design for health care in Michigan prisons.* Lansing, Mich.: Author, January 1975.

The Oregon lesson: Results of postelection research. *Journal of the American Dental Association,* May 1979, *98*(5), 749–754.

Quality assurance: Five experts examine the issues. *Journal of the American Dental Association,* May 1982, *104*(5), 608–617.

Rosenstein, D.I., Joseph, L.P., Mackenzie, L.J., & Wyden, R. Professional encroachment: A comparison of the emergence of denturists in Canada and Oregon. *American Journal of Public Health,* June 1980, *70*(6), 614–618.

Rosenstein, S.N., Bush, C.R., & Gorelick, J. Dental and oral conditions in a group of mental retardates attending occupation day centers. *New York State Dental Journal,* August–September 1971, *37*(7), 416–421.

Rossiter, L.F., & Lawson, W.R. *Charges and sources of payment for dental visits with separate charges* (U.S. Department of Health and Human Services, U.S. Public Health Service, National Center for Health Services Research, Office of Health Research, Statistics and Technology, Publication No. (PHS) 80-3275). Washington, D.C.: U.S. Government Printing Office, 1980.

Rozier, R.G., Kelly, T.W., & Slome, B.S. *Estimating dental care needs from disease prevalence.* Chapel Hill, N.C.: University of North Carolina, 1981.

Russell, A.L. A system of classification and scoring for prevalence surveys of periodontal disease. *Journal of Dental Research,* June 1956, *35*(3), 350–359.

Russell, A.L. International nutrition surveys: A summary of preliminary dental findings. *Journal of Dental Research,* January–February 1963, *42*(1), 233–244. (Supplement)

Ryge, G., & Snyder, M. Evaluating the clinical quality of restorations. *Journal of the American Dental Association,* August 1973, *87*(2), 369–377.

Schonfeld, H.K. *Description and documentation of the Veterans Administration dental delivery system* (U.S. Department of Health, Education, and Welfare, Health Resources Administration, Publication No. (HRA) 79-23). Washington, D.C.: U.S. Government Printing Office, 1979.

Sisty, N.L., Henderson, W.G., Paule, C.L., & Martin, J.F. Evaluation of student performance in the four-year study of expanded functions for dental hygienists at the University of Iowa. *Journal of the American Dental Association,* October 1978, *97*(4), 613–627.

Sisty, N.L., Henderson, W.G., & Paule, C.L. Review of training and evaluation studies in expanded functions for dental auxiliaries. *Journal of the American Dental Association,* February 1979, *98*(2), 233–248.

Spencer, A.J. The estimation of need for dental care. *Journal of Public Health Dentistry,* Fall 1980, *40*(4), 311–327.

U.S. General Accounting Office. *Increased use of expanded function dental auxiliaries would benefit consumers, dentists, and taxpayers* (GAO Publication No. HRD-80-51). Washington, D.C.: Author, March 1980.

U.S. Public Health Service. *Volume of dental visits, United States, July 1963–June 1964* (Department of Health, Education, and Welfare, National Center for Health Statistics,

PHS Publication Series 10, No. 23). Washington, D.C.: U.S. Government Printing Office, October 1965.

U.S. Public Health Service. *Group dental practice in the United States, 1971* (Department of Health, Education, and Welfare, National Institutes of Health, Publication No. (NIH) 72-189). Washington, D.C.: U.S. Government Printing Office, 1972. (a)

U.S. Public Health Service. *Ten-state nutrition survey, 1968–1970* (Department of Health, Education, and Welfare, Health Services and Mental Health Administration, Center for Disease Control, Publication Nos. (HSM) 72-8130, 72-8131, 72-8132, 72-8133). Washington, D.C.: U.S. Government Printing Office, 1972. (b)

U.S. Public Health Service. *Current estimates from the health intervention survey, United States, 1971* (Department of Health, Education, and Welfare, National Center for Health Statistics, PHS Publication Series 10, No. 78). Washington, D.C.: U.S. Government Printing Office, February 1973.

U.S. Public Health Service. *Ad hoc scientific evaluation panel: Evaluation of the NIDR periodontal disease research activity* (Department of Health, Education, and Welfare, National Institute of Dental Research). Bethesda, Md.: April 1976.

U.S. Public Health Service. *Dental delivery systems terminology.* (Department of Health, Education, and Welfare, Health Resources Administration, Bureau of Health Manpower, Division of Dentistry, Publication No. (HRA) 77-6). Washington, D.C.: U.S. Government Printing Office, 1977. (a)

U.S. Public Health Service. *Fluoridation census, 1975* (Department of Health, Education, and Welfare, Health Resources Administration, Center for Disease Control, Dental Disease Prevention Activity, Publication No. (HRA) 98-607). Washington, D.C.: U.S. Government Printing Office, April 1977. (b)

U.S. Public Health Service. *Projections of national requirements for dentists: 1980, 1985, and 1990* (Department of Health, Education, and Welfare, Health Resources Administration, Bureau of Health Manpower, Division of Dentistry, Publication No. (HRA) 78-70). Washington, D.C.: U.S. Government Printing Office, July 1977. (c)

U.S. Public Health Service. *Healthy people: The Surgeon General's report on health promotion and disease prevention* (Department of Health, Education, and Welfare, Publication No. (PHS) 79-55071). Washington, D.C.: Government Printing Office, 1979. (a)

U.S. Public Health Service. Barriers to attaining an effective dental health system. *Proceedings of the Region IX Dental Conference,* Department of Health, Education, and Welfare, Pacific Grove, Calif., August 30–September 1, 1979. (b)

U.S. Public Health Service. *Federal legislation affecting dentistry* (Department of Health, Education, and Welfare, Health Resources Administration, Bureau of Health Manpower, Division of Dentistry, Publication No. (HRA) 79-4). Washington, D.C.: U.S. Government Printing Office, 1979. (c)

U.S. Public Health Service. *The prevalence of dental caries in United States children, 1979–1980: The national caries prevalence survey* (Department of Health and Human Services, National Institute of Dental Research, National Dental Caries Program, Publication No. (NIH) 82-2245). Washington, D.C.: U.S. Government Printing Office, December 1981. (a)

U.S. Public Health Service. *Survey of dental benefits plans, 1978.* (Department of Health and Human Services, Health Resources Administration, Bureau of Health Professions, Division of Dentistry, Publication No. (HRA) 81-12). Washington, D.C.: U.S. Government Printing Office, 1981. (b)

Waerhaug, J. Epidemiology of periodontal disease—review of literature. In S.P. Ramfjord,

D.A. Kerr, & M.M. Ash (Eds.), *World workshop in periodontics: 1966.* Ann Arbor, Mich.: The University of Michigan, 1966.

Wilder, C.S. *Dental visits volume and interval since last visit: United States, 1978 and 1979* (U.S. Department of Health and Human Services, U.S. Public Health Service, Publication No. (PHS) 82-1566, Vital and Health Statistics, Series 10, No. 138). Washington, D.C.: U.S. Government Printing Office, April 1982.

W.K. Kellogg Foundation. *Annual report.* Battle Creek, Mich.: Author, 1979.

World Health Organization. *Application of the international classification of diseases to dentistry and stomatology.* Geneva: Author, 1978. (a)

World Health Organization. *Epidemiology, etiology, and prevention of periodontal diseases: Report of a WHO scientific group.* Technical Report Series 621. Geneva: Author, 1978. (b)

Young, W.O., & Striffler, D.F. *The dentist, his practice, and his community.* Philadelphia: W.B. Saunders Company, 1965.

Zacherl, W.A., & Long, D.M. Reduction in caries attack rate—nonfluoridated community. *Journal of Dental Research,* January 1979, *58* (Special Issue A), 227. (Abstract No. 535)

Chapter 13

The Changing Mental Health Scene

James W. Luckey

The years since the early 1950s have been marked by tremendous growth and change in the mental health field. Spurred by the rejection of more than 10 percent of potential draftees in World War II for psychiatric reasons, the nation focused increased attention and resources on its mental health needs. Immediately following the war, the National Institute on Mental Health (NIMH) was created as the first federal agency solely designated to address the country's needs in this field. Since its inception the NIMH has played an instrumental role in many changes through its support of research, training, and program development.

An event in the early 1950s that was critical to the changing mental health scene was the development of the major tranquilizers for use with psychotic patients. These psychotropic drugs greatly facilitated patient management in state hospitals, where a sizable proportion of the population was psychotic. In addition, these medications also permitted many patient discharges to the community. The watershed year for state- and county-supported hospitals was 1955, when their resident population peaked at 559,000 patients; by 1982, they had fewer than 170,000. Although it would be both simplistic and misleading to attribute this change solely to the development of the major tranquilizers, they certainly helped substantially.

The emergence of these medications coincided with the beginning of a general social period that was ripe for change in the mental health field. This was an economically prosperous time. Public attention returned to domestic matters following two wars. In 1955, a Joint Commission on Mental Illness and Health was appointed to examine the needs of the mentally ill. The timing of its final report, *Action for Mental Health* which was released in 1961, was propitious. The country was in a period of optimism, with a major concern being the welfare of fellow citizens. This era of positivism was reflected in the election of the youngest president ever, one who also held a personal and familial interest in mental health.

In response to the report's recommendations and a personal request to Congress by President Kennedy, the first Community Mental Health Centers Act was passed in 1963 (P.L. 88-164). As detailed later, the actual implementation of the concept fell well below the rhetoric, a failure as much from unrealistic expectations as from faulty implementation. Despite its shortcomings, this program had a profound effect on the delivery of mental health services. The outcome of this act was more than a program— it initiated a movement.

There were several key components of this movement.

- Emphasis shifted from a few severely disturbed individuals to the entire population. A whole range of problems, syndromes, and disorders of varying degrees of severity were beginning to be seen as appropriate for mental health intervention.
- Both the number of treatment approaches offered and the backgrounds of the persons providing them increased.
- Attention was paid to the prevention of problems and the promotion of mental wellness.
- The movement, probably most importantly, was at least partially responsible for fostering increasingly positive attitudes by the general public concerning mental health problems.

Another social trend beginning in the early 1960s that eventually affected the manner in which mental health services were delivered was an increased concern with equal treatment under the law. The attention being paid to the civil rights of various disadvantaged groups soon spilled over to mental patients. Beginning in 1965 in New York State with the creation of the Mental Health Information System to provide legal advocacy services to involuntarily committed patients, efforts were focused on protecting the rights of those under psychiatric treatment. Both the courts and state legislatures addressed key issues, including the methods and criteria for involuntary commitment, right to treatment, the right to refuse treatment and equal protection under the law. In addition to influencing treatment methods in institutions, these legal precedents helped foster the shift to community-based care.

Two of the major changes involving mental health since 1950 provide the underpinnings for the policy issues addressed in this chapter:

1. the expansion of the boundaries of the mental health field, with a rapid growth in the populations served, the number and types of providers, and the total number of episodes of care

2. the shift away from inpatient services, particularly in state- and county-supported institutions, as the primary locus of care

As discussed later, both events created dilemmas for the mental health field, the resolution of which could provide the major focus for the rest of the 1980s.

The changes highlight the importance of social factors in mental health, a crucial consideration to keep in mind in any analysis of the field. The presense or absence of a mental "problem" is determined on the basis of a normative evaluation of thoughts, feelings, or behaviors. Because of differing norms across settings for these actions or mental states, the evaluation of the degree of dysfunction involved is linked inextricably to the context in which the behavior is being assessed. The importance of social factors is even more pronounced when considering the type of intervention utilized. Although the patient's clinical level of distress is the best predictor of seeking services, the type and location of care is influenced strongly by both the availability and characteristics of the services and the client's social and economic status.

The social construction of mental illness is clearly evidenced by the changes since the 1950s. The enormous growth of situations now seen to be within the realm of mental health services is a prime example. Events previously regarded as normal reactions to a given situation now frequently precipitate a mental health intervention (e.g., reactions resulting from a divorce or other separation). Likewise, state and county hospitals, which once were praised as a great step forward, now are denounced by many as archaic and inhumane. The boundaries of what constitutes mental health problems and the response to these issues are sensitive to and a reflection of current values and beliefs (Magaro, Gripp, & McDowell, 1978). Any attempt at analysis of the mental health service system must pay close attention to the social milieu of the period.

Following two decades of growth and change, the early 1980s constituted a period for redefinition and consolidation of the mental health field. The trend was away from expanding services that attempted to meet the mental health needs of all persons, turning emphasis on specific groups or problems. Such focusing was necessary in an era of fiscal austerity and accountability.

Before discussing each of these issues in detail, it is important to describe the mental health scene. The task, seemingly as simple as a description of the field, can be overwhelming, as Kovel (1980) points out:

Any attempt to survey the pursuit in America of what is variously called mental health or emotional health runs up immediately against the sheer size of the territory and the ill-defined nature of the landscape (p. 72).

THE MENTAL HEALTH SCENE

An obvious starting point for this discussion is: What is mental health? It is notable that nowhere in the four volumes of the *Report of the President's Commission on Mental Health* (1978) is the term ever defined explicitly. This was not an oversight; rather, it was an attempt to avoid a debate where there were no answers, only informed opinions. Similarly, this chapter, rather than examining individual definitions of mental health or mental illness, takes a general approach, outlining the broad classes of models used to define, describe, and respond to these conditions.

Models of Mental Health/Illness

The lack of agreement on a model or models for mental illness is a reflection of both the amorphous nature of the problems and the immense range of conditions that are categorized under the rubric of those two words. This lack of clarity frequently has resulted in a lack of credibility for the field, problems for those attempting to make rational policy decisions that affect the subject, and reluctance by funding sources to involve themselves except in the most clear-cut of cases.

The three models analyzed here can be categorized as medical, psychological, or sociological/environmental. Few models or theories of mental illness fall precisely into one category. However, each does place relative emphasis on a particular point of view. This in turn defines the type and focus of the intervention and the qualifications of the intervenors.

The Medical Model

The term medical model as applied to mental illness must be defined explicitly and with care. The phrase has been used with various meanings that appear to be theoretically based but that have practical implications as well. Power, prestige, and financing factors often have clouded the arguments.

A medical model, as used here, specifically means a model for defining and explaining mental illness solely in terms of physiological, biochemical, or genetic processes. Early support for such a position developed around the turn of the century when it was discovered that a sizable portion of those in asylums were there as a result of advanced syphilis or the effects of pellagra. These conditions provided a clear-cut physiological basis for the disordered behavior.

Absolute proponents of this position, or of any of the three models, are indeed rare. Nonetheless, the influence of the medical model in practice is very strong. Patients are treated by physicians and medications often are prescribed. In more serious cases, the person is hospitalized despite the fact the diagnostic indicators are almost exclusively behavioral and, in most instances, medication is seen only as a facilitator rather than as the primary treatment.

This is not to detract from the efforts of the medical profession; rather, these practices demonstrate assumptions underlying patterns of care. The model alone does not determine these practices; there are many other reasons, including the credibility of the medical profession, the symptomatic relief afforded by medications, and the desire to remove explanation and evaluation of such behavior from the moral realm.

The Psychological Model

Similar to the medical model, a psychological model finds the locus of the problem within the person. That is, the abnormal behavior, feelings, or thoughts are a result of a disordered psyche. Psychoanalysis, first developed by Sigmund Freud, was one of the earliest theoretical frameworks in this tradition. Causal factors may have been external to the person (e.g., the parenting process) but the key consideration is that the problem resides within the individual.

As with a medical model, a psychological version focuses on the individual as the point of intervention. This may take many forms, including psychotherapy, behavior therapy, or a host of skill-building techniques (e.g., assertiveness training). Neither the actual setting nor the qualifications of the person or institution responsible for providing treatment are as clearly defined as with a medical model. The skills necessary for evaluation and treatment are in the behavioral or psychological sphere and do not require a medical background but, more likely, training in the social sciences.

The Sociological/Environmental Model

The sociological/environmental model posit that the type of disordered behavior called mental illness is a response to events external to the person and may even be a normal reaction to abnormal outside forces. The source of these external events may range from the person's immediate social network such as a spouse's or family's behavior all the way to global events such as a downturn in the economy.

The locus of intervention is equally broad and should focus on the disordered social unit. If it is a relationship problem, then the intervenor would act with the members of that relationship. Once beyond the level of the family as the social unit of concern, the discussion expands through personal health services and into some type of social action or community change. Many have argued convincingly that this is the direction mental health care should take if it is to have a significant impact.

In the sociological/environmental model, the setting for treatment is the context in which the disordered behavior occurs. This was part of the rationale of the community mental health movement, particularly in the early stages of conceptualization of the idea. Such a model also opens the possibility for a myriad of intervention agents in almost any setting imaginable.

Prevalence of Mental Health Problems

It should be evident from this discussion that an important factor in determining the extent of mental health problems is the choice of model and the stringency of the criteria used. Prevalence estimates vary markedly with the types of behaviors examined and the norms employed.

The first major attempt to determine the prevalence of mental disorders in this country was undertaken in Massachusetts by Edward Jarvis in 1855 (1971). Jarvis compiled information from hospital admission records and community leaders to estimate the extent of the problem. Based on those two sources, he reported 2,632 lunatics (the insane) and 1,087 idiots (the mentally retarded) in the Commonwealth needed care or custody, or about 0.3 percent of the population. Even more enlightening were his findings relating to the social characteristics and the role of treatment for these two groups. He found that:

1. insanity was much more frequent among paupers and immigrants
2. about half of both the lunatics and the idiots remained in the community despite the availability of institutional services, and
3. prognosis was best for those who received proper treatment soon after the first manifestation of their illness.

These findings have been "rediscovered" in many ensuing research efforts over the past 40 years.

Before World War II, most epidemiologic studies used indirect measures such as rates under treatment or opinions of community leaders to estimate the extent of the problem. One notable effort during this period was the work of Faris and Dunham (1967) in the late 1930s. Their study, although not intended to estimate the prevalence of mental disorders, was based on first admissions to all psychiatric hospitals in Chicago. Their results demonstrated the importance of social variables in mental disorders. They found that those given a diagnosis of schizophrenia were more likely to reside in the economically depressed sections of the city while those with a manic-depressive diagnosis were distributed randomly throughout the population. This finding set off a major discussion of the relative merits of social causality of mental disorders vs. downward social drift resulting from psychopathology.

Several key studies following World War II developed highly sophisticated community sampling techniques. The best known of these was the midtown Manhattan study by Srole, Langer, Michael, Opler, & Rennie (1962) who found 23 percent of the sampled residents were substantially impaired. Less than a quarter of their sample was found to be symptom free. Other key studies of the period including Gurin, Veroff, and Feld (1960) using a nationwide probability sample and Leighton, Harding, Macklin, Hughes, & Leighton in Nova Scotia (1963) reported similar startlingly high rates of mental disorder.

As important as the results from the psychiatric epidemiologic studies was the conceptual approach used. Most of the epidemiologic studies of that era focused on global impairment ratings rather than on psychiatric diagnoses. Diagnoses were not used because of concerns about both the reliability and the validity of a medical classification scheme for mental disorders. The social sciences had a strong influence on psychiatric epidemiology during this period, with most studies placing emphasis on social factors as causal variables. Anomie, social disintegration, stress and social class were considered prime etiologic determinants. The period of the 1950s and 1960s was marked by a rejection of the classical medical model with its discrete psychiatric disorders and specific physiologic causal factors.

Events since then began a dramatic shift in emphasis in psychiatric epidemiology. Bolstered by results suggesting a genetic component in schizophrenia and the bipolar affective disorders, the medical model with discrete nosological categories was on the ascendency. Considerable effort was expended to increase the reliability of the diagnostic process. After several years of debate and development, a third edition of the *Diagnostic and Statistical Manual of Mental Disorders* (APA, 1980) was produced. This revision, based heavily on the work of a research group of Washington University in St. Louis, provided more explicit criteria for the various diagnostic categories than the previous edition.

Summarizing the major studies, the *Report of the Task Panel on the Nature and Scope of the Problem* of the *President's Commission on*

Mental Health (1978) provided the following range of prevalence estimates for the major psychiatric disorders among the population as a whole:

Schizophrenia ....0.5 to 3.0 percent
Manic-depressive psychosis ....0.3 percent
Neurosis ....8.0 to 13.0 percent
Personality disorders ....7.0 percent

Estimates for substance abuse disorders provide an equally wide range of figures and the degree of overlap was not clear between those who were considered substance abusers and those who fall into the four psychiatric categories just listed, particularly the personality disorders. With these caveats in mind, studies generally have found that 5 to 8 percent of the total population abused alcohol (NIAAA, 1978). Data on the extent of abuse of other drugs, both legal and illegal, were difficult to interpret because most of the epidemiologic studies had emphasized use rather than defining patterns of use that would be considered as abusive. Because of this focus on use alone, only professional judgment of the prevalence of drug dependence was possible. The staff of the Alcohol, Drug Abuse, and Mental Health Administration (ADAMHA) used an estimate of 0.5 to 1.0 percent of the population to illustrate the general dimensions of the problem (ADAMHA, 1980).

Several major problems remain in determining the extent of the need for mental health services. Because of the range of estimates available and the question of the degree of overlap between the mental health and the substance abuse populations, the number of persons with such problems could range from 30 million to 70 million, a rather substantial spread. The situation is further complicated by the treatment-seeking patterns in the field. Extrapolation from the only complete psychiatric register in the country—Monroe County (Rochester area), New York—plus the most conservative estimate of prevalence indicate that only about 20 percent of those with a psychiatric disorder seek specialized treatment in a given year. Other studies have shown that this figure is dependent on both the availability and characteristics of services as well as the particularities of the population in need. Thus, even complete agreement on the extent of mental health problems would not translate directly into need for services.

AVAILABILITY OF MENTAL HEALTH SERVICES

A mental health service system as an organized structure of services does not exist. The characteristics of the population served constitute the only common denominator for services provided. This lack of coherence exists for a variety of reasons, including the absence of any agreement on the appropriate treatment mode or setting, vagaries of funding and reimbursement policies, the public's attitude toward these problems and on seeking help for them, and the multiple and sometimes contradictory functions of mental health services.

The variability in services for the emotionally disturbed was examined by Regier, Goldberg, & Taube (1978). They collected data from a variety of sources to ascertain where these persons actually received services. They estimated that less than 20 percent of this group obtained care from specialized mental health programs. The bulk of services were in the general health care sector. The analysis demonstrated the importance of not focusing solely on categorical mental health services when assessing how well the treatment needs of the mentally ill were being met. To obtain an accurate picture, it is necessary also to examine the role of the general health care system in meeting the needs of this population.

Inpatient Mental Health Services

Public Psychiatric Hospitals

Formal responsibility by the state for the care of the mentally ill dates to English common law under the parens patriae concept. However, specialized facilities for this group are a relatively recent phenomenon because throughout most of history no distinctions were made between the various indigent groups. The first real efforts in modern times at providing humane treatment for the mentally ill began in the late 18th century with the pioneering work of Pinel in France and Tuke in England. A few facilities for the mentally ill were opened in this country in the late 18th and early 19th centuries, often under religious auspices. Despite these early laudable efforts, however, the bulk of the mentally ill remained incarcerated with other indigents in local almhouses or were left to fend for themselves.

Beginning in the 1840s, reform efforts by persons such as Dorothea Dix brought attention to the plight of the mentally ill. In response to this publicity, most states built specialized facilities during the period from 1850 to 1870. These asylums, as they were called originally, were designed for relatively brief care, usually a year or less, in small facilities housing fewer than 250 patients. With the mass immigration of this period, the shift from an agrarian society to an industrialized one, and a changing view of insanity from treatable to untreatable, the small, short-stay facility no longer was possible. By 1872, when Pilgrim State Hospital was built in New York to house 10,000 patients, asylums had become custodial facilities, with deaths often exceeding discharges.

Despite some attempts at reform, this situation remained relatively unchanged over the next 80 years. Much of the care for the mentally ill was provided in large state- or county-operated facilities, with the primary focus on custodial care.

In the early 1950s several factors contributed to the shift in emphasis away from these facilities as the sole source of mental health care. The development of psychotropic medications, along with changing attitudes toward the mentally ill, facilitated the change. Another practical concern was the increased drain these institutions were creating on state coffers; existing facilities were not sufficient and expansion would have required massive capital expenditures.

With the shift away from institutions as primary providers of care, the role of these facilities changed. The reduction in patient population resulted in great part from a substantial decrease in the average length of stay rather than in the numbers of persons served. In 1955 the average stay was approximately six months; by 1975, it had decreased to 26 days (ADAMHA, 1980). These shorter stays required increased emphasis on the admission process and preparation of the patient for return to the community.

No longer could the institutions function as a self-contained community that addressed all the patients' needs over a long period of time. Successful implementation of the new role as crisis center required effective liaison and coordination with community-based programs in order to provide a continuum of services. However, many states created community programs under local control while institutions were operated by the state. One problem resulting from these parallel systems has been that of patients "falling between the cracks."

Another change is that these public institutions are providing care to a different clinical population. With the development of both publicly funded outpatient facilities and private inpatient services, the state and county institutions have been left with the most difficult cases. The types of persons admitted are those whose insurance coverage has expired at the private facilities or those who do not have the financial resources to afford private care. Both of these factors—failure to respond to treatment in a relatively brief period in private facilities and the lack of resources—are not indicators of a good prognosis.

Other Inpatient Facilities

Some of the decline in utilization of state and county hospitals since the 1950s has been offset by the increased availability and utilization of other inpatient facilities. It is difficult to determine the exact magnitude of this offset because of the lack of systematic data; however, some general indicators are available. For 1955, private psychiatric hospitals and general hospitals with psychiatric units had about 390,000 admissions, or approximately 30 percent of all inpatient episodes; state hospitals had 819,000 admissions that year, or 64 percent. By 1975, excluding federally funded community mental health center data that were not broken out by inpatient/outpatient episodes, the percentage of inpatient admissions by state and county hospitals had dropped to 33 percent (599,000) while those in private and general hospitals grew to 46 percent (731,000).

Even such relatively recent data may be misleading in underestimating the rapid growth of the private sector in providing inpatient mental health care. Between 1979 and 1980, proprietary hospitals added almost 2,300 psychiatric and substance abuse beds, a 38 percent increase. This situation led the president of one of the larger corporations to predict that by the end of this decade the private sector would have replaced most of the inpatient psychiatric services being offered under various governmental auspices (Kuntz, 1981).

Obviously, financial considerations made the venture into mental health attractive to the private sector. One motivating factor was the increased coverage for psychiatric and substance abuse treatment in health insurance policies. This reimbursement, coupled with declining occupancy rates in many hospitals, resulted in medical/surgical beds' being converted to psychiatric and substance abuse beds as a strategy for effective utilization of resources. The increased availability of third party coverage also prompted the development of new facilities, particularly since such services were less capital intensive than medical/surgical units, making them attractive to smaller corporations wishing to expand.

Although the private sector was replacing some of the beds being phased out in the public sector, it served a different population. Because insurance frequently limited care to 28 days a year, the private sector generally treated those who were acutely ill. In 1975, the median length of stay in state and county hospitals was 26 days; for general hospitals with psychiatric units, 12 days; and for private mental hospitals, 20 days. The diagnostic composition also was different, with about 40 percent of those in the private sector being diagnosed as depressive and 20 percent schizophrenic. For state and county hospitals, these percentages were reversed. In addition to the patient's clinical condition, the demographic characteristics also differed in that the private client or sponsor normally must be employed to have the insurance or other means to pay for the care. Financial considerations generally excluded the chronically disabled from private care.

Outpatient Services

The number of episodes of care in the mental health system increased tremendously from 1955, when the total was 1.7 million, to 1975, when it reached 7.1 million. This included a slight increase in the number of inpatient episodes but the vast majority of the expansion resulted from the growth of outpatient services. Several factors contributed to this, including:

- changing reimbursement and funding practices
- increased public acceptance of psychiatric care
- shorter inpatient stays requiring additional outpatient followup
- growth of the types of problems deemed to require psychiatric intervention
- increased reluctance by the legal system to commit persons involuntarily for long periods to an inpatient facility

The most visible symbol of these changing patterns of care was the community mental health movement.

Community Mental Health Centers

In response to the 1961 report *Action for Mental Health,* President Kennedy sought Congressional authorization for a system of community-based services for the mentally ill. The initial enabling legislation (P.L. 88-164) was passed in late 1963, providing construction grants for these facilities. The following year a program of staffing grants was approved. These funds were provided for eight years on a decreasing basis using the concept of seed funding. The original legislation required recipient institutions to provide five services (inpatient, outpatient, emergency, partial hospitalization, and consultation and education) in order to be eligible for federal funds. The 1975 amendments to the Community Mental Health Centers Act (P.L. 94-63) expanded this list to include specialized services for children and the elderly, screening, follow-up care for those discharged from state hospitals, alcohol and drug abuse services, and halfway houses.

The community mental health center movement was indeed a "bold new approach." However, funding was not commensurate with the charge. Originally, some 1,400 centers with a catchment area population of 75,000 to 200,000 persons each were envisioned. By 1982, only about half these were operational. Only about $2 billion of federal monies were allocated from 1963 to 1977 for a program initially designed to provide a comprehensive array of mental health services for everyone.

Given the relatively limited resources committed to the program, its accomplishments were notable. The *Report of the Task Panel on Community Mental Health Centers Assessment* of the *President's Commission on Mental Health* (1978) reported that in 1975, these centers provided for 29 percent of the total episodes of outpatient care in the nation, serving some 1.6 million persons, but expended only about 4 percent of the total mental health dollar.

The centers have been criticized repeatedly for a variety of reasons, including failure to meet the needs of the chronically mentally ill, inability to become financially independent, providing private practice care under the guise of being a community-focused agency, and the lack of real preventive efforts. All of these criticisms are justified; however, shortcomings of the effort should not detract from its accomplishments.

The major difficulty with the entire community mental health center program was undue optimism that resulted in its being oversold. Neither the resources nor the methods were available to accomplish all that the rhetoric promised. However, credit must be given to the movement for helping to drastically alter mental health service delivery patterns and to increase the public's acceptance of such problems.

The changes the centers effected include a dramatic reduction in the resident population of publicly supported institutions, increased emphasis on community-based treatment, attention to the environment as a contributing factor in both problems and responses, the importance of preventive efforts, increased accessibility of mental health services, and an enhanced community role.

Because of the importance of federal funds, the future of such centers was not clear under the Reagan Administration's block grant legislation. This was particularly true for centers in poverty areas where federal funds provided the bulk of support. In addition to the decline in or loss of fiscal support, removal of the service requirements (e.g., alcoholism services) could result in a dramatic change in the character of these centers.

Mental Health Providers

The final key ingredient in the categorical mental health services was the providers. They not only staffed the facilities, they also accounted for 20 percent of those treated in 1975 under private practice (ADAMHA, 1980). A major issue was the question of who was an appropriate provider of these services.

As noted, specialized treatment for the mentally ill is a relatively recent phenomenon. The early 19th century saw the growth of asylums, with the staffs being the first mental health personnel. During the 1830s and 1840s there was a trend toward requiring the superintendents of these facilities to be physicians. An association formed by these medical superintendents (the Association of Medical Superintendents organized in 1884) was the forerunner of the American Psychiatric Association (Rothman, 1971). A classification system for mental disorders developed by Kraeplin, a German neurologist in the latter part of the nineteenth century, and the realization in the early part of this century that nutritional deficits (i.e., pellagra) and advanced syphilis could result in disordered behavior, gave increased credence to psychiatry as a medical specialty.

Early efforts were focused on the severely disabled, with the vast majority of psychiatrists working in institutions. With the threat of Nazi Germany hovering over Europe in the 1930s, many followers of Freud fled to the United States. Their arrival was significant in diverting psychiatry's efforts away from institutional care.

Freud's theory and method were seen as applicable primarily to neurotic or less disabled individuals; more and more emphasis was put on outpatient care for this group. By 1982, it was estimated there were 25,000 trained psychiatrists in this country, the majority of whom devoted at least part of their time to office-based care. Most state hospitals encountered great difficulty recruiting psychiatrists and almost half of their staffs were foreign medical graduates (FMGs). However, recent restrictions subsequently imposed on FMGs and the decline in medical graduates entering psychiatric residencies made the availability of coverage in state hospitals an area of concern.

A profession with even a shorter history is clinical psychology. Although its origins can be traced to an earlier period, World War II provided the major impetus to the growth of this field. The acute need for methods and personnel to screen recruits and address the needs of psychological casualties of the battlefield resulted in academic psychologists' being pressed into clinical work. Based on this experience, the Veterans Administration in 1946 began supporting clinical training efforts. Its funds, along with training monies made available through NIMH beginning in the late 1940s, produced some 25,000 licensed clinical psychologists.

Besides increasing in numbers, the role of psychologists has expanded. They originally were relegated to the role of psychometricians or psychological testers while psychotherapy was seen as the responsibility of the physicians. However, this professional distinction no longer exists. This role blurring has been one factor in the lukewarm relationship between these two professions, which is compounded further by legal battles over access to the reimbursement dollar. Control traditionally has been in the hands of physicians; however, some 30 states have passed freedom-of-choice legislation allowing reimbursement for psychotherapy to qualified psychologists functioning without physician supervision.

The two other core mental health professionals are the psychiatric social workers and the psychiatric nurses. In 1976 there were more than 30,000 social work positions in mental health facilities, a 50 percent increase in four years (NIMH, 1977). More than 70 percent were for those holding at least a master's degree in social work (M.S.W.). It was estimated that an additional 12,000 social workers were engaged in private practice (NIMH, 1977), a trend that was on the increase.

Data on psychiatric nurses were sparse, primarily because official recognition of this group as a specialty was relatively recent. In 1975, the American Nurses' Association (ANA) established a Division of Psychiatric and Mental Health Nursing that certified qualified nurses. Of nurses who belonged to the ANA, 14 percent reported working in mental health settings (NIMH, 1977). As with social workers, psychiatric nurses were becoming involved in private practice. However, both professions suffered from lack of recognition by third party payers as independent providers of care.

The number of allied mental health professionals had grown to include, among others, vocational, pastoral, educational, and marriage counselors, and recreation, art, music, and occupational therapists.

The final group providing a sizable proportion of patient care was the paraprofessionals. This group generally was defined by exclusion (i.e., all those not listed above). Paraprofessionals' qualifications could be based on education, such as an associate degree from a community college; on experience (e.g., a recovering alcoholic), or just the desire to work with this population.

Several key issues in the mental health field related to personnel. One was the distribution of the four core professions: they tended to be clustered in metropolitan regions; rural areas, as with state hospitals, had difficulty attracting them. Another problem was role diffusion among the various professions. Psychotherapy, once the domain of the psychiatrist, now has no exclusive professional ownership. The ensuing conflicts created major administrative challenges. This lack of clear role differentiation also was a major obstacle to determining human resource requirements in mental health.

Mental Health in the Health Care Sector

The general health care sector by definition is not part of the mental health system; however, the majority of individuals with psychiatric problems only obtain services in the general health care sector. Data for 1975 indicated that, excluding visits to psychiatrists, more than 13 million persons seen by office-based physicians had some sort of emotional illness

(Regier, Goldberg, & Taube, 1978). This was almost twice the number seen by the entire speciality mental health sector that year. It was estimated that the typical primary care physician saw more mentally ill persons annually than did the average psychiatrist.

The other component of the health care system that bears a major portion of the mental health-related contacts are outpatient clinics and emergency rooms, where some 6.4 million persons were seen in 1975. Altogether, outpatient settings and inpatient units without specialized services provided care to some 20 million individuals with psychiatric problems in 1975, or about three times as many as the mental health specialty sector.

These staggering figures raised several important clinical and policy issues. At the individual level, the concern was whether persons with emotional problems were appropriately identified and treated in health care settings. The charge was made frequently that the health care sector provided only medication while failing to address the real problem. These accusations were supported by the high proportion of tranquilizing drugs prescribed in such settings, particularly Valium and Librium.

From the perspective of the primary health care sector, the mentally ill constituted a major drain on the available resources. The many individuals involved further exacerbated the situation by their excessive utilization patterns. Epidemiologic studies indicated that 10 percent of those seen in the health care sector were there because of an emotional or mental problem rather than a physical disorder; however, they constituted 20 percent of the visits (Hankin & Otkay, 1979). This disproportionately high rate of utilization arose in part because usual physiologic interventions did not provide effective relief from their problems.

It would be impossible for the mental health sector to address the needs of all those seen in the health care sector with emotional problems. This practical fact motivated efforts to develop methods to meet the needs of the emotionally disturbed more effectively in the general health care sector. Various models have been proposed, including referral to the mental health sector, psychiatric consultation, provision of a mental health specialist in the health care setting, and the training of health care personnel in psychiatric interventions. The majority of these efforts were in the initial stages of implementation in the early 1980s. No one model had been shown to be the best; rather, efforts had been focused on the most feasible and efficient method in a given setting.

THE FUTURE: CLARIFICATION AND CONSOLIDATION

The decades since World War II have seen phenomenal growth and change in the mental health field. The expansion of its boundaries and the shifting patterns of care both have created major challenges. Resolution of some of the resulting dilemmas will be necessary in the 1980s to consolidate and maintain the advances that have been made so far and to clarify future directions.

The most visible challenge was the care and treatment of the chronically mentally ill. Bolstered by a host of court decisions aimed at protecting patient rights and increasing treatment in the least restrictive alternative and changes in many states' involuntary civil commitment laws, the official policy from the mid-1970s was one of deinstitutionalization for this group. However, implementation of this policy was far from complete and it remained a major problem. The strong support for this movement in the mid-1970s was followed by a questioning of the desirability and feasibility of transferring all CMI patients to the community. Fiscal considerations, legal mandates, community reactions, patient and family concerns, and quality of care were just some of the forces that impinged on this question, frequently with contradictory needs and expectations.

A less visible but equally challenging issue lay in responding to the additional problems now considered within the purview of mental health. Despite the growth of public funds and increased third party coverage for mental health and substance abuse services, neither the financial resources nor the personnel in this speciality sector were sufficient to address the massive dimensions of emotional problems as now defined.

The attention in recent years to the role of the health care sector, particularly primary care providers, in offering mental health services illustrated one potential avenue for meeting these needs. Realization of the extent of emotional problems encountered in these settings, and the health care resources consumed by those with such difficulties, provide both fiscal and humane motivations for developing methods for responding to the mental health needs of those seeking service in the general health care sector.

Finally, and most difficult, were questions concerning the very nature of the field of mental health. Disagreements remained about the nature, cause, and scope of its problems and methods of responding to them. The long-range and most critical challenge is the clarification and at least partial resolution of these basic issues.

Care and Treatment of the Chronically Mentally Ill

The chronically mentally ill (CMI) are those with debilitating mental health problems of long duration. Estimates of the size of this population were based on various surrogate indicators. Epidemiologic surveys reported that 3 percent to 4 percent of the population was psychotic. However, not all of this group would be considered CMI, both because some did not meet the severity criterion and more importantly the duration criterion. A much more conservative estimate based on disability claims for mental disorder under Supplementary Security (SSI) under Social Security or Social Security Disability Insurance showed that in 1975 some 800,000 persons received such benefits for psychiatric reasons (Meier, 1981).

The care and treatment of these persons has a clear historical precedent as a public responsibility, primarily because of their indigent status. Until the early 1960s the publicly supported mental health speciality sector was almost solely concerned with the care of this group. The bulk of mental health funding was from the states and was used primarily to support large state hospitals; little federal monies were available and community-based services were almost nonexistent. Beginning in 1963, with the first infusion of federal funds in support of the Community Mental Health Centers program, increased attention was placed on the development of local programs to replace state and county hospitals for the care and treatment of the CMI.

The Trend to Deinstitutionalization

The deinstitutionalization movement received a significant boost in the late 1960s and early 1970s with the increased focus by the legal system on protecting the rights of psychiatric patients. Most states revised their commitment statutes to make it more difficult for patients to be admitted involuntarily. Many of these new laws also required that the care be provided in the least restrictive setting, which necessitated the development of community programs.

Even more critical to the move away from institutions was the new legal requirement for periodic review of involuntary stays. In the past, patients could be committed indefinitely and frequently were retained in the hospital for long periods. The shorter stays that resulted from this periodic review requirement placed increased emphasis on follow-up programs in the community. Finally, additional pressure was placed on state hospitals by several key court decisions that focused on their quality of care, the most famous being *Wyatt v. Stickney* (1971) which specified in great detail minimum facility standards and staff-to-patient ratios necessary to fulfill the right to treatment requirements for such patients.

Meeting minimum standards of care as defined in these rulings and fulfilling Medicare and Medicaid requirements required substantial additional funds to upgrade services. The result was that state hospitals no longer constituted the inexpensive solution they once had been; as average daily costs soared, community care often became a less expensive mode of treatment (Rubin, 1978).

For some, particularly elderly psychiatric patients, deinstitutionalization meant transfer from the state hospital to a nursing home, a trend bolstered by the availability of Medicare funds for such care. In 1977, 12.4 percent of all residents of nursing homes had psychiatric disorders as their primary diagnosis (National Center for Health Statistics, 1979). Some were lifelong disabilities, while others were the result of the aging process. Both types, however, would have received care in the state hospital prior to this movement.

This shift from psychiatric institutions to nursing homes, though not without its problems, was not the most troublesome aspect of the movement. The more difficult task was the shift of care from institutions to nonresidential community programs. Much debate ensued in both the professional literature and the public press about this effort. Although deinstitutionalization has been official policy in most states since about 1975, the task by no means has been completed. Structural, fiscal, and functional barriers hindered implementation of this policy and care of the CMI remained a major challenge.

Structural Barriers

One structural barrier was that the sheer size of the state hospitals made their dismantlement a complex task. Hundreds and even thousands of employees of any given facility relied on it for their economic sustenance. The power of this particular constituency often coalesced through strong unions that resisted efforts that could endanger their jobs. Alternative employment opportunities were necessary to reduce or phase out these facilities. Providing alternative employment was complicated by the fact that many of these institutions were located in rural settings and were the major job source for the area. Local options frequently were unavailable and most employees did not desire to relocate. These facilities also frequently were the economic mainstays of their areas and removal of those benefits could have spillover effects on the entire community and threaten many local businesses.

Another structural barrier to deinstitutionalization has been the existence of parallel organizational arrangements for institutional and community programs in many states. State hospitals receive their fiscal resources from the state and are under the jurisdiction of its mental health authority. Community programs, on the other hand, frequently have been structured so as to be clearly under local control. They may receive sizable support from the state but local autonomy has frequently been a guiding principle in their operation. Cooperation and coordination between the two systems has been hindered by this necessity of crossing organizational boundaries in order to accomplish these goals.

One problem in returning former patients to the community has been the transfer of responsibility for care from the state to the local system. Although efforts to provide for continuity of care have been made, it has not been an uncommon occurrence, as noted earlier, for the patients to get "lost between the cracks" in this transition.

Problems also have involved preventing inappropriate admissions to state hospitals. No single portal of entry into the mental health system exists; where services are received often hinges on the initial point of contact. Alternatives may exist in the community for a patient presented for admission to a state hospital but the logistic barriers of transferring such an individual to a local program may result in the decision to admit the person in the state facility. Without the presence of a clearly defined method for cross-organizational referrals and a single portal of entry into the system, patients will continue to be admitted to state hospitals who could receive community-based care.

The final structural barrier to the deinstitutionalization movement is the categorical separation of human service programs. Many of the CMI lack adequate personal, social, or financial resources and thus require the whole gamut of human services including housing assistance, vocational training, recreational opportunities, social skill building, medical services, and income supports, in addition to psychiatric care.

State hospitals are total institutions and can provide most of these services under a single organizational structure. No such comprehensive system exists in the community, requiring patients to seek services from a variety of agencies, each with its own eligibility requirements and methods for initiating contact. Such fragmentation has been   a formidable barrier for patients seeking the full array of services in the community.

One approach for dealing with this fragmentation is a case manager system for the CMI. One person, probably in the mental health system, would be designated as having primary responsibility for ensuring that the patient received all necessary services. This role would be quite different from that of a traditional mental health clinician and would require retraining of existing providers or the development of a new category of provider.

Fiscal Barriers

The latter two structural barriers—parallel mental health systems and the categorization of human services in the community—also have fiscal implications. There are no direct fiscal incentives for community-based programs to provide care for the CMI. Services for this group become an additional burden on agencies that already are overloaded. It makes intuitive sense to transfer savings accrued by state hospital to the communities that provide alternative care but mechanisms under which "funds follow the patient" have been difficult to institute.

Another barrier has been the contradictory federal policy of generally limiting Medicare and Medicaid reimbursement to residential facilities while simultaneously espousing a policy of deinstitutionalization. Problems also have been encountered with state monies, including transferring funds across organizational boundaries, determining when community-based care actually is an alternative to institutional care, and maintaining the fiscal solvency of the state hospitals.

Proponents of the state hospital system have resisted such a method because the loss of these funds could threaten the existence of their facilities. Relatively high fixed costs, particularly given the age of many of these institutions, and the increased expenses associated with fulfilling legal, regulatory, and accreditation requirements have driven the average cost per day up while total days of care decline. The actual saving to state hospitals by reduction in census frequently is not a significant amount because of the high fixed to variable costs ratio.

Functional Barriers

Finally, there have been functional barriers to implementation of deinstitutionalization. The mental health system, particularly the state hospitals, serves a dual social function. Their obvious role is the care and treatment of the mentally ill. However, it is not only the patient who benefits from these institutions. Although families do not relish the thought of a member's being in such a facility, the precipitating factor for admission often is their inability to continue to cope with that individual. State hospitals serve as a backstop for families when they no longer are able to care for mentally ill members.

A similar situation occurs at the community level. These patients' unusual or aberrant behavior frequently is seen as a threat to the social order of the community. Removal of the patient to a state hospital is met with a community sigh of relief. Amelioration of family or community disruption is an important function for these institutions. Efforts to replace them must take this role into consideration, either by providing for alternative buffering methods or by increasing family and community tolerance for certain forms of behavior.

No simple solution exists for such a complex problem as the care and treatment of the CMI, and a complete resolution was not expected in the 1980s. However, the deinstitutionalization movement will continue to consume a great deal of time, energy, and resources of the mental health system. Because of a host of legal precedents set in the 1970s relating to the requirement of minimum standards of care in the least restrictive alternative, this issue must continue to be addressed. Tremendous pressure from the community also is present to make such care as nonintrusive as possible.

Elements for a Successful Strategy

The optimistic hopes of a decade ago for closing down state hospitals no longer seem feasible. States have taken an incremental approach, moving the least disturbed and least disruptive patients into the community first. This skims the "cream" of state hospital populations, with the more difficult cases remaining there but still to be contended with in community placement later.

Success in deinstitutionalization is contingent on careful attention to several difficult technical details, including appropriate screening and preparation of patients, funding contingencies that favor community-based care, provision of transitional financing necessary to develop community programs, and timely flow of information across programs. These requirements are necessary but are not sufficient for success. The more amorphous and difficult tasks also must be tackled, including:

- community attitudes toward the CMI and its assumption of responsibility for their care
- bona fide interagency cooperation to ensure that all needs of this group are addressed
- clarification of the respective roles of the federal, state, and local governments
- protection of the rights of the mentally ill
- recognition of the community's right to be insulated from certain forms of disruptive or blatantly distasteful behavior

These difficult and sometimes contradictory requirements preclude an easy resolution of the problem but the dilemmas cannot be ignored. Courts and legislatures clearly have mandated such community treatment while at the same time local resistance to such placements remains. With any policy such as deinstitutionalization that is marked by a great deal of controversy, a key challenge is to go beyond a polarization of viewpoints and to examine the various assumptions and components of such an approach. Neither institutional-based or community-based care is inherently good or bad; both have their strengths and their weaknesses. The question is to determine what setting of care is most appropriate for what type of patient, given that person's needs, and the rights of both the individual's immediate social group and of the community.

The overriding principle is that the care and treatment of the CMI must be the number one priority of the public mental health sector in the 1980s. In the rush to community-based care and the focus on the mental health needs of the entire population, resources have been diverted from the CMI. Because of the indigent status of many members of this group, the state has clear responsibility for their care.

To meet this charge, that responsibility must be clearly delineated, either in the mental health system or in some other human service system. A major stumbling block has been a diffusion of responsibility among federal, state, and local governments and within the entire human service arena.

Linking Health and Mental Health

The mental health field's most clearly circumscribed policy issue in the 1980s is assessment and clarification of its role vis-à-vis the general health care system in the delivery of services to the emotionally disturbed. Mental health problems constitute a significant drain on the health care system. Over and above the many individuals involved, as a group they consume a disproportionately large share of the resources, as noted earlier. This group's members visit physicians more frequently than the average patient, they require more testing to rule out physical factors, and their typical office visit is 25 percent longer than for other types of clients (Hankin & Otkay, 1979).

Quality of Care

An equally important concern is the quality of treatment the mentally ill receive in the health care sector. The first issue is appropriate identification of the problem. Studies consistently have reported that 10 to 20 percent of those in outpatient settings have an emotional disorder as their primary problem but only about half of these receive a psychiatric diagnosis. However, this finding must be considered in light of the factors that mitigate against the use of such diagnoses, including reimbursement policies that frequently disallow outpatient mental health care, the stigma attached to such labels, and the potential negative implications for the patient.

Another area of concern is the prescription patterns of the psychoactive drugs, the most frequently prescribed group in this country. Concern about these prescription patterns include the potential for abuse or addiction, the appropriateness of the type and dosage, particularly with the anti-psychotics where idiosyncratic response requires special skill and monitoring, and a belief of many mental health personnel that drugs alone are not sufficient treatment but should be used in conjunction with verbal therapies.

This last point is based on the assumption that general health care personnel lack the skill, time, or inclination to provide psychotherapy. However, studies have reported anywhere from 25 to 96 percent of primary care physicians indicated they provided some form of counseling to patients with emotional problems (Hankin & Otkay, 1979). The actual amount provided to what types of patients still is in the realm of speculation, as is the efficacy of their efforts.

Clarification of the roles and responsibilities of the respective sectors in the delivery of care to the mentally ill is not an issue that has one answer or that can be addressed through a single course of action. Efforts need to focus on methods of augmenting existing approaches with the dual goals of optimal utilization of resources and provision of the highest quality of care. The actual approach taken to address this issue varies across settings and depends on many factors, including the availability of resources, both fiscal and personnel; the organizational structures of the agencies involved; the population served; and the values and attitudes of both the organizations and their staff.

Framework for Interaction

Pincus (1980) provided a useful framework to examine the various potential interorganizational or intraorganizational arrangements that could be implemented to address the needs of the emotionally disturbed in the health care sector. He listed potential factors in such efforts as including:

1. contractual elements—agreements between organizations specifying their respective roles and responsibilities
2. functional elements—the services actually encountered by the patient
3. educational elements—aimed at providing knowledge and skills to the staff.

Combinations of these elements result in six possible models of service delivery:

1. The *agreement* model is limited to contractual relationship between the two sectors while they continue to operate independently. An example would be a formal referral agreement between a mental health setting and a health care organization.
2. The *triage* model builds on the agreement model by adding some common service delivery component. An example would be staffing

a mental health specialist in a health care setting to provide evaluation and to facilitate referral to the mental health sector.

3. The *service delivery* model has a clearly defined speciality service delivery component within the larger organization. An example would be a mental health team within a prepaid medical practice plan.

4. The *consultation and service* model combines direct services with provider-focused consultation. An example would be the use of this model in prepaid plans where the mental health team provided both direct patient service and consultation to medical staff members in dealing with emotional problems encountered in their caseload.

5. The *education* model is limited to education and skill development of the caregivers. An example would be training physicians in the identification and treatment of emotional problems.

6. The *integrated health care team* involves combining organizational and functional health and mental health components. An example would be a health care team that included a mental health specialist as a team member.

The prepaid plans have led the way in the delivery of mental health services in the health care sector. Studies of prepaid plans' costs and of the potential benefits of their providing such care reported, with one exception, that medical utilization declined following mental health treatment (Jones & Vischi, 1979). The exception was with a medically underserved, low-income population where mental health services were instrumental in facilitating access to needed health care. Methodological and conceptual problems plagued these studies and the savings resulting from the reduction in health care costs did not offset the expense of these speciality services. However, this line of research helped to allay the fears about runaway costs if mental health services were to be made universally available through health insurance or prepaid plans.

The large number of persons with a primary psychiatric problem receiving service in the health care sector precludes specialized care for all in the mental health sector. Even if such treatment were feasible, it would not necessarily be desirable; advantages exist for including such treatment in general health care settings. Patients frequently do not see their problem as emotionally based; referral to a mental health practitioner can result in anger and resistance and may run the risk of losing the patient.

Similarly, there is not the stigma attached to receiving services in a health care setting as is found with mental health, thus facilitating access to treatment. The primary care physician frequently has an established relationship with the patient that facilitates a response to emotional problems and makes possible a continuing follow-up over a long period. Finally, reimbursement practices frequently preclude outpatient mental health treatment but will pay for services provided in a general health care setting.

In turn, the mental health field has special expertise to aid the health care system in treating patients whose emotional problems are secondary to their physical condition. Two categories of patients that have begun to receive more attention are those whose emotional factors play a role in the etiology, onset, course, or outcome of some physical problem (e.g., asthma) and those who have an emotional reaction as a result of some physical ailment (e.g., chronic or terminal illness).

The general health care sector and the mental health system clearly have overlapping areas, so the development of working relationships between them should be of mutual benefit. More important is the potential for significantly enhancing the quality of patient care in both settings.

Clarification of Focus and Function

As discussed earlier, the mental health field is beset by a host of seemingly irresolvable issues that concern the very nature of the field. At the heart of many of these controversies is a lack of agreement on a conceptual framework to define and describe mental health problems. Much rhetoric and research has been focused on such basic issues as what treatment should consist of, who should provide it, what are the most appropriate settings, and what is the anticipated outcome. Despite these efforts, the field still lacks a coherent structure either for evaluating existing undertakings or for guiding future endeavors.

This has been the major factor affecting both the credibility and the funding of mental health. Public and private financial sources clearly have relegated mental health to a secondary status in comparison to general health care for two related reasons: (1) the value of such care, which includes concerns about the efficacy of current efforts, and (2) the necessity for these services.

The more ominous concern for funding sources involves the unknown parameters of the mental health field. Third party payers particularly have a need to determine prospectively the fiscal implications of including a particular type of care as a reimbursable service. The two key variables that determine the costs for insurance coverage—the prevalence of the problem and the characteristics of the response to it—remain open to debate.

Many insurance carriers include psychiatric and substance abuse coverage but reimbursement frequently is marked by more constraints and limitations than medical/surgical coverage. Increasing fears of runaway costs led many companies to consider further measures to limit reimbursement for such treatment, including larger copayment schedules for psychiatric care, caps on yearly reimbursement per policy, limits on visits, and in some cases no coverage for outpatient care. Blue Cross and Blue Shield threatened to withdraw from the Federal Employees Health Benefits Program if not permitted to curtail some of its mental health benefits.

It was uncertain in the early 1980s whether the health insurance consumer—either the individual or the company paying for the policy—would acquiesce in curtailment of mental health coverage. Because such coverage often was viewed as an option or a luxury, the escalating costs of health insurance created opportunities for reducing or removing mental health coverage in policies in order to contain expenditures. To forestall this possibility, the mental health system faced the problem of how to justify its inclusion in health insurance plans.

A similar situation existed with federal and state entitlement programs, most notably Medicare and Medicaid. Discriminatory restrictions on mental health coverage strongly encouraged the utilization of more expensive care, particularly nursing homes and inpatient services. Coverage for less expensive day treatment and outpatient services was severely limited.

A long-range yet crucial policy challenge to the mental health field was the necessity of clarifying the focus and function of these services. An important first step would involve recognition of the key issues that needed to be addressed.

Need for Services

The usual starting point for the development of a rational policy or set of policies is to define the problem as clearly as possible. Based on such an explication, alternatives can be evaluated, using a variety of criteria. Numerical estimates of the various populations needing mental health services were lacking (Myers & Weissman, 1980). Over and above basic conceptual disagreements, the major epidemiologic studies in the field were more than 25 years old and by today's standards suffered from methodological deficiencies. Institutional populations were not included in community studies, incidence data were lacking and the studies often were done in isolation using differing criteria, making comparisons across studies difficult.

The NIMH recognized these problems and in 1979 committed significant resources to the Epidemiologic Catchment Area (ECA) program, funding half a dozen studies at various locations around the country. These large-scale community surveys included institutional populations in their sampling frame and consisted of two waves of interviews a year apart to obtain incidence data, with all of them using the same computer scored standardized instrument based on psychiatric nosology to permit comparisons across sites.

The ECA program was laudable in its design, focus and scope and was expected to make a major contribution to the field of psychiatric epidemiology. Disagreements about the reliance on psychiatric nosology aside, these studies alone could not define need for services. A complicating factor in the mental health field was that the presence of a disorder did not necessarily translate into a need for psychiatric care. Studies have shown that a host of personal, social, economic, and legal factors play a significant role in patients' seeking treatment and in the location of such care. No systematic framework existed to integrate all these factors into estimates of service need. This was further complicated by the lack of agreement on the appropriate response even if treatment was deemed necessary.

Appropriate Services

Disturbing questions also remained concerning the most efficient and effective manner in which to deliver services for the emotionally disturbed. Psychotherapy, the mainstay treatment, continued to be an enigma in that the process never had been explicated clearly and its efficacy still was a matter of public debate. This latter issue emerged with the publication of a treatment outcome review article by the British psychologist Hans Eysenk (1952) that called into question the effectiveness of psychotherapy. Since then, volumes of analyses, meta-analyses (e.g., Smith & Glass, 1977), and reviews of these studies have been written. Their general consensus has been that psychotherapy has some incremental positive effect. However, this debate has been confounded by the lack of consensus on the first question, namely: What is psychotherapy?

Although not completely an idiosyncratic endeavor, this mode of treatment varied a great deal from practitioner to practitioner. Many theoretical frameworks existed for describing this treatment; however, surveys of psychotherapists indicated that the vast majority used an eclectic approach. This inability to explicitly define the treatment made research on outcomes difficult and comparison across studies nearly impossible. This confusion was furthered by the lack of agreement on even what the outcome of such treatment should be.

There have been almost no studies that have examined an a priori specified outcome for a specific type of patients using a clearly defined method of psychotherapy. It has been estimated that some 150 mainstream schools of psychotherapy exist (Marshall, 1980). To examine the effectiveness of each of these would be an overwhelming task. However, some consensus on what constituted legitimate psychotherapy was becoming increasingly important as consumers became more sophisticated and third party payers more skeptical.

A related concern was the optimal intensity and duration of psychotherapy. Initially influenced by psychoanalytic theory, psychotherapy was conceived as a long-term endeavor focused on the individual as the treatment unit. When emotional problems began to be seen as interpersonal difficulties, group and family therapy began to be employed. This structural evolution was followed by a reconsideration of the outcome of such care. Amelioration of all emotional difficulties and maximization of patients' potential necessarily would be a long-term, if not a never-ending, process.

Practical considerations, most notably resource constraints, have resulted in the development of briefer, problem-specific types of treatment. An elaboration of such an approach would be intermittent therapy. As with brief therapy, this mode focused on a single problem or crisis. Development of this approach required a major conceptual shift concerning psychotherapy in that it entailed an acknowledgment that the effect of the intervention was limited and that the person would be likely to return for further treatment as other crises arose. Returning to treatment following services provided under the amelioration model would be considered a sign of failure for the initial effort. With intermittent therapy, seeking additional treatment at a later date would not be unexpected and could be one indication of a positive outcome of the first contact.

Psychotherapy has received the greatest amount of attention in the research literature but it was only one form of treatment and appeared to be of most benefit to those who were the least disturbed and who were most similar to the psychotherapist, generally those with middle and upper-class beliefs and values. For those with more severe conditions or from backgrounds that differed from those of current providers, traditional psychotherapy might not be the optimal treatment.

There are two potential problems in attempting to develop alternative models of treatment for these populations:

1. It is possible to create a two-tiered system of services with inferior care for those not deemed appropriate candidates for psychotherapy. This becomes a real possibility because providers with the greatest amount of training generally prefer providing insight-oriented verbal therapy.

2. Reimbursement policies generally do not cover alternative treatment modes such as skill-building or educational approaches, nor will they pay directly for care by nonprofessional providers.

Providers

A related and equally difficult series of questions related to who were the most appropriate providers of mental health care. Some functions, most notably the prescription of medications and the administration of electroconvulsive therapy, clearly were the responsibility of a physician. However, these treatments were only a portion of the interventions used. Psychotherapy, skill building, and educational approaches were functions that did not belong to any particular profession.

Third party payers generally sidestepped the question as to who was the most effective provider; instead, they focused on the therapists' educational credentials. For many years, only physicians or physician supervised providers were eligible for reimbursement. Freedom of choice legislation in some 30 states negated this tack by opening reimbursement to licensed clinical psychologists.

These efforts to permit direct reimbursement to professions other than psychiatry continued to be resisted in the court, most notably in the case of the two Blue Shield plans in Virginia that required that billing be through a physician. This practice, challenged by the Virginia Academy of Clinical Psychologists, was ruled arbitrary by the United States Court of Appeals for the Fourth Circuit. Clinical psychologists were the most active in seeking independent provider status, although the other two core mental health professions (psychiatric social workers and psychiatric nurses) also sought such recognition.

The disagreements over who was the appropriate provider of mental health services focused on the effectiveness issue but had direct implications for the efficiency of delivering such care. One argument for recognizing professions other than psychiatry was that this would expand the number of providers, resulting in increased competition and lowering of costs for mental health treatment.

Outcome

At the hub of many of these issues was the question of what the anticipated outcome of mental health treatment should be. For the purchasers of such services, be it the individual consumer, third party payers, or some governmental unit, the specification of the anticipated result should provide a basis for evaluating the value of the care. The vague justification of "helping" no longer is sufficient in times of fiscal constraint, as aptly pointed out by cartoon in Figure 13-1, first published in 1973 but even more appropriate today.

Resolution of the outcome question could provide the starting point for clearly defining the parameters of the mental health field. Determining

Figure 13-1 Plus Ça Change, Plus C'est La Même Chose

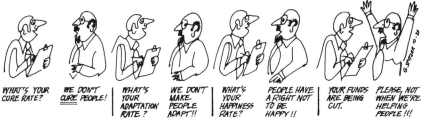

WHAT'S YOUR CURE RATE?   WE DON'T CURE PEOPLE!   WHAT'S YOUR ADAPTATION RATE ?   WE DON'T MAKE PEOPLE ADAPT!!   WHAT'S YOUR HAPPINESS RATE?   PEOPLE HAVE A RIGHT NOT TO BE HAPPY !!   YOUR FUNDS ARE BEING CUT.   PLEASE, NOT WHEN WE'RE HELPING PEOPLE !!!

Source: By Gil Spitzer, reprinted by permission from *APA Monitor,* American Psychological Association, © 1981.

specifically what services should accomplish would be the critical first step in designing studies to examine the relative efficacy of various treatment methods.

The *Report of the Task Panel on Research* to the *President's Commission on Mental Health* (1978) outlined four possible objectives for mental health services:

1. health goals that relate to the prevention, amelioration, or elimination of symptomatology associated with mental or emotional problems
2. rehabilitation goals that focus on the person's social role performance
3. humanistic goals that are aimed at the optimization of human potential
4. civil rights goals that address the community's protection from harmful or dangerous behaviors and protection of the patient's rights, including harmful treatment and unnecessary loss of freedom

The relative importance of each of these goals would vary with the population considered and the source of funding. For example, with the chronically mentally ill who relied primarily on publicly supported services, a balance must be reached between the civil rights and rehabilitation goals. At the other extreme, resources and technological constraints precluded using public or third party funds in efforts to realize humanistic goals.

Resolution of these issues will not be a simple task but a recognition of the need to address such problems would be a major step in the right direction. Such issues have received congressional attention as evidenced by a proposed amendment to the Social Security Act introduced by Senators Daniel K. Inouye and Spark M. Matsunga, both Democrats of Hawaii, in August 1980 to create a National Professional Mental Health Services

Commission. The task of this commission, if it had been approved, would have been:

> To determine on the basis of careful and thorough evaluation of the most credible and professional clinical and scientific information available (with formal expressions as to the adequacy and sufficiency of such information for purposes of making definitive recommendations), which combinations of patient characteristics (including the nature and severity of the patient's condition), therapeutic techniques, characteristics of mental health professionals, and types of settings are safe, effective and appropriate in treating specific mental problems (taking into account alternative types, methods, settings, and relative expense of treatment), and to make specific recommendations (including any conditions, restrictions, or other limiting considerations) based on these determinations, to the Secretary [of the U.S. Department of Health and Human Services] with respect to their reimbursement under this Act. (quoted in Greenberg, 1980)

The date for accomplishment of these gargantuan goals was set for January 1, 1984. Nicholas Cummings, then the president of the American Psychological Association, was quoted as saying such goals more realistically would take 10 to 20 years to accomplish (Greenberg, 1980). Despite the overwhelming nature of the task, these issues are critical for the mental health field if it is to systematically address in the rest of the 1980s.

CONCLUSION

The years ahead will be challenging for the mental health field as with all human services. Although this speciality sector has its unique strengths and problems, all such services in the foreseeable future will be required to operate in a restricted fiscal environment.

Such constraints will necessitate difficult decisions for both administrators and policy makers. Their decisions also provide opportunities to clarify and refine existing undertakings. Periods of scarcity require evaluation of past and current efforts that it is hoped will provide a refined basis for the next period of expansion.

REFERENCES

Alcohol, Drug Abuse, and Mental Health Administration (ADAMHA). *The alcohol, drug abuse, and mental health national data book* (Department of Health and Human Services Publication No. (ADM) 80-938). Washington, D.C.: U.S. Government Printing Office, 1980.

American Psychiatric Association (APA). *Diagnostic and statistical manual of mental disorders* (3rd ed.). Washington, D.C.: Author, 1980.

Eysenck, H. The effectiveness of psychotherapy: An evaluation. *Journal of Consulting Psychology.* 1952, *16*, 319–324.

Faris, R., & Dunham, H. *Mental disorders in urban areas: An ecological study of schizophrenia and other psychoses.* Chicago: The University of Chicago Press, 1967.

Greenberg, D. Reimbursement wars. *The New England Journal of Medicine,* 1980, *303*, 538–540.

Gurin, G., Veroff, J., & Feld, S. *Americans view their mental health: A nationwide interview.* New York: Basic Books, Inc., 1960.

Hankin, J., & Otkay, J. *Mental disorder and primary medical care: An analytic review of the literature* (Department of Health, Education, and Welfare, Alcohol, Drug Abuse, and Mental Health Administration, Publication No. (ADM) 78-661). Washington, D.C.: U.S. Government Printing Office, 1979.

Jarvis, E. *Insanity and idiocy in Massachusetts: Report of the Commission on Lunancy.* Cambridge, Mass.: Harvard University Press, 1971.

Jones, K., & Vischi, T. Impact of alcohol, drug abuse and mental health treatment on medical care utilization: A review of the research. *Medical Care,* 1979, *17*, 1–82. (Supplement)

Joint Commission on Mental Illness and Health. *Action for Mental Health.* Final report of the Joint Commission. New York: Basic Books, 1961.

Kovel, J. The American mental health industry. In D. Ingleby (Ed.), *Critical psychiatry: The politics of mental health.* New York: Pantheon Books, 1980.

Kuntz, E. Hospital chains grab psychiatric business from government facilities. *Modern HealthCare,* 1981, *11*, 90–91.

Leighton, D., Harding, J., Macklin, D., Hughes, C., & Leighton, A. Psychiatric findings of the Stirling County study. *American Journal of Psychiatry,* 1963, *119*, 1021–1026.

Magaro, P., Gripp, R., & McDowell, D. *The mental health industry: A cultural phenomenon.* New York: Wiley-Interscience Publications, 1978.

Marshall, E. Psychotherapy works, but for whom? *Science,* 1980, *207*, 506–508.

Meier, G. HMO experiences with mental health services to the long-term emotionally disabled. *Inquiry,* 1981, *18*, 125–138.

Myers, J., & Weissman, M. Psychiatric disorders and their treatment: A community survey. *Medical Care,* 1980, *18*, 117–123.

National Center for Health Statistics. *National nursing home survey: 1977 summary for the United States* (Department of Health, Education, and Welfare Pub. No. (PHS) 79-1794.) Washington, D.C.: U.S. Government Printing Office, 1979.

National Institute of Mental Health. *Staffing of mental health facilities, 1976.* Rockville, MD: National Institute of Mental Health, 1977.

National Institute on Alcohol Abuse and Alcoholism (NIAAA). *Third special report to the U.S. Congress on alcohol and health* (Department of Health, Education, and Welfare

Publication No. (ADM) 79-832.) Washington, D.C.: U.S. Government Printing Office, 1978.

Pincus, H. Linking general health and mental health systems of care: Conceptual models of implementation. *American Journal of Psychiatry*, 1980, *137*, 315–320.

Regier, D., Goldberg, I., & Taube, C. The de facto U.S. mental health service system. *Archives of General Psychiatry*, 1978, *35*, 685–693.

Report of the Task Panel on Community Mental Health Centers Assessment. President's Commission on Mental Health, Vol. II. Washington, D.C.: U.S. Government Printing Office, 1978.

Report of the Task Panel on the Nature and Scope of the Problem. President's Commission on Mental Health, Vol. II. Washington, D.C.: U.S. Government Printing Office, 1978.

Report of the Task Panel on Research. President's Commission on Mental Health, Vol. IV. Washington, D.C.: U.S. Government Printing Office, 1978.

Rothman, D. *The discovery of the asylum: Social order and disorder in the new republic.* Boston: Little, Brown and Company, 1971.

Rubin, J. *Economics, mental health and the law.* Lexington, Mass.: D.C. Heath & Co., 1978.

Smith, M., & Glass, G. Meta-analysis of psychotherapy outcome studies. *American Psychologist*, 1977, *32*, 752–760.

Srole, L., Langer, T., Michael, S., Opler, M., & Rennie, T. *Mental health in the metropolis: The midtown Manhattan study.* New York: McGraw-Hill Book Company, Inc., 1962.

Wyatt v. Stickney, 325 Federal Supp. 781 (M.D., Ala 1971).

Index

445

C

California, 189
California State Employees Health
Insurance Plan, 57
Camacho, T., 201
Cancer, 198
Capitalistic system, 3
Caries, 344, 345, 346-348, 353,
363-365, 366, 367, 368, 376, 378,
391, 392, 394
Carnegie Commission on Higher
Education (1970), 336
Carnegie Foundation, 176
Carter, President, 23, 56
Case manager system (mental
illness), 430
Cavities. *See* Caries
Center for Disease Control, 205, 394
Certificate of need (CON), 164, 178
health planning and, 101
P.L. 93-641 and, 117, 120-121, 123
regulation and, 52-53
Certification, 183
AMA and, 165
quality assurance and, 81-82
Change, organizational behavior and,
75-76
Children's Bureau, 9, 12
Chronically ill, regional organization
and, 181-182
Chronically mentally ill, 427-433
Cigarettes, 209, 210-211
Clinical Congress of Surgeons of
North America, 66
Code of Federal Regulations, 5
Code of Laws (Hammurabai, 1700
B.C.), 65
Codman, E. A., 66
Coelen, C., 53, 54, 55
Coffee, E. M., 335
Cojoint analysis, PHS informational
methodology and, 229-232, 250-252
Cole, K. O., 356
Colloton, J. W., 282
Colorado, 384

Commission on Hospital Care
(1947), 273
Commission on Public-General
Hospitals, 273
Committee on the Cost of Medical
Care (CCMC), 111, 168
Committee formation (regional
organization), 187
Committee on Health Planning Goals
and Standards (Institute of
Medicine), 126
Committee on Standardization of
Hospitals (1914), 66
Commonwealth Fund (N.Y.), 175
Community
dental health and, 355, 395, 397
education and, 119
health planning and, 113
hospitals, 280
mental illness programs and, 420,
429-430, 431, 432-433
centers for, 422-423, 428
public-general hospitals and,
272-273
regional organization and, 181
Community Health Services and
Facilities Act of 1961 (P.L.
87-395), 112
Community Mental Health Centers
Act of 1963 (P.L. 88-164), 412
Community mental health centers
(CMHC), 258, 260
Community Services Amendments
(Title VI of the Civil Rights Act
of 1964, P.L. 88-352), 101
Competence
certification and, 82
licensure and, 81, 91
Competition
certification and, 81-82
cost containment and, 56-62, 77
dental services and, 374
health planning and, 132-133
health services model and, 28-29
licensure and, 80, 81
physician and P.A., 336

D

regional organization and, 181
risk appraisal, 199-200, 205-207
State government, 209. *See also*
Government; Local government
  CCMC and, 111
  dental care and, 381
  early health departments and, 7-8
  fund use and, 166
  health services model and, 32-33,
    34
  Hill-Burton Act and, 111-112
  intergovernmental relationships
    and, 171-172
  licensure and, 80-81
  loan programs and, 325
  mental health care and, 419, 420,
    429-430, 432
  P.L. 93-641 and, 121, 131
  SHPDAs and, 120
  social welfare and, 13
State health coordinating council
  (SHCC), 117
State health planning and
  development agency (SHPDA),
  117, 120, 122, 123, 124
State medicine, 11-12
Steinwald, B., 53, 55
Steward Machine Co. v. Davis, 13
Stokey, E., 235
Striffler, D. F., 353
Structure, quality assurance and,
  80-84
Subsidies, risk appraisal and health,
  211
Substance abuse disorders, 418, 421
Sullivan, D., 53, 54, 55
Summers, R. L., 272
Suomi, J.D., 351
Supply
  health costs and, 28
  of health professionals, 292-297
Surface (S) Index, 346
Surgeon General's Consultant Group
  on Medical Education, 317
Survey method of performance
  evaluation, 74
Syphilis, mental illness and, 414

T

Taube, C., 419
Taxes, risk appraisal and health,
  210-212
Technological change, 168-170, 177
Technology, 167, 168, 187, 247
  adopting new, 139
  centralization and, 184
  dental, 364, 373
  health planning and, 140
  licensure and, 311
  national planning and cost
    inflation and, 162-163
  P.L. 93-641 and, 116
  risk and, 69
Ten-State Nutrition Survey, 386-388
*Texas ACORN et al. v. Texas
  Area V Health Systems Agency,
  et al.,* 121
*Texas Medical Association v.
  Mathews,* 87
Theilade, E., 394
Third-party payers. *See also* Blue
  Cross; Blue Shield; Health
  insurance; Medicaid; Medicare
  ambulatory care and, 282
  fees and financing and, 47-49
  mental health and, 421, 440, 441
  national health program and, 161
  prospective reimbursement and, 55
Thomas, T. W., 97, 105
Tranquilizers, 411, 415, 420, 426,
  433-434, 440
Transportation model (information
  study), 235-239
Treatment Priority Index (TPI), 346
Treiman, B. R., 390
Tuke, William, 419
Tychsen, S., 212

U

UAW dental benefit plan, 390
Unemployment insurance, 13
Unions, 9